VARIORUM COLLECTED STUDIES SERIES

Studies in the History of Modern Pharmacology and Drug Therapy

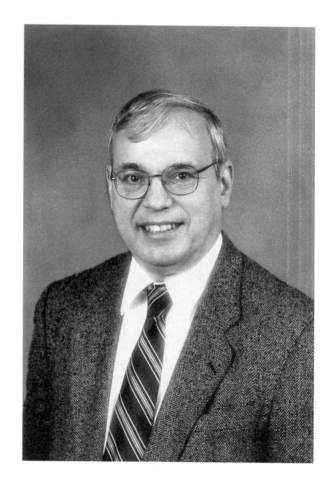

John Parascandola

John Parascandola

Studies in the History of Modern Pharmacology and Drug Therapy

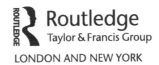

Routledge
Taylor & Francis Group

LONDON AND NEW YORK

First published 2012 by Ashgate Publishing

2 Park Square, Milton Park, Abingdon, Oxfordshire OX14 4RN
711 Third Avenue, New York, NY 10017

Routledge is an imprint of the Taylor & Francis Group, an informa business

First issued in paperback 2018

British Library Cataloguing in Publication Data
Parascandola, John, 1941–
   Studies in the history of modern pharmacology and drug therapy.
   – (Variorum collected studies series)
   1. Pharmacology – History. 2. Chemotherapy – History.
   I. Title II. Series
   615.1'09-dc22

ISBN 978-1-4094-1976-1 (hbk)
ISBN 978-1-138-37584-0 (pbk)

Library of Congress Control Number: 2011934461

VARIORUM COLLECTED STUDIES SERIES CS991

To my family

My wife Randee

My son Mark and his wife Christina

My son Adam and his wife Stephanie

CONTENTS

This volume contains xvi + 324 pages

PUBLISHER'S NOTE

The articles in this volume, as in all others in the Variorum Collected Studies Series, have not been given a new, continuous pagination. In order to avoid confusion, and to facilitate their use where these same studies have been referred to elsewhere, the original pagination has been maintained wherever possible.

Each article has been given a Roman number in order of appearance, as listed in the Contents. This number is repeated on each page and is quoted in the index entries.

PREFACE

A major portion of the research that I have undertaken in my career of more than forty years in the history of science, medicine and pharmacy has been devoted to the subject of the history of pharmacology and drugs. The present volume brings together what I consider to be the most important papers that I have contributed to the literature of this field. The works are divided into three categories, namely those dealing with the history of the science and theory of pharmacology, those dealing with the history of pharmacology as a discipline, and those dealing with the history of drug therapy.

The papers in the first section, on "Pharmacological Science and Theory," focus heavily on two of the major conceptual frameworks of modern pharmacology, the relationship of the pharmacological activity to the chemical structure of a drug and the receptor theory of drug action. From the time that scientists first began to draw structural formulas for chemical compounds in the nineteenth century, pharmacologists began to investigate the ways in which the chemical composition and structure of a molecule influenced its action on the body. At first they concentrated on relatively simple relationships, such as the effects of particular functional groups (e.g., the alcohol group) on the pharmacological activity of a substance. The early pioneers in this field were overly optimistic about how easy it would be to discover these relationships and to apply them to the design of drugs for specific therapeutic purposes, as illustrated by the article on "Structure-activity relationships: the early mirage."

As the difficulty of the task became more apparent, some pharmacologists questioned whether the physiological action of drugs was really determined directly by their chemical structure, or whether it might not actually be due to the physical properties (such as solubility and volatility) of the molecule. While they realized that physical properties were most likely ultimately determined by chemical structure, these pharmacologists believed it was the task of their discipline to focus on the physical properties that directly determine drug action, leaving the relationship between chemical structure and physical properties for chemists to explore. The article on "The controversy over structure-activity relationships in the early twentieth century" highlights this debate.

As chemistry and pharmacology advanced, practitioners of these disciplines were able to elucidate some of the more sophisticated relationships between structure and activity. For example, they began to examine the relationship between optical isomerism and pharmacological action, revealing that two compounds whose structures were almost identical except that they were mirror images of each other could have drastically different pharmacological properties. This topic is discussed in the papers on "The evolution of stereochemical concepts in pharmacology" and "Arthur Cushny, optical isomerism and the mechanism of drug action."

The article on "The theoretical basis of Paul Ehrlich's chemotherapy" bridges the two themes of structure-activity relations and receptor theory. The German physician Paul Ehrlich invented the science of chemotherapy, which he defined as the effort to synthesize drugs to combat specific microorganisms, in the early twentieth century. He began the modern science of drug design, synthetically altering the structure of molecules to alter their therapeutic and toxic properties. He was searching for "magic bullets" that could, by virtue of their specific chemical structure, seek out and destroy pathogenic microorganisms in the body without harming the host organism. His research was ultimately grounded in the receptor theory of drug action that was developed independently by Ehrlich and the English physiologist John Newport Langley in the first decade of the twentieth century.

This theory held that drugs and poisons exerted their physiological effects by attaching to receptors in the cells. The binding of a drug to a receptor was enabled by the specific chemical structure of both the drug and the receptor. The introduction of the theory by Ehrlich and Langley is discussed in the paper on "Origins of the receptor theory of drug action." The later development of this theory, which still (although in substantially modified form) provides the theoretical underpinning for pharmacology, is considered in the papers on "Carl Voegtlin and the 'arsenic receptor' in chemotherapy" and "The development of receptor theory."

The emergence of a distinct discipline of pharmacology and its later development are treated in the second section of the book, appropriately entitled "Discipline of Pharmacology." My own work has centered on the development of pharmacology in the United States, and consequently the four papers in this section are focused on this country. The "father" of pharmacology in this country is universally regarded to be John J. Abel, the first professor of pharmacology at the Johns Hopkins University. Trained in medicine in Germany, Abel brought the new science of pharmacology from that country, where it had first become established as a unique discipline, to America. In addition to occupying the first American chair in pharmacology, he founded a national society and a journal for the field and trained many of the next generation of American pharmacologists. His contributions are discussed in the article on "John J. Abel and the early development of pharmacology at the Johns Hopkins University."

After becoming established at a few progressive medical schools such as Johns Hopkins, pharmacology gradually came to replace the older didactic field of "materia medica" (which had focused heavily on the natural origin, physical description, and traditional therapeutic uses of drugs, mostly botanicals) at other medical schools across the country. In time, courses in materia medica at American pharmacy schools were also replaced by courses in pharmacology, as discussed in the article on "The development of pharmacology in American schools of pharmacy." The science of pharmacology also became established in industrial and government laboratories over the course of the twentieth century. These developments are discussed in the articles on "The beginnings of pharmacology in the Federal government" and on "The 'preposterous provision': The American Society for Pharmacology and Experimental Therapeutics' ban on industrial pharmacologists, 1908–1941."

The third and final section of the volume deals with "Drug Therapy." A variety of drugs and themes are considered in these papers. The article on "The search for the active oxytocic principle of ergot: laboratory science and clinical medicine in conflict," for example, illustrates (as the title indicates) the tension between laboratory researchers and clinicians as science began to take a more dominant role in medicine in the twentieth century. The article on "From germs to genes: trends in drug therapy, 1852–2002" provides a broad overview of changes in drug therapy over that 150-year period. "The introduction of antibiotics into therapeutics" reviews the early history of that most important class of drugs, with emphasis on penicillin.

The remaining four articles deal with the drug therapy of two specific diseases. As revealed by their titles, the articles on "Miracle at Carville: the introduction of the sulfones for the treatment of leprosy" and on "Chaulmoogra oil and the treatment of leprosy" discuss the drug therapy of leprosy. The articles complement each other nicely for chaulmoogra oil was the standard (if sometimes controversial) treatment for the disease for many years until it was replaced by the sulfones, the first really effective therapy for leprosy (now called Hansen's Disease), in the 1940s. Finally, the articles on "John Mahoney and the introduction of penicillin to treat syphilis" and "From mercury to miracle drugs: syphilis therapy over the centuries" obviously deal with the treatment of syphilis. These two papers also compliment each other. The latter article provides a broad overview of syphilis therapy, from the varied and largely unsuccessful efforts to treat the disease before the twentieth-century to the limited success of Paul Ehrlich's Salvarsan in the early twentieth century to the introduction of penicillin in the 1940s. The former paper provides a detailed look at the beginnings of modern antibiotic therapy for syphilis with the discovery of penicillin's effectiveness against the disease.

I am pleased to have the opportunity to bring these works together in one volume, where they will be more readily accessible to scholars with an interest in the history of drug science and therapy.

JOHN PARASCANDOLA

University of Maryland College Park, USA
April 2011

ACKNOWLEDGEMENTS

I would like to thank the following publishers for granting permission to reprint the articles in this volume: American Institute of the History of Pharmacy (for chapters I, III, X, XI, XII, XV, XVI, XVII, XVIII, XIX); Johns Hopkins University Press (II, IX); American Chemical Society (IV); Springer Netherlands (V); Oxford University Press (VI, VII); Elsevier (VIII); and Wissenschaftliche Verlagsgesellschaft (XIII).

I would also like to thank the following publishers and institutions for providing and/or granting permission to reprint the images in this book. When the source was not given or not correctly/completely given in the original publication, I have indicated the paper and page number of the image in parentheses below. Alan Mason Chesney Medical Archives of The Johns Hopkins Medical Institutions (IX-522 and IX-524); American Institute of the History of Pharmacy (for providing images and permissions for materials from the Kremers Reference Files, formerly of the F. B. Power Pharmaceutical Library, University of Wisconsin-Madison); American Society for Pharmacology and Experimental Therapeutics (XII-35); David H. Clark; Department of Health and Human Services; F.B. Power Pharmaceutical Library, University of Wisconsin-Madison; Food and Drug Administration History Office (XI-183); John Wiley and Sons (A.H. Beckett and A.F. Casy, *Journal of Pharmacy and Pharmacology*, 1955, 7:433-455) © 1955 (IV-156); Kremers Reference Files, School of Pharmacy, University of Wisconsin-Madison; Lasker Foundation (XVI-4 and XVI-11); Leprosy Mission International; Macmillan Publishers Ltd. (A.G. Ogston, *Nature*, 1948, 162: 963), © 1948 (IV-156); Massachusetts College of Pharmacy and Health Science (X-110); National Library of Medicine; National Museum of American History, Smithsonian Institution; Portland Press Ltd. (Leslie Easson and Edgar Stedman, *Biochemical Journal*, 1933, 27: 1257–1266), © the Biochemical Society (IV-150); Royal Society; Selman A. Waksman Papers, Special Collections and University Archives, Rutgers University Libraries (XVII-10); University of Washington School of Pharmacy (X-107).

Every effort has been made to trace all the copyright holders, but if any have been inadvertently overlooked the publishers will be pleased to make the necessary arrangement at the first opportunity.

Finally, I wish to thank Claire Jarvis, my editor at Ashgate, for her able assistance in seeing me through the process of publishing this book.

Structure-Activity Relationships

--*The Early Mirage* *

$\mathcal{T}$O CONSIDER the relationship between pharmacological activity and chemical structure, even crudely, one must possess at least the concept of a chemical formula and some knowledge of the general mode of action of certain drugs. Such studies thus had to await the nineteenth century, particularly the introduction of Dalton's atomic theory and the development of experimental pharmacology by men such as Magendie. The earliest investigators in this field understandably concentrated on relating physiological activity to the presence of certain elements or functional groups, not on more complicated questions involving the general structure of the molecule. In fact, the concept of the structural formula was only just emerging during the period we here consider.

James Blake (1815-1893) was probably the first man to make a

---

*Presented in the Section on Contributed Papers of the American Institute of the History of Pharmacy, Washington, D.C., April 13, 1970.

serious beginning in structure-activity relationships. Blake, an English physician who later emigrated to America, was a student of Magendie at Paris. While undertaking studies at the University of London, he came into contact with William Sharpey, the anatomist and physiologist. It has been said that Sharpey influenced young Blake to study the physiological action of substances introduced into the blood stream of living animals.[1]

In his first paper on this subject, Blake described his experiments with a wide variety of organic and inorganic compounds, including potassium nitrate, ammonia, strychnine, hydrocyanic acid, and morphine. He attempted to divide these substances into four different categories according to their pharmacological effects. In view of the diverse types of chemicals that he employed, it is not surprising that his classification scheme was somewhat general and that the fourth class consisted of substances that did not fit into one of the first three categories.[2]

Perhaps he decided that he could make more progress by narrowing the scope of his investigations, for his next paper, published in the same year, focused on a series of inorganic salts. In reviewing these experiments, Blake said, he was struck by the relationship that existed between chemical

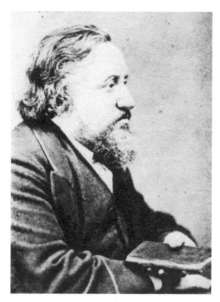

Sir Benjamin Ward Richardson, British physician and physiological investigator, in his middle years. (Courtesy of the National Library of Medicine)

composition and physiological action. The different salts of a given metal produced identical pharmacological effects. For example, sodium hydroxide, sodium nitrate, sodium sulfate and sodium carbonate exhibited identical pharmacological activity. Thus the metallic element of the salt seemed to be primarily responsible for its activity.[3]

Blake continued his experiments along these lines, and he began to divide the elements into various groups according to the physiological effects produced by their salts. In 1841, he announced his discovery that elements which were isomorphic generally had very similar pharmacological properties.[4] Eilhardt Mitscherlich had clearly established the relationship between chemical composition and crystalline form about twenty years earlier. His law of isomorphism stated that compounds which crystallize in the same form are similar in chemical composition.[5] Blake extended this similarity to include physiological effects. He commented:

"Should a more extended series of researches prove, that the identity which I have noticed in the physiological action of isomorphous compounds does not in all cases hold good, yet I think that the facts above are sufficient to show that there exists some intimate connection between the chemical properties of substances, and their physiological action, the investigation of which promises to furnish a rich field for physiological researches."[6]

By 1848, Blake had studied the physiological effects of the compounds of more than 25 elements, and he arranged them in groups on the basis of these effects. For example, the elements platinum, palladium, iridium and osmium were placed together in one group.[7] It is interesting to note that some of his groupings were very similar to those used and expanded by Mendeleev almost two decades later in constructing his periodic table of the elements.[8] Blake was not aware of any periodic relationship of the elements, however. He was impressed by the fact that when the elements were grouped according to their physiological properties, the elements within each group tended to be isomorphic. He concluded:

". . . that the physiological action of these substances depends upon some property they possess in connection with these isomorphous relations."[9]

Blake was later to extend these researches to show that within a given group of isomorphic elements, physiological activity increases with molecular weight.[10] His early work was important because it demonstrated that a relationship could be established between the pharmacological action and the chemical nature of a substance. He limited his investigations to inorganic compounds, however, because he felt that the composition and properties of organic compounds were only imperfectly understood.[11] It is certainly true that in the 1840's organic chemistry was virtually in a state of chaos. In the decade between 1850 and 1860, however, the development of the concept of valency, the introduction of the structural theory, and the revival of Avogadro's hypothesis all helped to bring a certain amount of order out of the confusion. Chemists then began drawing structural formulas for some organic compounds, e.g. Kekulé proposed a ring formula for benzene in 1865.[12]

While structural organic chemistry was still in its infancy, some attempts were made to relate the physiological action of organic compounds to their chemical structure. Perhaps the earliest systematic study of this kind was that of Benjamin Ward Richardson (1828-1896), the British physician and physiologist. In the years between 1864 and 1870, Richardson published a series of papers, in the *Report of the British Association for the Advancement of Science*, in which he described his experiments with a number of compounds of methane, ethane, butane, and pentane.[13] He compared the effects of different functional groups on the pharmacological action of these substances.

Richardson was able to associate certain functional groups with particular physiological properties. For example, the nitrite group was shown to be associated with vasodilation and quickening of the heart. The nitrites of all of the above - mentioned hydrocarbons possess these properties to some degree, although the degree and persistence of action increases with molecular weight (e.g. amyl nitrite is considerably more active than methyl nitrite). The hydrocarbons themselves, which may be considered to contain hydrogen as a functional group, all act as anesthetics. Their hydroxy derivatives, i.e. the alcohols, all depress the active functions of the cerebrospinal system. In this manner Richardson was able to establish at least a crude relationship between structure and activity.

The study that really drew attention to the field of structure-activity relationships, however, was the investigation by Alexander Crum Brown (1838-1922) and Thomas R. Fraser (1841-1920) of Edinburgh. Brown was a chemist and one of the pioneers in the development of structural formulas, while Fraser was a pharmacologist. The two men formed an appropriate team for research in the area of structure-activity relationships, and they began collaborating on such a project in 1867. Their first paper on the subject, published in 1869, began with a declaration of faith:

"There can be no reasonable doubt that a relation exists between the physiological action of a substance and its chemical composition and constitution, understanding by the latter term the mutual relations of the atoms in the substance."[14]

They went on to state that there were numerous indications of such a relation, and that attempts had been made to express it formally in certain cases (e.g. Blake's work on isomorphic salts). Beyond such limited generalizations, however, Brown and Fraser were not aware "that any approach has been made to the statement of a law connecting the physiological action of a substance with its chemical constitution." Some observers, they added, have tried to connect pharmacological action with composition, i.e., the presence and proportion of particular elements. The existence of isomers with very different physiological properties, however, shows that composition alone is not sufficient to explain biological activity. Constitution must also be taken into account, but unfortunately the structures of the majority of organic compounds were not known.

Refusing to allow such considerations to deter them, Brown and Fraser suggested utilizing a method resembling the "calculus of finite variations." They offered the following mathematical analogy to illustrate how they planned to proceed. Let $C =$ the constitution of a substance, which is unknown, and let $\phi =$ its physiological action, which is known. The physiological action is some unknown function of the constitution, i.e. $\phi = fC$. One could then produce a known change in C and observe the change that occurs in ϕ. If the method were applied to a sufficiently large number of substances, and if the type of change produced in C were varied, one might hope to determine what function ϕ is of C. The method is not strictly mathematical, because one cannot express the known quantities with sufficient definiteness to make them the subjects of calculation. One can hope, however, to discover the nature of the relation between constitution (C) and activity (ϕ) in an approximate manner.

To implement this approach, Brown and Fraser needed a chemical operation that would produce a known change in structure which would be the same in a number of different compounds. They considered both substitution and addition reactions, but decided on the latter because they felt that such reactions generally produced a more marked change in physiological activity. They understood by the term "addition" any reaction in which new constituents enter a molecule without displacing anything already there. An examination of the data available in the literature led them to speculate that physiological activity was often associated with an unsaturated valence, i.e., with an atom that could undergo further addition. Substances which were highly condensed or saturated were generally inert, and activity seemed to be removed or diminished by chemical addition. For example, they pointed out, carbon monoxide is highly toxic, while carbon dioxide is much less so. The valency of carbon in carbon monoxide is not saturated, but addition of another oxygen atom produces a more saturated, hence relatively inert, compound. As another example, they cited the work of Stahlschmidt, who demonstrated in 1859 that the addition of methyl iodide to strychnine and brucine apparently destroyed their physiological action.[15]

Stahlschmidt's results prompted Brown and Fraser to extend this work on alkaloids and their methylated derivatives. Although the structures of the alkaloids were unknown, it was believed that they generally belonged to the class of "nitrile" bases. The term "nitrile" was not used in the modern sense, i.e., to indicate the presence of a cyano group, but rather to describe a tertiary amine. "Nitriles" were

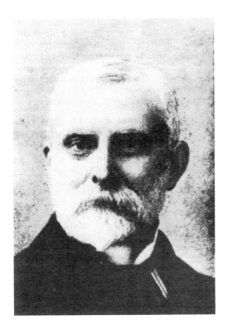

Sir Thomas Lauder Brunton, who speculated in 1877 that physicians would soon be able to predict the pharmacological action of any compound from its chemical constitution. (Courtesy of the National Library of Medicine)

compounds of the type $N + R_3$, such as trimethylamine, $N + 3$ (CH_3).[16] The addition of methyl iodide produced a known change in structure in such "nitrile" bases, i.e., the formation of an ammonium salt. According to Brown and Fraser, the formation of the salt involved the conversion of triatomic nitrogen to pentatomic nitrogen.[17]

In their first experiments on this subject, the two Scottish scientists studied the pharmacological action of strychnine, brucine, thebaine, codeine, morphine, and nicotine, as well as that of their methylated derivatives. They found that upon methylation the ability of these alkaloids to produce convulsions disappeared.[18] The narcotic property of morphine was also diminished,

and that of codeine was essentially destroyed. At the same time, the methylated compounds still exhibited toxic effects, although generally only at doses many times greater than those required by the alkaloids themselves. The pharmacological action of the methyl compounds, however, was drastically different from that of the alkaloids. The methylated derivatives all exhibited a paralyzing, curare-like action. In fact, Brown and Fraser showed that, like curare, these compounds acted at the neuro-muscular junction. These results were rather dramatic. A small change in structure produced a spectacular change, both quantitative and qualitative, in the pharmacological properties of the alkaloids.[19]

Brown and Fraser extended these studies to other compounds, such as atropine and trimethylamine. It was shown that, in general, the ammonium salts of such compounds, i.e., what we would call quaternary ammonium salts, were associated with a paralyzing action.[20] They had been quite fortunate in choosing the right compounds to study, because such clear-cut relationships between structure and activity are not that common. Their results undoubtedly encouraged other investigators to undertake research in this area.

At first, there was considerable optimism that a general law, or perhaps a few generalizations, describing the relationship between structure and activity would be discovered. James Blake had, after all, classified the pharmacological properties of many inorganic substances on the basis of his "law of isomorphism." Benjamin Richardson hoped that further studies on the effects of different functional groups would lead to a physiological law similar to the law of substitution in chemistry.[21] As previously mentioned, Brown and Fraser hoped to approximate the "functional relationship" between structure and activity. They felt that the degree of condensation or saturation of a substance, while not the only factor contributing to physiological action, was at least a key factor in this respect.

High hopes were also held out for the therapeutic applications of structure-activity research. Some investigators felt that a therapeutic millennium was at hand. In 1869, Benjamin Richardson declared that the study of remedies must be based on structure-activity considerations, and he added:

"I am certain the time must soon come when the books we call 'Pharmacopoeias' will be everywhere constructed on this basis of thought, and when the chemist and physician will become one and one."[22]

A decade later, Thomas Lauder Brunton (1844-1916), the eminent physician and pharmacologist, echoed these sentiments when he suggested that the time might not be far off when scientists would be able to synthesize substances that would act on the body in any desired way. He hoped that therapeutics would soon be placed on a completely rational basis, with physicians being able to predict the pharmacological action of any compound from its chemical constitution.[23] Brunton himself became involved in some researches on structure - activity relationships.[24] In 1889, he again emphasized his hopes for therapeutics when he stated:

"The prospects of therapeutics appear to me very bright . . . I think it is highly probably that before long we shall have a series of drugs which will stimulate the biliary secretion of the liver or modify its glycogenic function, arranged in order of comparative strength, in much the same way we

have now the class of antipyretics. We may also look for a series of remedies which will modify the circulation by dilating the blood vessels not only temporarily but more or less permanently . . . We may also, I think, fairly expect to obtain a series of remedies having an action upon the heart and vessels. . ."[25]

The noted biologist Thomas Huxley was also very much impressed by the advances made in experimental pharmacology during his lifetime, and in 1881 he wrote:

". . . . there surely can be no ground for doubting that, sooner or later, the pharmacologist will supply the physician with the means of affecting, in any desired sense, the functions of any physiological element of the body. It will, in short, become possible to introduce into the economy a molecular mechanism which, like a very cunningly contrived torpedo, shall find its way to some particular group of living elements, and cause an explosion among them, leaving the rest untouched."[26]

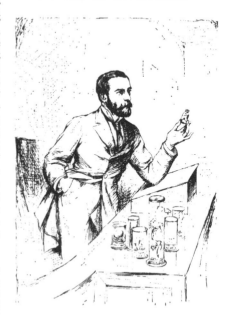

Sir Thomas R. Fraser, about 1884, lecturing about drugs. An etching by William Brassey Hole. (Courtesy of the National Library of Medicine)

It is true that some synthetic drugs were developed in the last few decades of the nineteenth century as a result of structural considerations. For example, Carl Duisberg was able to modify the structure of *para*-nitrophenol, a by-product of the dye industry, in such a way as to produce a useful antipyretic, phenacetin. He consciously synthesized a compound with a structure similar to that of acetanilid, a drug whose antipyretic and analgesic properties had been discovered by accident.[27] Often, however, success in synthesizing new drugs was due more to luck than to correct reasoning. Ludwig Knorr, for example, attempted to synthesize a quinine-type structure in 1883, although the structural formula of quinine was not completely known. He did succeed in preparing a new antipyretic, antipyrine, but its structure was not what he had predicted and did not resemble that of quinine.[28]

The introduction of chloral hydrate into medicine by Oscar Liebreich in 1869 also seemed to support those who saw great therapeutic possibilities in the structure-activity approach. Yet this important discovery is another example of incorrect reasoning leading to useful results. Liebreich predicted that since chloral hydrate decomposes to chloroform in caustic alkaline solutions, it should undergo a similar decomposition in the alkaline body fluids. Chloroform would thus be slowly released, and eventually would induce a state of unconsciousness. Chloral hydrate did prove to be a successful hypnotic, but it was soon shown that Liebreich's theory concerning its mode of action was incorrect. The alkalinity of the body was not strong enough to decompose the chloral hydrate to chloroform.[29]

By the end of the nineteenth century, the early optimism concerning structure-activity relationships began to waver. Determining the relationship between structure and activity was turning out to be more difficult than had originally been anticipated. In many cases, the relationship was not at all clear-cut. No general law correlating structure and activity had emerged and Brunton's dream of the physician having at his command drugs to produce any desired effect did not seem very close to fulfillment. In 1901, F. Gowland Hopkins summed up the situation when he wrote:

". . . . it is a matter for some disappointment, and perhaps for surprise, that we should, today, after thirty years, be able to point to very few general relations bearing the stamp of such definiteness and simplicity as are found in the case brought to light by Crum Brown and Fraser; and that even now the results obtained by these investigators may be quoted as the most satisfactory instance to hand, of obvious relation between chemical constitution and physiological action."[30]

It is interesting to note that the fifth edition of *May's Chemistry of Synthetic Drugs* (1959) reproduced the above quotation and commented: "Over half a century has elapsed and these remarks still remain true."[31] A great deal of research has been devoted to the question of structure-activity relationships in the twentieth century. There is no doubt that many valuable results have emerged from these studies, and that a number of generalizations of limited application have come to light. However, the early hope that some kind of general law completely correlating structure and activity would be discovered before long, and that consequently one would soon be able to predict the pharmacological activity of any substance by merely inspecting its structural formula,

I

turned out to be a mirage. In spite of the impressive advances made in chemical pharmacology during the present century, we have yet to achieve the goals set forth by men such as Benjamin Ward Richardson and Thomas Lauder Brunton.

AUTHOR'S NOTE: *After this paper was in type for this issue of* PHARMACY IN HISTORY, *an article on early structure-activity studies was published by William Bynum, "Chemical Structure and Pharmacological Action: A Chapter in the History of 19th Century Molecular Pharmacology." Bull. Hist. Med., 44, 518-538 (1970).*

Footnotes

1. Sister Mary Ambrose Devereux, Hugh Donahoe and Kazuo Kimura, "A Physiological Basis for the Grouping of the Elements—James Blake (1815-93)," *J. Chem. Ed.*, 33, 340 (1956).

2. James Blake, "Observations on the Physiological Effects of Various Agents Introduced into the Circulation, as Indicated by the Haemadynamometer," *Edinburgh Med. Surg. J.*, 51, 330-345 (1839).

3. James Blake, "Memoire sur les Effets de Diverses Substances Salines Injectees dans le Systeme Circulatoire," *Arch. Gen. Med.*, 3rd series, 6, 289-300 (1839).

4. James Blake, "On the Action of Certain Inorganic Compounds When Introduced Directly into the Blood," *Edinburgh Med. Surg. J.*, 56, 104-124 (1341).

5. A. J. Ihde, *The Development of Modern Chemistry*, New York: Harper and Row, 1964, pp. 147-149.

6. *Ibid*, p. 124.

7. James Blake, "On the Influence of Isomorphism in Determining the Reactions that Take Place between Inorganic Compounds, and the Elements of Living Beings," *Am. J. Med. Sci.*, new series, 15, 63-76 (1848).

8. Devereux, et. al., *op. cit.*, p. 341; Chauncey Leake, "Gold Rush Doc," *Gesnerus*, 8, 117 (1951).

9. Reference 7, p. 72.

10. James Blake, "On the Connection between the Atomic Weight of Substances and Their Physiological Action," *Proc. California Acad. Sci.*, 5, 75-77 (1873-1874).

11. Reference 7, p. 64.

12. For a discussion of the development of organic chemistry in the nineteenth century, see A. J. Ihde, *Development of Modern Chemistry*, pp. 161-230, 304-362.

13. Benjamin Ward Richardson, "Report on the Physiological Action of Nitrite of Amyl," *Brit. Assoc. Rep.*, 34, 120-129 (1864); "Second Report on the Physiological Action of Certain of the Amyl Compounds," *ibid.*, 35, 272-281 (1865); "Report on the Physiological Action of the Methyl Compounds," *ibid.*, 37, 47-57 (1867); "Report on the Physiological Action of the Methyl and Allied Compounds," *ibid.*, 38, 170-186 (1863); "Report on the Physiological Action of the Methyl and Allied Series," *ibid.*, 39, 404-421 (1969); "Report on the Action of the Methyl and Allied Series," *ibid.*, 40, 155-170 (1870).

14. A. Crum Brown and Thomas Fraser, "On the Connection between Chemical Constitution and Physiological Action. Part I—On the Physiological Action of the Salts of the Ammonium Bases, Derived from Strychnia, Brucia, Thebaia. Codeia, Morphia, and Nicotia," *Trans. Roy. Soc. Edinburgh*, 25, 151 (1869).

15. The discussion of the methodological approach and theoretical views of Brown and Fraser is a summary of their account in *ibid.*, pp. 151-155.

16. See William Gregory, *A Handbook of Organic Chemistry*, third edition, London: Taylor, Walton, and Maberly, 1852, pp. 327-333. See also Thomas Fraser, "Connection between Chemical Properties and Physiological Action," *Pharm. J.*, 32, 404-405 (1872).

17. Reference 14. pp. 155-156.

18. Brown and Fraser claimed that they found some degree of convulsant action for all of these alkaloids, although they admitted that their results were not perfectly clear with alkaloids such as morphine, whose narcotic properties tend to obscure the situation. See *ibid.*, pp. 182-186.

19. For a summary and discussion of their results. see *ibid.*, pp. 192-193.

20. See, for example, A. Crum Brown and Thomas Fraser, "On the Connection between Chemical Constitution and Physiological Action. Part II—On the Physiological Action of the Ammonium Bases derived from Atropia and Conia," *Trans. Roy. Soc. Edinburgh*, 25, 693-739 (1869), and A. Crum Brown and Thomas Fraser, "On the Connection between Chemical Constitution and Physiological Action:—On the Physiological Action of the Salts of Ammonia. of Tri-methylamine, and of Tetra-methyl-ammonium; of the Salts of Tropia, and of the Ammonium Bases Derived from It; and of Tropic, Atropic, and Isatropic Acids and their Salts. With Further Details on the Physiological Action of the Salts of Methyl-strychnium and Ethyl-strychnium," *Proc. Roy. Soc. Edinburgh*, 6, 556-561 (1869). They also showed that sulfonium salts have the same paralyzing property exhibited by quaternary ammonium salts. See Crum Brown and Thomas Fraser, "On the Connection between Chemical Constitution and Physiological Action—Continued. On the Physiological Action of the Salts of Trimethylsulphin," *Proc. Roy. Soc. Edinburgh*, 7, 663-665 (1872).

21. Benjamin Ward Richardson, "Second Report on Physiological Action of Certain of the Amyl Compounds," *Brit. Assoc. Rep.*, 35, 280-281 (1865).

22. Benjamin Ward Richardson, "Report on the Physiological Action of the Methyl and Allied Series," *Brit. Assoc. Rep.*, 39, 421 (1869).

23. T. Lauder Brunton. *Pharmacology and Therapeutics* (Gulstonian Lectures for 1877), London: Macmillan. 1980, pp. 194-196.

24. See, for example, T. Lauder Brunton and J. Theodore Cash, "Contributions to Our Knowledge of the Connection Between Chemical Constitution, Physiological Action, and Antagonism," *Phil. Trans.*, 175 (I), 197-244 (1884).

25. T. Lauder Brunton, *An Introduction to Modern Therapeutics* (Croonian Lectures for 1889), London: Macmillan, 1892, p. 4.

26. Thomas Huxley, "The Connection of the Biological Sciences with Medicine," *Nature*, 24, 346 (1881).

27. Hans-Joachim Flechtner, *Carl Duisberg*, Dusseldorf: Econ Verlag. 1959. pp. 103-110; Carl Duisberg. "Zur Geschichte der Entdeckung des Phenacetins," *Z. cnnew. Chemie*, 26 (I), 240 (1913).

28. Milton Silverman, *Magic in a Bottle*, New York: Macmillan, 1941, pp. 180-182; anon., "Discoverer of Antipyrin. A Note on Ludwig Knorr (1859-1912)," *Chemist and Druggist*, 172, 508 (1959).

29. See M. P. Earles, "Introduction of Chloral Hydrate into Medicine," *Pharm. J.*, 202, 457-459 (1969), and Rudolph Zaunick, "Vom Anbruch Moderner Arzneimittel-Forschung. Zur Erinnerung an die klassichen Arbeiten von Alexander Crum Brown, (Sir) Thomas Richard Fraser. (Sir) Benjamin Ward Richardson und Oscar Liebreich im Jahre 1869," *Veroeffentlichungen Internat. Gesellsch. f. Gesch. d. Pharm.*, 13, 31-38 (1958).

30. F. G. Hopkins, "On the Relation between Chemical Constitution and Physiological Action," in W. Hale-White, ed., *Textbook of Pharmacology and Therapeutics*, Edinburgh: Young J. Pentland, 1901, p. 3.

31. G. Malcolm Dyson and Percy May, *May's Chemistry of Synthetic Drugs*, fifth edition, London: Longmans. 1959, p. 11.

II

ORIGINS OF THE RECEPTOR THEORY OF DRUG ACTION

JOHN PARASCANDOLA AND RONALD JASENSKY *

In modern molecular pharmacology, the effects of drugs on biological systems are explained in many cases in terms of the interaction between the drug molecule and specific molecules or complex macromolecular structures in the cell which are termed "receptors." Although it was suggested by several investigators in the nineteenth century that the action of drugs might be due to a reaction between the drug and some constituent of the cell, the concept of drug receptors was first clearly developed at the beginning of the twentieth century by John Newport Langley (1852-1925) in England and by Paul Ehrlich (1854-1915) in Germany. Beginning with different problems, each elaborated a theory which he was able to use to explain certain pharmacological phenomena. The purpose of this paper is to examine the origins of the receptor theory in the work of these two men.

Nineteenth-Century Background

By the second half of the nineteenth century, some investigators were attempting to study the relationship between the pharmacological action of a drug and its chemical structure and properties. Even before the middle of the century, in the 1840s, James Blake demonstrated that elements which were isomorphous generally had very similar pharmacological properties. The studies of Benjamin Ward Richardson and especially of Crum Brown and Fraser in the 1860s were really responsible for opening up the field of structure-activity relationships.[1] In this period of emerging interest in the application of chemistry to pharmacology, it is not surprising that interest in the nature of the reaction between

* A preliminary version of this paper was presented to the American Institute of the History of Pharmacy, Section on Contributed Papers, Houston, Texas, April 24, 1972. The authors wish to thank the National Science Foundation for support of this research under grant number GS-28549 and under Undergraduate Research Participation grant number GY-8817. We also express our gratitude to the Wellcome Institute of the History of Medicine for permission to examine the Ehrlich papers deposited in the Institute's Library, and to the Library staff for their able and courteous assistance.

[1] For a discussion of these early structure-activity studies, see John Parascandola, "Structure-activity relationships: the early mirage," *Pharmacy in History*, 1971, *13:* 3-10; also William F. Bynum, "Chemical structure and pharmacological action: a chapter in the history of 19th century molecular pharmacology," *Bull. Hist. Med.*, 1970, *44:* 518-538.

the drug and the body was stimulated. To pharmacologists such as Thomas Fraser and T. Lauder Brunton, who were themselves involved in structure-activity studies, it seemed likely that the physiological action of drugs is usually due to a chemical reaction between the drug and some constituent of the cell or tissue. Oscar Loew postulated in 1893 that certain poisons exert their actions by combining with aldehyde or amino groups of protoplasm. At the turn of the twentieth century, Sigmund Fränkel argued that the selective action of drugs can only be understood by assuming that certain groups in the drug molecule enter into a chemical union with the cell substance of a particular tissue. Once fixed in the cell in this manner, the drug can then exert its pharmacological action.[2]

Some pharmacological evidence for the view that certain drugs exert their influence by forming compounds with substances in the cells was provided by the experimental work of John Newport Langley. In 1874, while still a student of physiology at Cambridge University, he began to investigate the action of pilocarpine on the heart at the suggestion of the noted physiologist Michael Foster.[3] He also studied its effects on secretion, especially on the secretion of saliva by the sub-maxillary gland. During the course of his work, he observed that atropine and pilocarpine were mutually antagonistic in their actions on the gland. In a paper published in 1878, he explained this antagonism by assuming that these drugs compete for a specific substance in the body. He commented:

. . . we may, I think, without much rashness, assume that there is a substance or substances in the nerve endings or gland cells with which both atropin and pilocarpin are

---

[2] Fraser felt that "physiological action is often, if not always, the result of a chemical reaction between the foreign body and certain of the constituents of the vital structures whose action is modified by it." Thomas Fraser, "Lectures on the connection between the chemical properties and the physiological action of active substances," *Brit. Med. J.*, 1872, 2: 403. Brunton suggested that certain chemical compounds, e.g., curare, enter into a reversible combination with the cell, thus altering its physical character and functional properties. T. Lauder Brunton, "Lectures on the experimental investigation of the action of medicines," *Brit. Med. J.*, 1871, 1: 414. For Loew's views, see Oscar Loew, *Ein natürliches System der Gift-wirkungen* (Munich: E. Wolff and H. Lüneburg, 1893), especially pp. 38-62. The theory mentioned above applied only to what Loew called "substituting poisons" (his elaborate classification scheme for poisons is beyond the scope of this paper). The concept of "substituting poisons" could not explain the selective action of drugs, since presumably the protoplasm of all cells contains aldehyde and amino groups. Sigmund Fränkel, in his *Die Arzneimittel-Synthese auf Grundlage der Beziehungen zwischen chemischem Aufbau und Wirkung* (Berlin: Julius Springer, 1901), especially pp. 13-41, offered perhaps the clearest expression of the view that drugs combine with specific substances in the cell before the elaboration of the receptor theory by Ehrlich and Langley.

[3] W. M. Fletcher, "John Newport Langley. In memoriam," *J. Physiol.*, 1926, 61: 2-3.

capable of forming compounds. On this assumption then the atropin or pilocarpin compounds are formed according to some law of which their relative mass and chemical affinity for the substance are factors.[4]

This statement contains the germ of the receptor theory, but Langley did not follow it up for another quarter of a century.

The Side Chain Theory of Paul Ehrlich

In the same year that Langley published the above-mentioned paper, 1878, Paul Ehrlich received his medical degree from the University of Leipzig. His thesis dealt with histological staining. This interest in dyes was to influence much of his later work, and it is necessary to note here the views expressed in this dissertation concerning the mechanism of binding of dyes to the tissues. Ehrlich suggested that the process was more than merely physical adhesion, but he saw it as involving a chemical interaction similar to that involved in the formation of so-called "double salts" (i.e., the linking together of two apparently saturated compounds, such as silver chloride and mercurous chloride). The reaction might be non-stoichiometric, but nevertheless it was chemical in nature.[5] He also recognized that the chemical group on the dye molecule which was responsible for its color was generally not the same as the group responsible for the molecule's affinity for the tissues.[6]

In his "Habilitationsschrift" for his appointment as "Privatdocent" in the University of Berlin (1885), Ehrlich investigated the ability of different tissues to reduce certain dyestuffs. This study is relevant to our present concern because it contains the first indication of his famous "side chain" theory.[7] Ehrlich pointed out that recent studies on the

---

[4] J. N. Langley, "On the physiology of the salivary secretion. Part II. On the mutual antagonism of atropin and pilocarpin, having especial reference to their relations in the sub-maxillary gland of the cat," *J. Physiol.*, 1878, *1*: 367.

[5] Paul Erlich, "Contributions to the theory and practice of histological staining," in *The Collected Papers of Paul Ehrlich*, edited by F. Himmelweit (London: Pergamon Press, 1956-1960), vol. 1, p. 68-73 (previously unpublished Inaugural Dissertation, University of Leipzig, 1878). All references to Ehrlich's published works will be cited from the *Collected Papers* (as it will be referred to hereafter) except in the case of works which were not included in this collection. If an English version of the publication appears in the *Collected Papers*, the reference will be to this version. For bibliographical purposes, the place and date of the first published version of all works will be given in parentheses after each citation (e.g., in this note the original version, in this case an unpublished dissertation, of Ehrlich's paper on staining is cited).

[6] *Ibid.*, pp. 73-74.

[7] Paul Ehrlich, "The requirement of the organism for oxygen: an analytical study with the aid of dyes," *Collected Papers*, vol. 1, pp. 435-438 (Berlin: Hirschwald, 1885). For a discussion of the concept of protoplasm as a "giant molecule" ("biogen"), see Thomas

connection between chemical constitution and function, e.g., in dyes, showed that particular properties depend upon the presence of specific atom groups. This concept can also be applied to protoplasm. He adopted Eduard Pflüger's view that protoplasm can be envisioned as a giant molecule consisting of a chemical nucleus of special structure which is responsible for the specific functions of a particular cell (e.g., a liver cell or a kidney cell), with attached chemical side chains. These side chains are more involved in the vital processes common to all cells than in the specific functions of a particular type of cell. It was likely, he felt, that the side chains were the site of cellular oxidation. Some side chains have the ability to fix oxygen (or, more accurately, to give up hydrogen to oxygen and thus become oxidizing agents themselves).[8] Other side chains are concerned with nutrition. Ehrlich imagined that there were probably certain sites on the chemical nucleus which had the capacity to attract and fix "combustible molecule-groups," thus building up nutritive side chains. These nutritive chains are consumed during the process of oxidation and then regenerated.

It was this side chain concept which Ehrlich later used to explain the neutralization of bacterial toxins by antibodies. In 1890, he joined the staff of Robert Koch's newly founded Institute for Infectious Diseases, and became actively involved in the problems of immunotherapy. In 1897, he published the first account of his influential side chain theory of immunity.[9] His experiments with toxins such as ricin and diptheria toxin indicated that the interaction between a toxin and its antitoxin is chemical in nature. Perhaps influenced by his earlier work on dyes, he suggested that the neutralization of a toxin by an antitoxin or antibody may involve the formation of a double salt, although the evidence seemed to indicate that the reaction was stoichiometric (a molecule of toxin combined with a definite quantity of antibody in accordance with the proportions of a simple equivalence). He further noted:

It must be assumed that this ability to combine with antitoxin is attributable to the presence in the toxin complex of a specific group of atoms with a maximum specific

---

Hall, *Ideas of Life and Matter* (Chicago: University of Chicago Press, 1969), vol. 2, pp. 351-353.

[8] Ehrlich, "Requirement" (n. 7 above), pp. 482-485.

[9] Paul Ehrlich, "The assay of the activity of diphtheria-curative serum and its theoretical basis," *Collected Papers*, vol. 2, pp. 113-115 (*Klin. Jb.*, 1897).

affinity to another group of atoms in the antitoxin complex, the first fitting the second easily, as a key does a lock, to quote Emil Fischer's well-known simile.[10]

Ehrlich was referring, of course, to Fischer's "lock and key theory" of enzyme action, which was first published in 1894.[11] In attempting to explain the structural specificity exhibited by certain enzymes towards their substrates, Fischer utilized the analogy of a lock and key to emphasize the close relationship which must exist between the configuration of the enzyme and the configuration of the substrate.

The organism has the ability to neutralize a multiplicity of different toxins, yet Ehrlich found it hard to believe that the body had the "inventive activity" to create as needed antitoxins with the appropriate chemical structure to combine with specific toxins. This idea probably seemed to him to border on vitalism, and he dismissed it as a return to the concepts current in the days of "Naturphilosophie."[12] It seemed more likely that the enhancement of a normal cell function was involved, and that physiological analogs of the antibodies must exist beforehand in the organism.

To explain the process of immunization, he called upon the side chain theory which he had earlier used to explain cellular oxidation (Fig. I). Assume, he postulated, that one of the side chains possesses an atom group with a specific combining property for a particular toxin, such as tetanus toxin (No. 1). This side chain is normally involved in ordinary physiological processes, and it is merely coincidental that it has the ability to combine with tetanus toxin. Later,[13] he tended to identify this normal physiological function as a nutritive one, the taking up of foodstuffs (which thus become assimilated into protoplasm). He noted that toxins are complex, protein-like substances, hence it would not be surprising if they possessed a combining group corresponding to that of a foodstuff. Combination with the toxin, however, renders the side chain

[10] *Ibid.*, p. 114.

[11] Emil Fischer, "Einfluss der Configuration auf die Wirkung der Enzyme." *Ber. dtsch. chem. Ges.*, 1894, 27: 2992.

[12] In the original German version of the paper cited in note 9 above, Ehrlich uses the term "Zeiten der Naturphilosophie." See Paul Ehrlich, "Die Wertbemessung des Diphtherieheilserums und deren theoretische Grundlagen." *Collected Papers*, vol. 2, p. 94. This phrase is translated in the English version (n. 9 above, p. 114) as the "days of [an obsolete] natural philosophy." It appears to us, however, that Ehrlich is probably referring specifically to the German "Naturphilosophie" of Oken. Goethe and others in the early nineteenth century.

[13] Paul Ehrlich, "On immunity with special reference to cell life." *Collected Papers*, vol. 2, pp. 184-185 (*Proc. Roy. Soc.*, 1900).

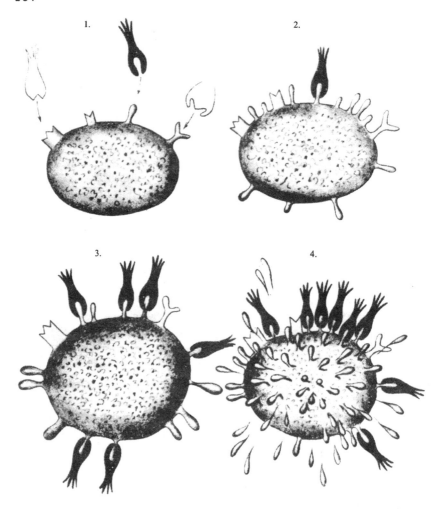

Fig. I

Diagrammatic Representation of Ehrlich's Side Chain Theory
Ehrlich emphasized that these diagrams were merely a pictorial method of presenting his
views and were not supposed to represent morphological structures. (*Proc. Roy. Soc.*, 1900.
With the permission of the Royal Society.)

incapable of performing its physiological function (No. 2). The cell
then produces more of these side chains to make up for the deficiency,
but it overcompensates (No. 3). Excess side chains are produced, and
these break away from the cell and are released into the bloodstream
(No. 4). These excess side chains in the blood are what we call anti-

bodies or antitoxins, and they neutralize the toxin by combining with it. If the toxin cannot be fixed to the cell by combining with a side chain attached to the chemical nucleus, it cannot exert its poisonous effects.[14] Ehrlich later distinguished clearly between the "toxophore" and the "haptophore" groups of the toxin. The haptophore group is the atom group involved in binding the toxin to the side chain. Once the toxin is thus anchored to the cell, the cell comes under the influence of the toxophore group, which is responsible for the poisonous properties of the toxin.[15] This concept may have derived from an analogy with dyes, where the chemical grouping responsible for color is different from that responsible for fixing the dye to the fabric or tissue.

Ehrlich's theory became more elaborate as he struggled to explain various immunological phenomena, but it is not necessary for us to discuss these modifications here.[16] This paper is concerned with his views about the mechanism of action of drugs, and his work on immunity has been considered here, in brief outline, only because of its influence on his thinking about drugs.

Ehrlich's Reluctance to Apply the Side Chain Concept to Drugs

Accounts of Ehrlich's work generally stress the similarity of his view of "chemoreceptors" for drugs to his side chain theory of immunity. The obvious relationship between these two concepts should not mislead us, as it has some authors, into assuming that the former followed directly and immediately from the latter. For when we examine Ehrlich's work, we find that it took him about ten years to apply his side chain theory to the problem of drug action. Indeed, he at first specifically denied that drugs were bound to the cell in a manner similar to the binding of toxins, a fact generally overlooked in the historical literature.[17]

---

[14] Ehrlich, "Assay" (n. 9 above), p. 115.

[15] Ehrlich, "Immunity" (n. 13 above), pp. 181-182, 185-186.

[16] For further information on Ehrlich's elaboration of his theory of immunity, see his *Collected Studies in Immunity*, translated by Charles Bolduan (New York: John Wiley, 1906); also Ernest Witebsky, "Ehrlich's side-chain theory in the light of present immunology," *Ann. N.Y. Acad. Sci.*, 1954, *59*: 168-181.

[17] T. S. Work, "The work of Paul Ehrlich and his position in the history of medical research," *Int. Arch. Allergy*, 1954, *5*: 103 claims that Ehrlich's "Habilitationsschrift" (1885) contains the idea that drugs are fixed to receptors because they are chemically similar to the foodstuffs normally fixed by these receptors. Adrien Albert, "The relationship between structure and biological activity: some fundamental aspects," *Ergeb. Physiol.*, 1957, *49*: 426 discusses Ehrlich's theory of immunology and then adds that "Ehrlich soon applied the concept of receptors to explain the action of drugs." We provide evidence in

In an address delivered in 1898, for example, he stated that it is not likely that a firm combination is formed between a drug and the cell, such as in the case of toxins. He pointed out that many drugs can easily be extracted from tissues by solvents, thus they cannot be firmly bound. In addition, the action of many drugs is of a transitory character. Barring a few exceptions, chemically defined drugs and poisons, as opposed to foodstuffs and toxins, are not incorporated into the protoplasmic molecule by a chemical union. They do not possess haptophore groups and are not capable of evoking the production of antibodies.[18]

In his Croonian Lecture of 1900, Ehrlich stated:

If alkaloids, aromatic amines, antipyretics, or aniline dyes be introduced into the animal body it is a very easy matter, by means of water, alcohol, or acetone, according to the nature of the substance, to remove all these things quickly and easily from the tissues . . . . We are therefore obliged to conclude that none of the foreign bodies just mentioned enter synthetically into the cell complex; but are merely contained in the cells in their free state. The combinations into which they enter with the cells, and notably with the not really living parts of them . . . are very unstable, and usually correspond only to the conditions obtaining in solid solutions, while in other cases only a feeble salt-like formation takes place. . . .

Hence with regard to the pharmacologically active bodies in general, it was not allowable to assume that they possessed definite atom groups, which entered into combination with corresponding groups of the protoplasm.[19]

Yet Ehrlich was well aware of the fact that drugs exhibit a selectivity for certain tissues. In fact, he argued that the distribution of a substance in the organism plays an essential part in determining pharmacological activity. His own experimental work had demonstrated to him the affinities of various dyes for specific tissues, such as nerve tissue or fat tissue, and he was convinced that drugs act in a similar manner.[20] This

---

this paper, however, which contradicts these statements and demonstrates that Ehrlich did not apply the receptor concept to drugs until much later. Even when such claims are not specifically made, accounts of Ehrlich's work generally seem to overlook the fact that he deliberately refused to apply the side chain theory to drugs for some ten years. See, for example, Hans Loewe, *Paul Ehrlich: Schöpfer der Chemotherapie* (Stuttgart: Wissenschaftliche Verlagsgesellschaft, 1950), especially pp. 182-187, and Claude Dolman, "Paul Ehrlich," *Dictionary of Scientific Biography* (New York: Charles Scribner's Sons, 1971), vol. 4, pp. 295-305.

[18] Paul Ehrlich, "The relations existing between chemical constitution, distribution and pharmacological action," *Collected Papers*, vol. 1, pp. 608-611, 613-614 (*v. Leyden Festschrift*, Berlin: Hirschwald, 1902). In this connection, Ehrlich criticized Lowe's theory of the action of "substituting poisons" (*ibid.*, pp. 610-611).

[19] Ehrlich, "Immunity" (n. 13 above), p. 184.

[20] See, for example, his "Constitution, distribution and pharmacological action" (n. 18 above), pp. 602-608.

specificity had to be explained, and here his work on dyes once again influenced his thinking.

The fixing of dyes, he noted, is not merely a mechanical or physical process involving surface attraction and adsorption. He discussed two current theories of the mechanism of dyeing or staining, each of which might be correct, he felt, in certain cases. The first of these involved the combination of the dye with a constituent of the fabric to form an insoluble, salt-like compound called a "lake." A similar process might occur, he felt, in the tissues of the organism and might be involved in fixing drugs. Cells which possessed constituents capable of forming a "lake" with a particular drug could thus localize the drug. Although this process involves chemical combination, it is quite different from his side chain or receptor concept. The drug is not thought to combine with the cellular protoplasm (note Ehrlich's reference in the above quotation from his Croonian Lecture to the "not really living parts" of the cell). Instead, it is believed to react with a free substance in the cell, such as an acid, to form an insoluble complex which precipitates out of solution and is thus fixed in the cell.

The second theory of dyeing discussed by Ehrlich involved the formation of solid solutions, where the dye forms a homogeneous mixture with the substance of the fabric. He suggested that certain drugs might be fixed in cells through a similar process, which he associated with the lipid portions of the cell. We must assume, he stated, "that certain fat-like substances of the nervous system, as well as the fat of fat cells, possess a high solvent power, by means of which these soluble substances are anchored or accumulated in the tissue, just as the alkaloids are taken up by the ether in the Stas-Otto procedure." Again, this mechanism (based upon the physicochemical property of solubility) is quite different from the side chain theory, and does not involve chemical combination between an atom group of the drug and an atom group of a receptor. Hence while Ehrlich felt that the interaction between a drug and the cell involved "chemical affinities in the widest meaning of the term" (i.e., the formation of "lakes" and solid solutions), he did not believe that drugs (barring a few exceptions) entered into a "chemical union" with the "protoplasmic molecule." [21]

In the case of drugs, Ehrlich believed, there was no single definite

[21] *Ibid.*, pp. 608, 614-616. Ehrlich noted that of the hundreds of different compounds which he investigated, he only found convincing evidence, in his view, for the formation of a chemical synthetic union with protoplasm in one case (*ibid.*, p. 611).

group, no haptophore group, which was responsible for the distribution of the substance in the organism (i.e., responsible for fixing it in specific cells). Instead, the distribution of a drug depended upon "the combined action of the separate components," and hence upon the "entire constitution" of the molecule. On the other hand, he felt that drugs did possess toxophore or "therapeutically active" groups which were responsible for their pharmacological action once they were fixed in the cell (although he did not offer any suggestions as to the mechanism involved).[22]

In defending his views of the essential difference between the mode of action of toxins and that of drugs, Ehrlich argued in 1903 that whereas the haptophore groups of toxins exhibit a specific combining power towards certain atom groups of protoplasm, the ordinary functional groups of organic chemistry possess affinities for a large number of other groups. For example, aldehyde groups can unite with amino groups, methylene groups. etc. Their combining power is not specifically limited, and hence the lock and key analogy (and the receptor concept) does not apply to drugs.[23]

Ehrlich's doubts about the probability of a "true chemical combination" taking place between the drug and the cell were shared by many of his contemporaries. The fact that so little was known about the nature of chemical bonding must certainly have played an important role in creating such doubts. Chemical combination was generally thought of essentially in terms of covalent bonds, which are not easily broken. Such concepts as hydrogen bonds and Van der Waals bonds had not yet been developed, nor was the electronic nature of bonding recognized. It was thus hard to reconcile phenomena such as the ease with which many drugs could be washed out of tissues by solvents with the contemporary concepts of chemical bonding.

By the end of the nineteenth century, some of the early enthusiasm about studying the relationship between pharmacological activity and chemical structure had begun to wane. The task had proved far more difficult than some investigators had imagined, and no general laws had emerged from such studies.[24] There was also a growing awareness of the

---

[22] *Ibid.,* pp. 617-618.

[23] Paul Ehrlich, "Toxin and antitoxin: a reply to the latest attack of Gruber," in his *Collected Studies on Immunity* (n. 16 above), pp. 531-533 (this paper was originally published in *Münch. med Wochensch.,* 1903; the German version was reprinted in Ehrlich's *Collected Papers,* vol. 2, pp. 391-394).

[24] See Parascandola, "Structure-activity" (n. 1 above), p. 9.

importance of such physical properties as solubility in determining the action of drugs, and the advances made in physical chemistry during this period no doubt stimulated interest in such factors. Some pharmacologists preferred to attribute most drug actions to general physicochemical properties of the molecule rather than to the presence of specific structural features which would enable the molecule to combine with the cell. While it was recognized that physical properties depended ultimately on chemical structure, such questions were in the realm of the chemist and the physicist rather than the pharmacologist. As Arthur Cushny noted in 1903, if the pharmacological effects of drugs are due to the formation of chemical compounds in the tissues, then the pharmacologist must be concerned with the molecular structure of drugs. If, on the other hand, the action is due more to the physical properties of the drugs as "uncombined foreign bodies," then structure is of less immediate interest to the pharmacologist.[25] He himself felt that:

. . . many facts . . . can be explained more satisfactorily by assuming that structure is only the ultimate fact, and that the physical factors depending on structure are the immediate determinants of the action in the organism.[26]

By the end of the nineteenth century, it had become obvious that chemicals of widely different structures can sometimes produce the same pharmacological effect. The best known example of this phenomenon involved narcosis, which can be produced by such diverse compounds as ether, chloroform, pentane, etc. (which are generally rather inert chemically). At the turn of the twentieth century, Meyer and Overton independently pointed out that the depressant activities of these narcotic agents was directly proportional to their partition coefficients between a lipid and water, i.e., dependent upon a physical property only indirectly related to structure.[27] The role played by chemical combination in determining pharmacological activity was thus further called into question.

[25] Arthur Cushny, "The pharmacologic action of drugs. Is it determined by chemical structure or by physical characters?" *J. Amer. Med. Assoc.*, 1903, *41*: 1253.

[26] *Ibid.*, p. 1255. For a discussion of this controversy over the nature of drug action, see John Parascandola, "The controversy over structure-activity relationships in the early 20th century," *Pharmacy in History*, 1974, *16*: 54-63.

[27] Hans Meyer, "Zur Theorie der Alkoholnarkose. Erste Mittheilung. Welche Eigenschaft der Anästhetica bedingt ihre narkotische Wirkung?" *Arch. exp. Path. Pharmakol.*, 1899, *42*: 109-137; E. Overton, *Studien über die Narkose, zugleich ein Beitrag zur allgemeinen Pharmakologie* (Jena: Gustav Fischer, 1901). Adrien Albert has pointed out that the Overton-Meyer rule was very disturbing to those investigating the relationship between

Ehrlich Changes His Mind

As late as September of 1906, in an address delivered at the dedication of the Georg-Speyer-Haus, Ehrlich discussed the question of the affinity of drugs for various tissues or various types of organisms without utilizing the receptor concept. He stressed the fact that drugs must be "fixed" in the cell before they can act, and he suggested that the action of drugs depends upon the presence of two structural features, a selective group which governs distribution and a pharmacophore group which is responsible for pharmacological activity (the same type of dualism which appears in his thinking about dyes and toxins).[28] Ehrlich had thus moved a step closer to accepting the side chain theory for drugs by adopting the view that a specific chemical group (the "selective group"), rather than the entire structure of the molecule, is responsible for its distribution in the body (i.e., for its being fixed in particular cells). There is no mention, however, of a specific chemical combination between the drug and a receptor or side chain in the cell. Yet by June of 1907, when he delivered his Harben Lectures in London, he was able to state:

> I have now formed the opinion that some of the chemically defined substances are attached to the cell by atom groupings that are analogous to toxin-receptors; these atom groupings I will distinguish from the toxin-receptors by the name of "chemo-receptors." [29]

---

structure and activity. See his "Relations between molecular structure and biological activity: stages in the evolution of current concepts," *Ann. Rev. Pharmacol.*, 1971, *11*: 15-16. Ehrlich, incidentally, felt that he had been the first to point out the pharmacological importance of the distribution of a substance between tissues in his discussion of neurotropic, lipotropic, etc. properties, and to emphasize the importance of lipid solubility. He complained that Meyer had overlooked his work. See Paul Ehrlich, "Address delivered at the dedication of the Georg-Speyer-Haus," *Collected Papers*, vol. 3, pp. 56-57 (previously unpublished).

[28] Ehrlich, "Georg-Speyer-Haus" (n. 27 above), pp. 54-58.

[29] Paul Ehrlich, "Experimental researches on specific therapy: chemotherapeutic studies on trypanosomes. Third Harben Lecture," *Collected Papers*, vol. 3, p. 132 (*The Harben Lectures for 1907 of the Royal Institute of Public Health*, London: Lewis, 1908). Martha Marquardt, Ehrlich's secretary, recounts that when Professor Erich Hoffmann of Bonn came to visit him in the autumn of 1906, Ehrlich mentioned that his experiments had convinced him that chemical substances such as atoxyl are fixed by receptors in the cell. See Martha Marquardt, *Paul Ehrlich* (London: Heinemann, 1949), pp. 151-152. Her recollection of this meeting, written many years later, may not be accurate in every detail, but this story is not incompatible with the views presented in this paper. It would appear that Ehrlich became firmly convinced of the receptor theory of drug action somewhere between September 6, 1906 (when he delivered the Speyer-Haus speech) and early June of 1907 (when he delivered his Harben Lectures).

What had happened to change Ehrlich's mind about the mechanism of action of drugs? Two important factors appear to have played a role in altering Ehrlich's attitude, the work of J. N. Langley and Ehrlich's own studies on drug resistance. In 1913, Ehrlich, looking back at this period, said:

> For many reasons I had hesitated to apply these ideas about receptors to chemical substances in general, and in this connexion it was, in particular, the brilliant investigations by Langley, on the effects of alkaloids, which caused my doubts to disappear and made the existence of chemoreceptors seem probable to me.[30]

We must thus turn back to Langley and consider these investigations to which Ehrlich refers.

Langley and Receptive Substances

Since the late 1880s, Langley had been involved in a detailed study of the autonomic nervous system, the work for which he is best known. During the course of this research, he found that the drug nicotine was a useful tool in the investigation of the structures and functions of the autonomic system. Some of his early experimental work with Dickinson suggested to him that the paralysis of sympathetic nerves caused by nicotine was due to a direct action of the drug on the nerve cells of the superior cervical ganglia, rather than on the peripheral endings of the sympathetic nerves.[31] In 1901, he was able to demonstrate more convincingly that the stimulation of sympathetic ganglia by nicotine, which preceded paralysis of the nerves, was due to a direct action on the nerve cells. Langley severed the pre-ganglionic fibers and allowed their nerve endings to degenerate, yet nicotine still had its usual stimulating effect, thus indicating that it did not cause stimulation by acting on the nerve endings.[32]

In the same year, he reported on a study of the effects of supra-renal extract, which contained adrenalin as its active ingredient.[33] His interest

---

[30] Paul Ehrlich, "Chemotherapy," *Collected Papers,* vol. 3, p. 507 (*Proc. 17th Int. Congr. Med.,* 1913, published 1914).

[31] J. N. Langley and W. Lee Dickinson, "On the local paralysis of peripheral ganglia, and on the connexion of different classes of nerve fibres with them," *Proc. Roy. Soc.,* 1889, *46:* 423-431; J. N. Langley and W. Lee Dickinson, "On the progressive paralysis of the different classes of nerve cells in the superior cervical ganglion," *ibid.,* 1890, *47:* 379-390.

[32] J. N. Langley, "On the stimulation and paralysis of nerve-cells and of nerve-endings. Part I," *J. Physiol.,* 1901, *27:* 228-229.

[33] J. N. Langley, "Observations on the physiological action of extracts of the supra-renal bodies," *J. Physiol.,* 1901, *27:* 237-256.

in this substance was probably motivated by the fact that it was known to produce certain effects similar to those resulting from stimulation of the sympathetic nerves, such as contraction of the unstriated muscle of the eye.[34] Supra-renal extract thus seemed like another potential tool in his investigation of the autonomic nerves. Langley was able to demonstrate other effects of the extract, such as the constriction of the blood vessels of the sub-maxillary gland, which were also similar to the effects produced upon stimulation of certain sympathetic nerves. The evidence thus suggested that the extract exerted its action through stimulation of the sympathetic nerve endings which terminated in the various glands or muscles affected. On the other hand, Langley confirmed and extended the earlier observation of Lewandowsky [35] that supra-renal extract continued to exert its effects after degeneration of the post-ganglionic sympathetic nerves had taken place. To Langley, this was strong evidence that the action must be directly on the tissues affected, such as unstriated muscle, and not on the nerve endings.[36]

Langley's studies generated a certain amount of controversy, for since Claude Bernard's work on curare there had been a tendency to view the nerve endings as being especially sensitive to the action of various drugs. Brodie and Dixon challenged Langley's conclusions about the action of supra-renal extract (adrenalin), and offered evidence that it acted on the nerve endings or on the "connection link" between nerve and muscle.[37] Elliott elaborated upon this latter suggestion and developed a theory of the action of adrenalin on the "myo-neural junction." [38] But Langley was convinced that there was more or less satisfactory evidence that a number of drugs and poisons act directly on tissues such as muscle and gland, rather than through the nerve endings or through a hypothetical myo-neural junction.[39] It was in an attempt to provide further evidence for this point of view that he was led to develop the recep-

[34] For example, Langley (*ibid.*, pp. 244-245) called attention to the studies of Lewandowsky on supra-renal extract. See M. Lewandowsky, "Ueber die Wirkung des Nebennierenextractes auf die glatten Muskeln, im Besonderen des Auges," *Arch. Physiol.*, 1899, 360-366.

[35] Lewandowsky, *ibid.*

[36] Langley, "Observations" (n. 33 above), p. 256.

[37] T. G. Brodie and W. E. Dixon, "Contributions to the physiology of the lungs. Part II. On the innervation of the pulmonary blood vessels; and some observations on the action of suprarenal extract," *J. Physiol.*, 1904, *30:* 491-501.

[38] T. R. Elliott, "The action of adrenalin," *J. Physiol.*, 1905, *32:* 427-441.

[39] J. N. Langley, "On the reaction of cells and of nerve-endings to certain poisons, chiefly as regards the reaction of striated muscle to nicotine and to curari," *J. Physiol.*, 1905, *33:* 379-380.

tor theory, which was first described in a paper published in 1905 and in his Croonian Lecture of the following year.

Langley decided to test his hypothesis on another tissue besides unstriated muscle or gland tissue, and he chose striated muscle for his experiments.[40] In 1903, in the course of investigating the sympathetic nervous system of birds, he had devoted some attention to the muscular contraction which was known to be produced in fowl by injection of nicotine. At that time, this contraction appeared to him to be largely due to a stimulation of the nerve endings.[41] In 1905, however, he decided to examine this phenomenon in greater detail in connection with the developing controversy about the site of action of drugs such as nicotine and adrenalin. The injection of nicotine into the fowl caused certain muscles to contract, in fact to pass into a state of tonic rigidity. Nicotine, of course, also exerts a paralyzing action, when administered in sufficient quantities, by preventing stimulation of the motor nerve from having any effect upon the muscle. Yet Langley found that even after the nervous-muscular connection had been blocked by relatively large doses of nicotine, further administration of the drug still continued to cause muscular contraction.[42] Could it be that nicotine acts upon two different parts of the neuro-muscular mechanism, paralyzing the nerve endings (thus preventing nervous stimulation of muscle) while at the same time directly stimulating the muscle? Since the paralyzing effect of curare, like that of nicotine, was believed to be due to an action on the nerve endings, Langley reasoned that if the contraction caused by nicotine in fowls was really due to a direct action on the muscle cell it should not be antagonized by curare. He found to the contrary, however, that curare had a marked antagonizing effect; a sufficient dose of curare completely annulled the contraction produced by a small amount of nicotine and diminished that caused by a large amount. Further injection of nicotine once again resulted in contraction.[43]

Langley's next step was to investigate the effects of these drugs when no nerve endings were present, i.e. after cutting the nerves to the muscle and allowing them to degenerate. He found that nicotine still produced

[40] *Ibid.*, p. 380.

[41] J. N. Langley, "On the sympathetic system of birds, and on the muscles which move the feathers," *J. Physiol.*, 1903, *30:* 239.

[42] Langley, "On the reaction" (n. 39 above), pp. 380-385; J. N. Langley, "On nerve endings and on special excitable substances in cells," *Proc. Roy. Soc.*, B, 1906, *78:* 174-176.

[43] Langley "On the reaction" (n. 39 above), pp. 387-393; Langley, "On nerve endings" (n. 42 above), pp. 176-178.

contraction after section of the nerves, and, in fact, that curare continued to antagonize this contracting action. He could only conclude that both substances were capable of a direct action on the muscle cell.[44]

To explain the observed antagonism between nicotine and curare, he returned to the suggestion he had made in 1878 when discussing the antagonism between atropine and pilocarpine. The two drugs must act on the same protoplasmic substance or substances in the muscle, and presumably this involved a combination of the alkaloid with protoplasm. In the presence of both nicotine and curare, which muscle-alkaloid compound is formed depends upon the amount of each alkaloid present and on their relative chemical affinities for the muscle substance.[45]

Since the contracting effect of nicotine and the antagonistic effect of curare were apparently due to an action on the muscle, Langley questioned whether there was any justification for the accepted view that the paralyzing action of these compounds occurred at the nerve endings. He saw no need to postulate two different sites of action. Since the curare decreased the irritability of the muscle to the nicotine stimulus, he felt that it was not unreasonable to assume that it also decreased the irritability of the muscle to nervous stimuli, inducing paralysis in this fashion. Nicotine prevented stimulation of the nerves from causing contraction in the same manner, but it also had the ability of itself stimulating the contraction of muscle (hence explaining its double action of stimulation and paralysis).[46]

After a muscle had been paralyzed by curare or nicotine and it no longer reacted to nervous stimulation, the muscle could still be directly stimulated to contract, e.g., by an electrical current. The muscle substance with which these drugs combine, Langley reasoned, could thus not be the substance which actually contracts. Instead, nicotine and curare must combine with some other constituent of the muscle cell, and he called this unknown constituent "receptive substance." He postulated that the normal function of this receptive substance is to receive the stimulus from the nerve and transmit it to the contractile substance. By combining with the receptive substance, curare and nicotine might diminish its excitability or irritability, hence preventing nervous stimuli

[44] Langley, "On the reaction" (n. 39 above), pp. 393-397; Langley, "On nerve endings" (n. 42 above), pp. 178-180.

[45] Langley, "On the reaction" (n. 39 above), pp. 392-393 (on p. 393, Langley specifically refers to his earlier work on atropine and pilocarpine); Langley, "On nerve endings" (n. 42 above), pp. 181-182.

[46] *Ibid.*

from having any effect.[47] In 1906, he suggested alternatively that it was also possible that the transmission of an impulse from nerve to muscle does not take place via an electrical discharge, but involves the secretion of a special chemical substance at the end of the nerve. The receptive substance in the muscle cell combines with the chemical transmitter, forming a compound which stimulates the contractible substance. If curare or nicotine combine with the receptive substance, they prevent it from uniting with the transmitter substance and thus block the passage of nervous impulses.[48] Since the contractile substance itself is not altered by these drugs, however, it can still be directly stimulated. The nicotine-receptive substance compound, although blocking nervous transmission, must have a certain ability to stimulate the contractile substance and cause contraction.

Langley felt that there was evidence to suggest that many other drugs and poisons, such as adrenalin, acted by combining with specific constituents of the cell. He generalized:

I conclude then that in all cells two constituents at least must be distinguished, (1) substances concerned with carrying out the chief functions of the cells, such as contraction, secretion, the formation of special metabolic products and (2) receptive substances especially liable to change and capable of setting the chief substance in action. Further, that nicotine, curari, atropine, pilocarpine, strychnine, and most other alkaloids, as well as the effective material of internal secretions produce their effects by combining with the receptive substance, and not by action on axon-endings if these are present, nor by a direct action on the chief substance.[49]

The fact that drugs produce different effects in different cells indicates that all cells do not possess the same receptive substance or substances. One would expect, however, that the receptive substances of the cells within a given class would be similar. Consequently, Langley argued, the fact that the effects of adrenalin on different tissues are always like those produced by stimulation of the sympathetic nerves does not mean that it acts by stimulating these nerves. The relationship of adrenalin to the sympathetic system could be explained by assuming that the presence of sympathetic nerves during the development of certain tissues created a certain chemical environment which led to the

---

[47] Langley, "On the reaction" (n. 39 above), pp. 393, 399; Langley, "On nerve endings" (n. 42 above), pp. 181-183.

[48] Langley, "On nerve endings" (n. 42 above), p. 183.

[49] Langley, "On the reaction" (n. 39 above), pp. 400-401.

formation in these tissues of similar receptive substances, substances which had the ability to combine with adrenalin.[50]

Langley also suggested that the receptive substances and the other substances responsible for carrying out the function of the cell need not actually be separate compounds. It is possible, he commented, that the receptive substance is a side chain on the contractile molecule.[51] In his Croonian Lecture of 1906, he leaned towards the more general idea that all of these different substances (receptive substance, contractile substance, etc.) are radicles or side chains of the protoplasmic molecule.[52] He recognized [53] and specifically mentioned the similarity of such views to Ehrlich's side chain theory of immunity, and we must now return to Ehrlich and his adoption of the concept of chemoreceptors for drugs.

Ehrlich's Receptor Theory of Drug Action

Ehrlich himself has indicated, as previously mentioned, that Langley's work was instrumental in changing his mind about drug receptors. An entry in one of his notebooks indicates that he was aware of Langley's concept of receptive substances by February of 1906, although his failure to mention this theory in his address at the dedication of the Speyer-Haus in September of that year suggests that he was not yet convinced of its validity.[54] It is questionable, however, whether Ehrlich would have been receptive to Langley's theory if the studies being carried out in his own laboratory at about that time on drug resistance had not provided him with another reason for altering his ideas. It was in dealing with the phenomenon of drug resistance that he first applied the receptor concept to drugs.

About 1903, Ehrlich and his coworkers had begun in earnest their work in chemotherapy with a study of the effects of various chemicals in treating infections caused by trypanosomes, the microorganisms responsible for sleeping sickness. Over the next few years, their work and that of other investigators established that there were three different classes of compounds which could attack trypanosomes:

1) arsenical compounds, such as atoxyl;

---

[50] *Ibid.*, pp. 402-404.

[51] *Ibid.*, p. 399.

[52] Langley, "On nerve endings" (n. 42 above), p. 194.

[53] Langley, "On the reaction" (n. 39 above), p. 399.

[54] Paul Ehrlich's Copybooks, MS, Series IV, No. III, p. 127, February 20, 1906, Wellcome Institute of the History of Medicine Library, London, England.

2) azo dyes, such as trypan red; and

3) basic triphenylmethane dyes, such as fuchsin.[55]

Experiments carried out in Ehrlich's laboratory by Franke, Röhl and Browning in the period 1905-1907 led to the first clear recognition of the phenomenon of drug resistance. The results of these studies were published by Ehrlich and by Browning in 1907.[56]

During the treatment of trypanosome-infected animals by drugs, in some cases the trypanosomes would disappear from the blood for a time and then reappear again at a later date. When the animal was treated again with the same drug, a larger dose was necessary to banish the microorganism from the blood stream for a second time. The trypanosomes might then reappear again, and a still greater quantity of the drug would be required to remove them. Eventually, the drug was virtually ineffective and the animal succumbed to the disease. Was this diminishing effect of the drug due to an alteration of the trypanosome strain or to some change occurring in the host animal? Franke and Röhl were able to demonstrate that in such cases the recurrence was due to the fact that the trypanosome strain had acquired a resistance to the drug. They treated mice infected with the nagana strain of trypanosomes with parafuchsin, and produced a strain in certain animals which no longer responded to treatment by the drug. When the parasites were isolated from these mice and inoculated into a normal animal, the resulting infection did not respond in the least to parafuchsin. Hence the resistance resided in the microorganisms themselves rather than in the original host animal. Once acquired, this resistance persisted from generation to generation as the trypanosome strain was passed through normal untreated animals.

Browning then developed a strain of trypanosomes resistant to atoxyl, as well as strains resistant to trypan red and trypan blue. Resistance was found not to be limited to the compound used to develop it, but to extend also to other compounds within the same chemical class. For example, the atoxyl-resistant strain exhibited a significant degree of

---

[55] For a discussion of these studies, see Paul Ehrlich, "Chemotherapeutische Trypanosomen-Studien," *Collected Papers*, vol. 3, pp. 81-93 (*Berlin klin. Wochensch.*, 1907). See also Carl Browning, "Chemotherapy in trypanosome-infections: an experimental study," *J. Path. Bact.*, 1908, *12:* 169-176.

[56] Ehrlich, "Trypanosomen-Studien" (n. 55 above), pp. 98-103; Carl Browning, "Experimental chemotherapy in trypanosome infections," *Brit. Med. J.* 1907, *2:* 1405-1409. Our discussion of the drug resistance studies is based upon these two sources.

resistance towards other arsenical compounds, such as acetyl-atoxyl, and the trypan-red resistant strain exhibited some resistance towards other azo dyes, such as trypan blue and trypan violet. The development of resistance towards one group of compounds (e.g., the arsenicals), however, did not increase resistance towards compounds of the other classes (i.e., azo dyes and basic triphenylmethane dyes). A strain with triple resistance, i.e., resistance against all three of the classes of drugs which attacked trypanosomes, was produced by Browning, but each type of resistance had to be developed separately.

In his first published report of these results in 1907, Ehrlich offered a brief and somewhat vague explanation for this specificity, but one which would seem to suggest an acceptance of the receptor concept for drugs. He argued that one must imagine that the protoplasm of trypanosomes (and, in general, of all cells) must possess different "places of attack" ("Angriffsstellen") for which specific types of drugs have particular affinities.[57]

Ehrlich's first clear exposition of his concept of "chemoreceptors" was in his previously mentioned Harben Lectures in London in June of 1907. As we have already noted, he pointed out in these lectures that he had come to believe that at least some drugs are bound to the protoplasm by certain atom groupings in a manner somewhat analogous to the binding of toxins. Yet he stressed the fact that there are fundamental differences between the binding of drugs and the binding of toxins. The chemoreceptors for drugs, he felt, must be assumed to possess a simpler structure than toxin receptors, and they do not show the same independence (i.e., they are not separated from the cell and released into the blood as antibodies).[58] In order for an organism to be acted upon by a given poison, it must possess chemoreceptors which combine with the poison. He further explained (using arsenicals as an example):

If now a mouse infected with trypanosomes is injected with the arsenical medicament, this substance will be distributed between the parasites and the organism of the mouse. If the receptivity of the parasites is the stronger, they will be killed in the organism; in the alternative case, they will not be destroyed. Consequently the curative result obtained when experimenting under normal circumstances represents also the differential between two avidities; i.e., if a mouse infected with the normal strain of trypanosomes is injected with the arsenical preparation, the "trypanotropic" force

[57] Ehrlich, "Trypanosomen-Studien" (n. 55 above), p. 103.
[58] Ehrlich, "Third Harben Lecture" (n. 29 above), p. 132.

of the drug is stronger than the "organotropic" force; we therefore obtain a curative effect with doses which are not injurious to the organism of the mouse.[59]

The studies on drug resistance, Ehrlich argued, supported the concept of chemoreceptors. The atoxyl-resistant strain, for example, was resistant to a number of arsenic compounds which otherwise possessed significant differences in their chemical characteristics. The arsenic acid radicle, however, represents a common point of attack in this series. It is bound to the cell by chemoreceptors. The trypanosome cell possesses other chemoreceptors which represent the points of attack for other poisons.[60] In a lecture to the German Chemical Society and in his Nobel Prize Lecture, both delivered in 1908, Ehrlich emphasized further the indirect evidence which the studies on drug resistance provided for the receptor theory. The specificity of resistance made it clear, he felt, that one was dealing with three separate functions, i.e., there are different receptors for each of the three different known classes of trypanocidal drugs.[61]

The development of resistance, he noted in his Harben Lectures, could be readily explained in terms of the receptor concept. The chemoreceptors of resistant trypanosome strains have somehow developed a reduced affinity for the drug, so that the distribution of the drug between the microorganisms and the host animal is shifted in the direction of the latter (the cells of the host animal, of course, also possess chemoreceptors).[62] Or, in other words, the "organotropic" force of the drug becomes greater than its "trypanotropic" force.

Thus Ehrlich had come to accept the receptor theory of drug action. In 1908, at a Congress of the German Dermatological Society, he admitted that he had earlier believed that drugs, as opposed to toxins, were not bound to specific receptors in the cell, but that the study of

---

[59] Paul Ehrlich, "Experimental researches on specific therapy: on athreptic functions. Second Harben Lecture," *Collected Papers*, vol. 3, p. 121 (*The Harben Lectures for 1907 of the Royal Institute of Public Health*, London: Lewis, 1908).

[60] Ehrlich, "Third Harben Lecture" (n. 29 above), p. 132. Browning, in his 1907 paper (n. 56 above), p. 1408, stated that the results of the resistance studies "can only be explained on the basis of Ehrlich's theory, according to which toxic action depends upon a direct chemical relationship between the toxic agent and particular atom groups of the protoplasm, the chemoreceptors." He added that Langley had recently developed a similar concept. ·

[61] Paul Ehrlich, "Über den jetzigen Stand der Chemotherapie," *Collected Papers*, vol. 3, pp. 159-161 (*Ber. dtsch. chem. Ges.*, 1909) ; Paul Ehrlich, "On partial functions of the cell," *Collected Papers*, vol. 3, pp. 190-191 (*Les Prix Nobel*, 1909).

[62] Ehrlich, "Second Harben Lecture" (n. 59 above), p. 121.

trypanosomes had caused him to change his mind. He now found himself, he added, in agreement with the views of Langley.[63]

Conclusion

The concept of drug receptors was first clearly stated by J. N. Langley in 1905 and by Paul Ehrlich in 1907. Langley's concept developed out of his investigations on the actions of nicotine and adrenaline on the body, which were occasioned by his interest in the sympathetic nervous system. Ehrlich's theory developed out of his studies on drug resistance, which were a result of his interest in the chemotherapy of trypanosomes, and ultimately out of his side chain concept of cellular function. While their ideas were developed separately and from different sources, their thoughts did interact. Langley recognized the similarity of his concept of receptive side chains of protoplasm (an idea which he developed further in his later work) to Ehrlich's side chain theory of immunity. Ehrlich admitted to being influenced by Langley's work in his decision to apply the side chain or receptor concept to drugs.

Both Ehrlich and Langley further developed the concept of drug receptors in the period following the origin of the theory. For Langley, the receptor idea played an important part in his understanding of the interaction of nerves and other cells such as muscles. For Ehrlich, the theory formed the theoretical basis for his work in chemotherapy.

[63] Paul Ehrlich, "Über moderne Chemotherapie," *Collected Papers*, vol. 3, p. 146 (*Verh. 10. Kongr. dtsch. derm. Ges.,* 1908). In a statement written in one of his notebooks in October, 1907, Ehrlich also clearly stated that he had earlier accepted the "lipoid theory," especially in view of the fact that dyestuffs can easily be removed from cells by alcohol. He indicated, however, that on the basis of the work on drug-resistant strains of trypanosomes, he had come to accept the idea of chemoreceptors. See Paul Ehrlich's Copybooks, MS, Series IV, No. IV, p. 132, October 15, 1907, Wellcome Institute of the History of Medicine Library, London, England. By the "lipoid theory" Ehrlich meant the view that substances are fixed in the cell through their solubility in lipids (discussed above).

The Controversy over Structure-Activity Relationships in the Early Twentieth Century *

𝒯HE study of the relationship between pharmacological activity and chemical structure had its beginnings in the nineteenth century. The investigations of James Blake, Benjamin Ward Richardson, Alexander Crum Brown and Thomas Fraser and others demonstrated that a relationship could often be established between certain chemical properties or components of a drug molecule and its physiological action. For example, Crum Brown and Fraser demonstrated that quaternary ammonium compounds were, in general, associated with a paralyzing action. These results led to a feeling of optimism on the part of certain physiologists and pharmacologists that a general law, or perhaps a few generalizations, describing the relationship between structure and activity would soon be discovered, ushering in a therapeutic millenium. Such hopes were doomed to disappointment. By the end of the century, it had become apparent that determining the relationship between structure and activity was more difficult than had originally been anticipated, and no laws of a very general nature had emerged (although a number of generalizations of limited application had come to light).[1]

By the early twentieth century, the significance of the study of structure-activity relationships for pharmacology and drug therapy was being questioned by some scientists on more serious grounds than the difficulty of the task. The fundamental issue was raised as to whether pharmacological activity generally depended directly upon chemical structure, or rather more upon physical properties and thus only indirectly upon structure. The purpose of this paper is to examine the controversy over structure-activity relationships in phar-

* Presented in the Section on Contributed Papers of the American Institute of the History of Pharmacy, Boston, July, 1973. The author wishes to thank the National Science Foundation (under Grant number GS-28549), and the Wisconsin Alumni Research Foundation and the University of Wisconsin Graduate School, for support of this research.

macology in the first quarter of the twentieth century.

The Controversy

In 1901, Cambridge biochemist F. G. Hopkins, in a review of research on the relationship between chemical constitution and physiological action, expressed disappointment that progress in elucidating general laws in this area had been very slow. Yet he was convinced that such a relationship existed, and that the difficulties involved in investigating the question did not render the study unprofitable. Hopkins discussed in some detail the facts which had come to light in nineteenth century studies on various groups of compounds indicating relationships between certain structural features and specified pharmacological actions (such as the characteristic intoxicant and narcotic properties of primary alcohols).[2]

Research on structure-activity relationships continued to be actively pursued in the early twentieth century in spite of the disappointment over the failure to develop broad generalizations. At the Wellcome Chemical Research Laboratories, for example, Frank Lee Pyman and Hooper Jowett investigated structure-activity relationships in the tropeines and other substances. Charles Marshall, at St. Andrew's University, performed structural studies on organic halogen compounds (such as the chlorhydrins), nitro compounds, etc. As one other example, the work of the French pharmaceutical chemist Ernest Fourneau on the relationship of the structure of amino alcohols to their local anesthetic properties may be cited.[3] A number of significant monographs and textbooks on structure-activity relationships,

chemical pharmacology, and drug synthesis were also published in the first quarter of this century.[4] These works summarized the available knowledge of specific relationships between structure and activity in given families of compounds (such as hydrocarbons, amines, related alkaloids, etc.) and emphasized the importance of structural organic chemistry for pharmacology.

Not all drug researchers, however, were enthusiastic about the structural approach. The rise of physical chemistry as a distinct discipline at the end of the nineteenth century apparently led to a greater interest in the influence of physicochemical factors (such as solubility) upon drug action.[5] A controversy began to develop over whether physical (or physicochemical) or chemical properties played more of a part in determining pharmacological activity. Although it was recognized by many that one could not always clearly distinguish between physical and chemical factors,[6] there was a tendency among pharmacologists and others concerned with the question of drug action to emphasize either one or the other approach. Thus, for example, Leopold Spiegel, while admitting that physical properties must be taken into consideration, favored the theory that drugs generally act by forming a chemical union with the protoplasm of the cell. The chemical view also formed the basis of the receptor theories developed by John Newport Langley and by Paul Ehrlich in the first decade of the twentieth century.[7] On the other hand, Walther Straub is an example of a pharmacologist who leaned towards the view that the action of drugs is determined largely by their physical or physicochemical

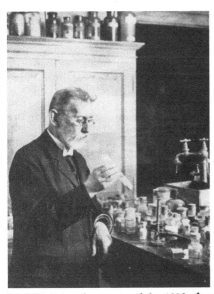

Paul Ehrlich, who suggested in 1898 that the distribution of a drug in the organism is the link between its chemical structure and its pharmacological activity. (Courtesy of the National Library of Medicine).

mulas ("which adorn so many pharmacologic treatises but which I fear fail to enlighten as many readers as they repel") represent. These formulas, he stated, may be regarded as "a sort of shorthand statement of a series of reactions which the compound has been found to present." The formula indicates such things as the origin of the molecule and what compounds it is likely to react with, but it gives one no information about the physical properties of the molecule. Only in so far as the pharmacological action of a drug depends upon its ability to enter into chemical combinations can the structural formula indicate its action. The molecular structure, however, gives no clue to effects which depend upon volatility, solubility, etc., and yet such factors play a crucial role in determining the action of drugs.[9] One cannot then expect to accurately predict the physiological effects of a drug from its structure. As he so quaintly phrased it in a lecture to his students: "In breeding racers one pays attention to relationships, but one would not back a horse for the Derby on the ground of his pedigree only. One must experiment with him by racing him in minor races."[10] Cushny summarized his views as follows:

"In other words, a doubt has arisen whether the pharmacological effects are due to the formation of chemical combinations in the tissues or the presence of the drugs as uncombined foreign bodies in the cells and fluids. If chemical compounds are formed, then the molecular structure is the direct determining factor, though it may be modified by the physical characters, while, on the other hand, if no true chemical combinations are formed, the structure is of less immediate interest to the pharmacologist, and the physical characters ought to receive his chief attention, while the connection between the structure and the physical properties scarcely comes within his sphere of action."[11]

properties.[8] Those who supported the physical view argued that drugs generally induce their effects by altering the surface tension, electrolytic balance, osmotic pressure, etc., of cells, rather than through the formation of chemical bonds with the protoplasm.

The supporters of the physical view tended to criticize the structure-activity approach to pharmacology, with its emphasis on structural organic chemistry. The challenge was clearly stated in 1903 by Arthur Cushny, then Professor of Materia Medica and Therapeutics at the University of Michigan, who was to become one of the most prominent pharmacologists of his generation. In discussing the question of the relationship between molecular structure and pharmacological action, Cushny first analyzed what structural for-

In many cases, Cushny felt, the facts could be more satisfactorily explained by assuming that physical properties were the immediate determinants of the action of a drug, although these properties ultimately depended upon the structure of the molecule (a question outside the pharmacologist's "sphere of action").[12] This view was not uncommon among pharmacologists, physiologists and chemists in the early decades of this century. While it was not denied that changes in chemical constitution affected pharmacological activity, it was often argued (for example, by physiologist William Bayliss, biochemist Carl Alsberg, physical chemist Isidor Traube, and pharmacologist Walther Straub) that since altering the structure of a substance alters its physical properties as well as its chemical reactivity, one could relate the change in physiological action to the former as well as to the latter. Chemical constitution and configuration were thus only important in so far as they determine physical properties.[13]

In Cushny's case, one can clearly see his development of a skeptical attitude toward the structural approach in the pages of his influential *Textbook of Pharmacology and Therapeutics* (the first true textbook of pharmacology in the English language). In the first edition (1899), for example, Cushny wrote:

"*As* the effects of drugs in living matter is conceived to be due to a chemical reaction between them, it might be inferred that those drugs which present a close resemblance in their chemical properties and composition must induce similar changes in the organism. And *this is true as a general statement*, although the relation existing between chemical constitution and pharmacological action can be followed only a short distance as yet." [italics mine].[14]

Cushny did not bother to change this statement through the next three editions of the book even though, as we have seen, he had become quite critical of the chemical view of drug action by 1903.[15] In the fifth edition (1910) of his textbook, however, one can observe significant changes in the wording of his statement on the relationship between structure and activity.

"*If* the effects of drugs on living matter were due to a chemical reaction between them, it might be expected that those drugs which present a close resemblance in their chemical properties and composition would induce similar changes in the organism. And *in a number of instances this has proved correct . . .*" [italics mine].[16]

He then went on to discuss how the relation breaks down when one attempts to follow it in detail, and inserted a new paragraph which clearly revealed his bias towards the physical viewpoint and his

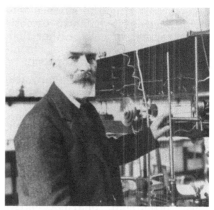

Arthur Robertson Cushny (in his newly-equipped pharmacological laboratory at the University of Edinburgh in 1920), who was one of the critics of the structure-activity approach to pharmacology. (Courtesy of the National Library of Medicine).

doubts about the structural approach.

"As a matter of fact the physical properties of drugs appear to have a more direct bearing upon their action than the chemical structure; that is, the properties of the molecule as a whole determine its effects more than any of its constituent parts. For such properties as solubility in the fluids of the tissues, volatility, and diffusibility in colloid solutions determine whether a drug can be absorbed and come into contact with the living cells; thus, if two drugs differ in solubility in water their effects may be very different, although they are nearly related chemically. These physical characters depend ultimately upon the chemical structure, but as yet little has been done to correlate them with it and it is impossible to deduce them from the structural formulae."[17]

This statement further clarifies the main criticism of the advocates of the physicochemical view against the structure-activity approach. If drug action depended primarily upon physical properties, which appeared to be determined by the structure of the molecule as a whole rather than by the presence of particular functional groups or specific structural features, and if these physical properties could apparently not be predicted from the molecular structure, then why should the pharmacologist concern himself very much with structural chemistry? Even if one desired to attempt to relate physical properties to structure, was this not a task (as Cushny had indicated) for the chemist rather than for the pharmacologist?[18]

The concept that the entire structure of the molecule determines its physiological action through its physicochemical properties seems to have its roots in the work of Paul Ehrlich. Although in the early twentieth century Ehrlich established a theory of "chemoreceptors," which was criticized by those supporting the physical viewpoint, his earlier work contributed to the recognition of the significance of physicochemical properties, such as solubility, in determining pharmacological activity. In 1898, Ehrlich suggested that pharmacological action is only indirectly related to chemical constitution, that there is a link between the two, namely, the distribution in the organism. In order to exert an action on some specific organ, a drug must reach that organ and be localized or concentrated there. At this point in time, Ehrlich felt that drugs were not localized in specific tissues by chemically combining with protoplasm. Rather, he conceived of drugs as being anchored in cells through physicochemical processes such as solid solution. For example, nerve cells contain significant quantities of lipids and hence tend to concentrate lipid-soluble materials. Changing the structure of a drug would alter such properties as its solubility in lipids, and thus its pharmacological activity (by changing its distribution in the body). The distribution of a substance in the body depends upon its entire constitution, Ehrlich argued, and not upon the presence of a single, specific chemical group. Although Ehrlich did mention the need for a drug to possess a "therapeutically active group" in order to exert pharmacological action, his emphasis was on the distribution of the substance in the organism, a factor which depended upon structure, but in a rather general and somewhat obscure fashion.[19] While he stressed the need for structure-activity studies in order to predict selective distribution, his work challenged the direct relationship between constitution and action and emphasized physicochemical mechanisms, such as solution, over chemical combination.

The physicochemical view was probably given its greatest boost, and the structure-activity approach its greatest challenge, by the Meyer-Overton theory of narcosis. By the late nineteenth century, it was obvious that a number of chemicals of widely different chemical composition (such as ether, chloroform, pentane, ethanol, and urethane) all had the ability to produce narcosis in the organism. This situation was difficult to explain from a structural viewpoint, as one could not associate any particular grouping of atoms in these molecules with the narcotic or anesthetic properties. Many anesthetics, in fact, were rather inert chemically. At the turn of the twentieth century, Hans Horst Meyer and Charles Ernest Overton independently concluded that the depressant activities of these narcotic agents was directly proportional to their partition coefficients between lipids and water (i.e., dependent upon a physical property only indirectly related to structure.) [20] Their theory was widely accepted, and even its critics found it hard to deny that lipid solubility apparently played an important part in the action of anesthetics. [21] As Adrien Albert has remarked, the Meyer-Overton hypothesis was deeply disturbing to those attempting to relate structure and activity. [22]

The general anesthetics may have been the most obvious example of substances of very different structures producing a similar physiological effect, but other cases could also be cited. For example, it was recognized that such structurally unrelated substances as cocaine, benzyl alcohol, antipyrine, and certain inorganic salts all exhibit some local anesthetic action. [23] Carl Alsberg, who supported the physical view, argued that for such substances "we may be sure that their action depends upon their physical rather than their chemical properties." [24]

On the other hand, it was observed that substances which were very closely related in structure sometimes differed markedly in their physiological action. Substances as similar in chemical structure as pairs of optical isomers, for example, were shown to exhibit significant differences in pharmacological activity. [25]

Supporters of the structural chemistry approach, of course, responded to these criticisms with arguments defending their views. They challenged the view that drugs generally acted through the physical properties (although admitting that these properties played some part in determining pharmacological activity), and pointed to cases which seemed to illustrate a clear relationship between structure and activity. [26] Even in the case of narcosis, some staunch advocates of the chemical viewpoint believed that while lipid solubility might be responsible for the active agent reaching the site of action, some chemical factors were probably responsible for the actual activity. [27]

Even if physicochemical interactions, rather than "true" chemical combinations, were involved in the fixing of certain drugs in cells, the structural approach would not be negated, argued its defenders. One textbook of chemical pharmacology pointed out that whether the interaction between the drug and the cell was of a physical or a chemical character, the action of a drug appeared to depend on its possessing some specific group of atoms capable of such interaction with the cell, and the pharmacologist must thus concern himself with the correlation of physiological action with molecular structure.[28] Leopold Spiegel also argued that the action of a drug, whether of a chemical or a physical nature, depends upon its chemical constitution, hence structure-activity researches were of great practical value in pharmacology and therapeutics.[29] The practical importance of structural studies was underscored by others, such as Frank Lee Pyman, who emphasized that drugs could be chemically modified in order to eliminate side reactions, improve stability, etc. He added that the relation between chemical constitution and physiological action "has a significance in the discovery of new drugs similar to the relation between chemical constitution and colour in the discovery of new dyes."[30] Percy May, in his *Chemistry of Synthetic Drugs* (1911), suggested that even if pharmacological activity did largely depend upon physical properties, that would be all the more reason for studying the relationship between structure and activity.

"At this point it may be advisable to indicate the relation between the chemical composition and the physical properties of a substance. It is held by some pharmacologists that the physiological action of a drug is conditioned solely by its physical properties, but even if this were always the case, it would not exclude a connection between the physiological action and the chemical constitution. It may be that the effects of some drugs is due to a subtle combination of various physical properties; these cannot, however, be readily ascertained in the majority of cases, but we can endeavour to correlate the chemical constitution—which is the foundation of these properties — with the physiological action."[31]

May thus turned the argument of the supporters of the physical view on its head by implying that it might be easier to correlate physiological action with chemical constitution than with physical properties, even in cases where the latter were directly responsible for the pharmacological effects of the drug.

Conclusion

The controversy over structure-activity relationships was never resolved during the first quarter of the twentieth century. There were no "crucial" experiments which could have been performed to distinguish between the physical and chemical viewpoints. Each side reviewed the same mass of data, but stressed different aspects of and chose to give different interpretations to the "facts." In a sense, both sides were right, since both the physical and the chemical properties of a drug influence its action. The borderline between "physical" and "chemical" has also become more blurred as our understanding of molecular interactions has progressed. In a period when little was known of the biochemistry of the cell, and when the concept of the electronic nature of chemical bonding was only just emerging, however, it is not difficult to understand how a distinction developed between physical and chemical factors which may seem to us to be too rigid and artificial. To scientists at the beginning of the twentieth century, a chemical bond or union implied a covalent bond, as the concepts of hydrogen bonding, Van der Waals forces, etc. had not yet been developed. While some investigators clearly recognized that the term "chemical" might be interpreted more broadly (e.g., it was pointed out by Bayliss that adsorption was not a purely physical process but that "chemical relationships" played a part in it),[32] there was still a lack of agreement about the involvement of "true chemical bonding" in drug action and about the relative importance to pharmacology of physical chemistry as opposed to structural organic chemistry.

Since structure-activity relationships have continued, up to the present time, to be an area of great interest in pharmacology, and since a number of important drugs have been developed in the twentieth century as a result of structural considerations, one might be tempted to conclude that those who challenged the structural approach in the early part of this century impeded the progress of pharmacology. While the doubts that the supporters of the physicochemical theory expressed concerning the value of structure-activity studies may have had a negative influence on this area of research, the questions that they raised also had a positive side which exerted a healthy influence on the relatively young discipline of pharmacology.

The skepticism of the supporters of the physical theory towards structure-activity studies helped to balance overzealous efforts to correlate structure and activity. Some of the chemically-oriented pharmacologists and medicinal chemists of the nineteenth (and even of the twentieth) century tended to oversimplify the complicated relationship between structure and activity by striving too hard to directly relate a particular pharmacological activity to the presence of a specific chemical grouping in the molecule. For example, Benjamin Ward Richardson in the 1860's associated the nitrite group with vasodilation and quickening of the heart, the hydroxyl group with depression of the active function of the cerebrospinal system, etc.[33] While there is, of course, some correlation between certain functional groups and certain pharmacological properties, there was perhaps too much emphasis on attempting to assign anesthetic, depressant, etc. properties to particular chemical groups,[34] and defenders of the physicochemical viewpoint criticized this approach.[35]

In challenging the structural approach, those who favored an emphasis on physical chemistry made pharmacologists more aware of the influence of physical properties on drug action. Even the advocates of the chemical viewpoint were forced to admit the need to take physicochemical factors into account.[36] One textbook of chemical pharmacology, published in 1908, acknowledged that it was necessary to extend to the word "chemical" a very wide significance, i.e., to include all those changes commonly called physicochemical.[37]

Critics of structure-activity research made it clear that altering the structure of a drug might change its physiological action through modification of some physical property, such as solubility, rather than through modification of its chemical reactivity. As Adrien Albert has recently pointed out, a modern scientist is able to glean many of the physical as well as the chemical properties of a substance from an inspection of its molecular formula. As an example, he indicated that with the aid of various "rules" which have been developed, one can predict from the formula of phenol its acid strength, its relative solubility in water as compared to lipoids, its likelihood of being attacked by electrophilic and nucleophilic substances at various positions on the aromatic nucleus, etc.[38] He summarized as follows:

" . . . the discoveries of this century have trained our minds to read out many kinds of chemical and physical properties (many more, in fact, than the above sampling) by mere inspection of the printed structure. There are some kinds of drug action where the structure itself plays an outstanding part, namely in the use of metabolite analogs. In many other kinds of action, a physical property is its main source, and this property could be provided by many kinds of structure."[39]

The debate over structure-activity relationships helped to sharpen the focus of questions relating to the mechanism of drug action. Proponents of both views were no doubt forced to reexamine their thinking and clarify their views as they responded to each other's criticisms. Agreements were even reached on certain key points. De-

spite their differences in outlook, reasonable men on both sides had to admit that both physical and chemical properties were involved in drug action (and that it was not always easy to distinguish between them) and that pharmacological activity was at least ultimately, even if not necessarily directly, related to molecular structure. The discussion of these questions helped pave the way for a broader view of drug action, a view which essentially absorbed both positions and thereby made the controversy no longer meaningful. While there is still ample room for controversy, and still much to be learned about the molecular mechanisms of drug action, pharmacologists are generally agreed upon the importance of both physical chemistry and structural organic chemistry in probing this subject.[40]

Footnotes

1. On nineteenth-century attempts to relate structure and activity, see John Parascandola, "Structure-Activity Relationships: The Early Mirage," *Pharmacy in History*, 13, 3-10 (1971); William Bynum "Chemical Structure and Pharmacological Action: A Chapter in the History of the 19th-Century Molecular Pharmacology," *Bull. Hist. Med.*, 44 518-538 (1970).

2. F. G. Hopkins, "On the Relation between Chemical Constitution and Physiological Action," in William Hale-White, ed., *Textbook of Pharmacology and Therapeutics*, Edinburgh: Young J. Pentland, 1959, pp. 1-39.

3. See, for example, H. A. D. Jowett and F. L. Pyman, "Relation between Chemical Constitution and Physiological Action in the Tropeines," *J. Chem. Soc.*, 91, 92-98 (1907); F. L. Pyman, "The Relation between Chemical Constitution and Physiological Action," *J. Chem. Soc.*, 111, 1103-1128 (1917); C. R. Marshall, "Studies on the Relation between Chemical Constitution and Pharmacological Activity," *Pharm. J.*, 90, 622-626 (1913); E. Fourneau, "Sur quelques aminoalcools à fonction alcoolique tertiare du type," *Compt. rend. Acad. Sci.*, 138, 766-768 (1904); E. Fourneau, "Aminoalcools er dérivés à properiétés thérapeutiques," *J. Pharm. Chim.*, 7th ser., 2, 56-64 (1910).

4. For example, Sigmund Fränkel, *Die Arzneimittel-Synthese auf Grundlage der Beziehungen zwischen chemischen Aufbau und Wirkung*, Berlin: Julius Springer, 1901; Francis Francis and J. M. Fortesque-Brickdale, *The Chemical Basis of Pharmacology*, London: Edward Arnold, 1908; Leopold Spiegel, *Chemical Constitution and Physiological Action*, translated from the German edition (Stuttgart, 1909) by C. Luedeking and A. C. Boylston, New York: D. Van Nostrand, 1915; Hugh McGuigan, *An Introduction to Chemical Pharmacology: Pharmacodynamics in Relation to Chemistry*, Philadelphia: P. Blakiston's Sons, 1921; Percy May, *The Chemistry of Synthetic Drugs*, London; Longmanns, Green, 1911.

5. Physical chemistry was making its influence felt in many areas of biological science during the late 19th and early 20th centuries, e.g., biochemistry. For examples of this influence see Ferenc Szabadváry, "Development of the pH Concept," translated by Ralph Oesper, *J. Chem. Ed.*, 41, 105-107 (1964); John Parascandola, "L. J. Henderson and the Theory of Buffer Action," *Medizinhistorisches J.*, 6, 297-309 (1971).

6. Francis and Fortesque-Brickdale, *op. cit.* (n. 4), p. 23; McGuigan, *op. cit.* (n. 4), p. v; H. H. Dale, "Chemical Structure and Physiological Action," *Bull. Johns Hopkins Hosp.*, 31, 377-379 (1920).

7. Speigel, *op. cit.* (n.4), pp. 6-16. On the receptor theory see John Parascandola and Ronald Jasensky, "Origins of the Receptor Theory of Drug Action," *Bull. Hist. Med.*, in press.

8. Walther Straub, "Die Bedeutung der Zellmembran," *Verhandl. Ges. Deutsch. Naturforscher Arzte*, 84, 192-214 (1912).

9. Arthur R. Cushny, "The Pharmacologic Action of Drugs: Is it Determined by Chemical Structure or by Physical Characters?" *J. Amer. Med. Assoc.*, 41, 1252-1253; the quotations are from p. 1252.

10. Arthur R. Cushny, MS notes for lectures on materia medica at Edinburgh University (1918-1926), Lecture I, p. 6, Manuscripts Division, University of Edinburgh Library, Edinburgh, Scotland. I am grateful to the Library for permission to use the Cushny manuscripts.

11. Cushny, "Pharmacologic Action," (n. 9), p. 1253.

12. *Ibid.*, p. 1255.

13. William Bayliss, *Principles of General Physiology*, London: Longmans, Green 1915, pp. 723-727; Carl Alsberg, "Chemical Structure and Physiological Action," *J. Washington Acad. Sci.*, 11, 323-324 (1921); Isidor Traube, "Die physikalische Theorie der Arz-

neimittel—und Giftwirkung," *Biochem. Z.*, **98**, 177-178 (1919). In discussing camphor, Walther Straub, "Camphor and the Modern Analeptics," in *Lane Lectures on Pharmacology*, Stanford: Stanford University Press, 1931, p. 80 argued that this medicament had previously been unreliable because of its conditions of solubility, rather than because of "the mysterious connection between chemical consitution and pharmacological action," and that it had been necessary to improve the "physicochemical constants" of the drug to make it more reliable. See, also Straub, "Bedeutung der Zellmembran" (n. 8). In their early studies on arsenicals, pharmacologist Carl Voegtlin and his colleagues argued that the chemical constitution of these drugs determined their chemotherapeutic action only indirectly through their physical properties. See, e.g., Carl Voegtlin, Helen Dyer, and Dorothy Miller, "Quantitative Studies in Chemotherapy. VII. Effects of Ligation of the Uterers or Bile Duct upon the Toxicity and Trypanocidal Action of Arsenicals," *J. Pharmacol. Exp. Ther.*, **20**, 129-130 (1922).

14. Arthur R. Cushny, *A Textbook of Pharmacology and Therapeutics; Or, The Action of Drugs in Health or Disease*, London: Rebman, 1899, p. 23.

15. Cushny did, in the 4th edition (1906) of his textbook (n. 14), give more emphasis to the influence of physical properties on drug action than he had done in earlier editions (see especially p. 20).

16. Cushny, *Textbook* (n. 14), 5th edition, London: Churchill, 1910, p. 24.

17. *Ibid.*, p. 25.

18. Alsberg, *op. cit.* (n. 13), p. 324.

19. Paul Ehrlich, "The Relations Existing between Chemical Constitution, Distribution, and Pharmacological Action," in F. Himmelweit, ed., *The Collected Papers of Paul Ehrlich*, vol. I, London: Pergamon Press, 1956, pp. 596-618, especially pp. 602-603 and 614-618. (English translation by C. Bolduan, which first appeared in Paul Ehrlich, *Collected Studies in Immunity*, New York: John Wiley and Sons, 1906; original German version of this address, delivered to the Verein für innere Medicin on December 12, 1898, was published in the *v. Leyden-Festschrift*, 1902). See also Parascandola and Jasensky, *op. cit.* (n. 7).

20. Hans Meyer, "Zur Theorie der Alkoholnarkose. Erste Mittheilung. Welche Eigenschaft der Anästhetica bedingt ihre Narkotische Wirkung?" *Arch. exp. Path. Pharmacol.*, **42**, 109-137 (1899); E. Overton, *Studien über die Narkose, zugleich ein Beitrag zur allgemeinen Pharmakologie*, Jena: Gustav Fischer, 1901.

21. Spiegel, *op. cit.* (n. 4), pp. 9-12; Francis and Fortesque-Brickdale, *op. cit.* (n. 4), pp. 83-88. Percy May, an advocate of the structural chemistry approach, admitted (*op. cit.*, n. 4, p. 45) that physical theories of narcosis were superior to any "purely chemical theory."

22. Adrien Albert, "Relations between Molecular Structure and Biological Activity: Stages in the Evolution of Current Concepts," *Ann. Rev. Pharmacol.*, **11**, 15-16 (1971).

23. Alsberg, *op. cit.* (n. 13), p. 338.

24. *Ibid.*, p. 324.

25. Walter Dixon, *A Manual of Pharmacology*, London: Edward Arnold, 1906, p. 19 stated that: "No two bodies can be more closely related chemically than the two hyoscyamines (optical isomers), yet some of the most characteristic features in the action of the one are almost entirely wanting in the other." I have dealt with the relationship of optical isomer-

ism to theories of drug action in this period in a paper entitled "Arthur Cushny, Optical Isomerism and the Mechanism of Drug Action," delivered to the History of Chemistry Division of the American Chemical Society, Chicago, August, 1973.

26. Spiegel, *op. cit.* (n. 4), pp. 12-16; May, *op. cit.* (n. 4), p. 4; Fränkel, *op. cit.*, (n. 4), pp. 15-17, 25-27.

27. For example, Spiegel, *op. cit.* (n. 4), pp. 9-10.

28. Francis and Fortesque-Brickdale, *op. cit.* (n. 4), p. 23.

29. Spiegel, *op. cit.* (n. 4), p. 16.

30. F. L. Pyman, "The Relation between Chemical Constitution and Physiological Action," *J. Chem. Soc.*, **111**, 1104 (1917).

31. May, *op. cit.* (n. 4), p. 3.

32. Bayliss, *op. cit.* (n. 13), pp. 324-327, 726; William Bayliss, *The Nature of Enzyme Action*, London: Longmanns, Green, 1908, pp. 18, 61-62; William Bayliss, "The Nature of Enzyme Action," *Science Prog.*, **1**, 303 (1906). Paul Ehrlich, *op. cit.* (n. 19), p. 608 felt that such processes as solution of substances in lipoids, while not involving the formation of true chemical combinations, did involve "chemical affinities in the widest meaning of the term."

33. See, for example, Benjamin Ward Richardson, "Second Report on the Physiological Action of Certain of the Amyl Compounds," *British Assoc. Rep.*, **35**, 272-281 (1855). See also the references in note 1 for a fuller discussion of Richardson's structure-activity studies, as well as John Parascandola, "Benjamin Ward Richardson's Studies on Structure-Activity Relationships and His Theory of Disease," *Actes XIIIe Cong. Int. Hist. Sci.*, 1971, in press.

34. See M. Tiffeneau, "De groupements atomiques actifs au point de vue pharmacodynamique," *Rev. gén. Chim.*, **14**, 85-96 (1911) for an example of an attempt to classify chemical groups or radicals as hypnotic groups, local anesthetic groups, etc. Spiegel, *op. cit.* (n. 4), pp. 152-154 also emphasizes the specific pharmacological properties of particular functional groups (e.g., alkyl groups are associated with a narcotic effect, carboxyl groups with a neutralization or weakening of the effects of other groups, etc.). Pharmacologist Daniel Leech of Manchester, in his Croonian Lectures for 1893, argued that individual constituent elements or functional groups (such as the nitro group) in a molecule often act separately (i.e., independently of the over-all structure of a molecule) in exerting their pharmacological effects. See Daniel Leech, *The Pharmacological Action and Therapeutic Uses of Nitrites and Allied Compounds*, ed. by R. B. Wild, Manchester: Sherratt and Hughes, 1902, pp. 65-161.

35. For example, Carl Alsberg, *op. cit.* (n. 13), pp. 322-323 criticized the attempt to label particular groupings of atoms in the molecule as anesthetic groups, toxophore groups, etc.

36. For example, Spiegel, *op. cit.* (n. 4), pp. 9-12; May, *op. cit.* (n. 4), pp. 2-4, 45.

37. Francis and Fortesque-Brickdale, *op. cit.* (n. 4), p. 19.

38. Albert, *op. cit.* (n. 22), pp. 14-15.

39. *Ibid.*, p. 15.

40. There now exists, of course, an entire field or subdivision of organic chemistry known as "physical organic chemistry." See, for example, Jack Hine, *Physical Organic Chemistry*, 2nd edition, New York: McGraw-Hill, 1962.

IV

The Evolution of Stereochemical Concepts in Pharmacology

The purpose of this paper is to examine the historical
development of the application of stereochemical concepts to the
field of pharmacology. It is not possible, however, to present
an exhaustive treatment of so broad a subject within the confines
of the present paper, and thus it will be necessary to focus the
discussion on selected aspects of the topic. Particular attention
will be devoted to the attempts to explain the observed difference
in activity between optical enantiomers (compounds which are nonsuperimposable mirror images of each other).

The study of the stereochemical factors involved in drug
action developed out of an attempt to explain the mechanism of
drug action in chemical terms. Although the iatrochemists of the
seventeenth century had already attempted to relate the physiological action of certain substances to their chemical properties
(especially acidity and basicity), chemistry and pharmacology had
not developed sufficiently enough to allow for significant advances in this direction before the nineteenth century. The first
serious attempt to relate chemical composition to physiological
action in a systematic manner seems to have been made by James
Blake, an English physician who later emigrated to America. In
1839, Blake showed that the different salts of a given metal
tended to produce the same physiological effect, thus indicating
that the metallic element of the salt seemed to be largely responsible for its activity. He later found that elements which were
isomorphic generally had similar pharmacological properties.
Blake's work demonstrated that a relationship could be established
between the pharmacological action and the chemical nature of a
substance (1,2).

While structural organic chemistry was still in its infancy
in the 1860's, some attempts were made to relate the physiological
action of certain organic compounds to their chemical structure.
These early studies understandably concentrated largely on relating physiological activity to the presence of certain elements or
functional groups in a molecule, not on more complicated questions
involving the general structure or the stereochemistry of the

molecule. Thus Benjamin Ward Richardson, the British physician and physiologist, attempted to assign specific pharmacological properties to certain functional groups (e.g., he associated the nitrite group with vasodilation and quickening of the heart) (1, 2).

Probably the most influential of these early studies on structure-activity relationships was the investigation of alkaloids and amines by two Edinburgh scientists, Alexander Crum Brown, the chemist, and Thomas Fraser, the pharmacologist, beginning in 1867. They clearly recognized that the constitution or structure of a molecule was as important as its chemical composition in explaining biological activity (e.g., two isomers may have very different physiological properties), but unfortunately the structures of most organic drugs and poisons were not known. Although the exact structures of many of the compounds they studied were unknown, they were able to establish a relationship between a specific structural feature of a molecule and a particular pharmacological property. Brown and Fraser demonstrated that the quaternary ammonium salts of various alkaloids (such as strychnine and morphine) and of various amines always seemed to be associated with a paralyzing action similar to that of curare. They attributed this action to the presence of a pentavalent nitrogen atom in all of these substances (1,2).

The work of Brown and Fraser stimulated interest in the application of structural organic chemistry to pharmacology and encouraged research on structure-activity relationships. It is also of significance in our present discussion because it led to one of the early examples of the attempt to take stereochemical factors into account in considering drug action. In 1872, Brown and Fraser extended their work on nitrogen compounds to show that sulfonium salts possess the same paralyzing properties exhibited by quaternary ammonium compounds (3). The studies of other investigators soon revealed that arsonium, phosphonium and stibonium salts all exhibited a curare-like action (4,5,6). In other words, the nature of the central atom in the onium salt, whether nitrogen, arsenic, sulfur, etc., did not seem to affect the pharmacological properties of the compound. The paralyzing action seemed in some way to be associated with the whole structure of these onium compounds.

At the close of the nineteenth century an understanding of the stereochemistry of elements other than carbon began to emerge. In the 1890's for example, Alfred Werner and his co-workers investigated the stereochemistry of nitrogen compounds (7). William Pope and Stanley Peachy established in 1900 that the asymmetric quadrivalent sulfur atom acts as a center of optical activity (8). Chemists and pharmacologists began to associate the paralyzing properties possessed by onium salts with the change from a planar structure to a three-dimensional structure (9,10,11). For example, it was argued that the molecule

$$R_1-S-R_2$$

must have a planar configuration, since there are only three groups involved. A sulfonium salt of structure

$$R_1-\overset{\overset{\displaystyle R_2}{|}}{\underset{\underset{\displaystyle X}{|}}{S}}-R_3$$

must, however, have a tetrahedral configuration, since such compounds possess optical activity when four different groups are attached to the sulfur atom. No explanation was offered as to exactly why this change from a planar to a three-dimensional configuration resulted in the introduction of paralyzing properties, but it was generally assumed that this alteration in the stereochemistry of the molecule was somehow responsible for the development of curare-like effects.

H. R. Ing and his associates were to show many years later that the curare-like action of onium salts was actually due to their ionic character (12). They apparently act, as does curare, by antagonizing acetylcholine (itself a quaternary ammonium compound) by competing for the receptor site. The possibility that the action of quaternary ammonium salts might depend upon their strong basicity was suggested early in the century (12), but this view does not seem to have been widely accepted before Ing's work. Thus this "classic" case which was frequently pointed out in the early twentieth century as an example of the importance of stereochemistry for pharmacology turned out to depend upon an ionic effect rather than upon a stereochemical effect.

Other examples of the importance of stereochemical effects in the action of certain drugs also came to light in the late nineteenth and early twentieth centuries. For example, in the 1890's the geometric isomers maleic and fumaric acid were shown to differ significantly in their toxicity towards various microorganisms (13,14,15). Other examples of differences in pharmacological activity among geometric isomers were later uncovered (16,17).

Geometric isomerism, however, never received nearly as much attention from pharmacologists and medicinal chemists as did optical isomerism, probably because so many interesting and important drugs, especially the alkaloids, existed in optically isomeric forms. In addition, optical isomers probably had a certain theoretical appeal, since they seemed to be essentially identical in their physical and chemical properties; hence, it was a difficult challenge to explain differences in physiological activity.

The fact that optical isomers may differ in their biological effects had been known since about 1860 when Louis Pasteur demonstrated that certain microorganisms preferentially destroy one member of a pair of optical isomers over the other. These studies were later extended by others to show that this differentiation also applied to oxidation by animal tissues. Other observations revealed that certain ferments could distinguish between optical isomers, and that optical isomers may differ in taste. It thus became clear that living organisms could, at least in some cases, distinguish between enantiomers (18,19).

A number of attempts were made in the late nineteenth century to compare the pharmacological and toxicological properties of pairs of optical isomers, but the first convincing examples of differences in pharmacological activity between enantiomers was provided by the work of Arthur Cushny. I have already discussed Cushny's work on this subject in some detail in a previous paper presented before the Division of History of Chemistry (20), and here I will just briefly review the material most pertinent to our present discussion.

In the period from 1903 through 1909, Cushny (who began his work on optical isomers at the University of Michigan and later continued it at London and at Edinburgh) demonstrated that one member of a pair of optical isomers could in some cases exhibit a much greater pharmacological activity than its mirror image. For example, l-hyoscyamine appeared to be twelve to fourteen times as potent as d-hyoscyamine with respect to their action on the motor nerve endings (21,22,23,24).

In the rest of this paper, I would like to focus on the attempts to explain this phenomenon, for this difference in activity of optical isomers was a clear example of how the spatial arrangement of the atoms within a molecule could influence its pharmacological effects. It helped to stimulate pharmacologists and medicinal chemists to take stereochemical factors into account in considering drug action.

We should begin by asking how Cushny himself interpreted the results of his work on optical isomers. It is interesting to note that he did not really emphasize the stereochemical configurations of the molecules, and that he placed more emphasis on physical properties than on chemical structure. Before discussing his views, however, I must provide some brief background about theories of the mechanism of drug action at the turn of the century.

In the early part of the twentieth century there was considerable discussion and controversy over the question of whether physical (or perhaps it would be better to say "physicochemical") or chemical properties played more of a part in determining drug action. I have discussed this subject in more detail elsewhere (25). Although it was recognized that both chemical and physical factors were probably involved to some extent, and that one could not always clearly distinguish between them, there was a tendency among pharmacologists and others concerned with the question of drug action to emphasize one or the other approach. The supporters of the chemical viewpoint held that drugs generally exerted their effects by forming a chemical union with the cell or with some component of the cell. This view received its clearest exposition in the receptor theory developed by John Newport Langley

in England and by Paul Ehrlich in Germany. Ehrlich emphasized
that for a drug or poison to act on a cell, it must possess a
specific group cf atoms which have a specific affinity for and
can combine with another group of atoms on a chemical side chain
of the protoplasmic molecule, so that it can be fixed or anchored
in the cell (26). Supporters of the physical or physicochemical
viewpoint, on the other hand, argued that drugs did not generally
unite chemically with the cell, but rather induced their effects
by altering the surface tension, electrolytic balance, osmotic
pressure, etc. of the cell (25).

While Cushny recognized that both physical properties and
chemical reactions can play some part in pharmacological action,
he gave much more emphasis to the former in his writings (25). It
is not surprising then that his theory of the action of optical
isomers reflects this bias. Yet he had to admit that a chemical
reaction was in some way involved in the ability of organisms to
distinguish between enantiomers, for enantiomers have identical
physical properties (except for the direction in which they rotate
the plane of polarized light). So Cushny postulated that the two
optical isomers combined with an optically active receptive substance in the cell, probably an acid or a base, to form two dia-
stereomers (stereoisomers which are dissymmetric, at least in
part, and hence are not mirror images of each other). So, for
example, if the receptive substance was levorotatory, the reaction
would be as follows:

d - isomer + ℓ - receptor = d - isomer - ℓ - receptor

ℓ - isomer + d - receptor = ℓ - isomer - d - receptor

The two diastereomeric products differ in their properties, of
course, since they are not mirror images, and Cushny argued that
it is the difference in physical properties, such as solubility,
of these diastereoisomers which leads to their difference in
pharmacological activity (27,28,29).

Note that while Cushny admitted the involvement of a chemical
reaction, he emphasized that it was the difference in physical
properties of the compounds formed by the reactions which determined the difference in pharmacological activity. In all of his
discussions on the subject, he emphasized the difference in optical rotation between two enantiomers, rather than speaking of
their different configurations. Structural formulas play almost
no role in his treatment of the subject. In fact, he separated
out the influence of the asymmetric carbon atom from that of the
general configuration or structure of the molecule (20).

Cushny specifically rejected the possiblity that the difference in pharmacological activity of two enantiomers might be due
to a difference in their ability to combine with the receptor. It
was true, he stated, that some chemical reaction occurred between
the drug and the receptor, but this followed whether the d-isomer

or the ℓ-isomer was present. He added that the "difference in action lies not in the facility with which the chemical combination is formed, but in the physical characters of the resultant compound" (29). Perhaps Cushny found it difficult to imagine that the receptor could differentiate between two substances so identical in structure as optical enantiomers.

It must be remembered that in the early twentieth century, chemical reactions were thought of largely in terms of covalent and ionic bonds. Concepts of hydrogen bonding, van der Waals forces, etc. had not yet been developed, nor had an understanding of the secondary and tertiary structure of proteins and other macromolecules yet emerged. I find that the pharmacological and pharmaceutical chemical writings of this period still tend to be largely concerned with two-dimensional chemistry. Chemical interactions were thought of largely in terms of the reaction of a specific functional group on one molecule with a specific functional group on another molecule, although admittedly the term "chemical" was beginning to be interpreted more broadly by some (the question of whether relatively nonspecific processes such as adsorption might involve chemical forces as well as physical forces was, for example, being discussed) (25).

Some investigators in the early twentieth century did attempt to explain the difference in activity between enantiomers in terms of the stereochemical configurations of the drug and the receptor, but these early attempts were rather vague. The chemist Alfred Stewart, author of a 1907 book on Stereochemistry, argued that spatial or three-dimensional factors play a part in many chemical reactions involved in vital processes. He suggested that the speed of reaction of an optically active drug with an asymmetric tissue substance sometimes depends upon the spatial arrangements of the atoms (30). Stewart noted that it was probable that the tissues, which are themselves asymmetric, select the substances whose stereochemical configurations best fit in with their own (18), a view which reminds one of Emil Fischer's well-known "lock and key" analogy for the reaction between an enzyme and its substrate. Stewart did not, however, suggest any specific mechanism which could explain how the tissues were able to "select" one optical isomer in preference to another.

The dependence of the pharmacological action of a molecule upon its stereochemistry was stressed by others such as the German medicinal chemist Sigmund Fränkel, who argued that the orientation of the atoms or radicals of a molecule in space is at least as important as their chemical nature in determining physiological activity (31). Suggestions as to the mechanism of action involved, however, did not really go beyond the "lock and key" analogy, or, as one pharmacologist suggested, a "glove and hand" analogy (i.e., just as the glove from the left hand cannot fit the right hand, so perhaps an ℓ-isomer could not "fit" a d-receptor) (32).

No satisfactory three-dimensional explanation as to how a receptor could distinguish between optical isomers seems to have

been offered until 1933. In that year, Leslie Easson and Edgar
Stedman of the Department of Medicinal Chemistry at the University
of Edinburgh expounded an alternative to Cushny's theory (33).
They criticized Cushny for considering optical activity to be a
factor which was quite distinct from general structure in determining the magnitude of the specific pharmacological activity of
the molecule, a view which they believed was commonly held. They
felt that the difference in activity between optical isomers, just
as the difference in activity between any two different substances,
depended upon their molecular arrangement, and suggested a specific mechanism which could explain the difference. Easson and
Stedman assumed that three of the four groups surrounding the
asymmetric carbon atom of the drug are involved in the reaction
with the receptor. For the drug to produce the maximum physiological effect, they hypothesized, it must be attached to the
receptor in such a way that groups B, C, and D (Figure 1) in the
drug coincide with B', C', and D' on the receptor. This alignment
can be achieved by only one of the enantiomers, and hence one
enantiomer would exhibit greater activity than the other.

They reasoned that if their theory were correct, i.e., if it
were not optical activity per se but the general structure of the
molecule which was important in determining pharmacological activity, than a molecule such as V (Figure 1), which has the same
configuration of the three binding groups as does the active
isomer III, should have about the same activity as the active
isomer even though V is optically inactive (it does not contain
an asymmetric carbon atom). They recognized, however, that one
would have to take into account any changes in the physical properties of the molecule associated with the substitution of B for
A. Changes in the solubility of the molecule, for example, could
significantly alter its pharmacological activity.

Easson and Stedman offered evidence from the literature and
from their own experimental work to support their views, and I
will just mention one example. Compound VII (Figure 2) contains
an asymmetric carbon atom and hence exists in two optically active
forms. One of these, the ℓ-isomer, possesses exceptional miotic
activity (i.e., it constricts the pupil of the eye), five times
that of the corresponding d-isomer. Compound VIII, if R is a hydrogen atom, possesses very little miotic activity. The introduction of a methyl group into compound VIII, converting it to VII,
thus greatly increases the miotic activity, while at the same time
introducing an asymmetric carbon atom into the molecule.

One might be tempted to associate this increased activity
with the optical asymmetry. Suppose, however, postulate Easson
and Stedman, that the drug (VII) is attached to the receptor by
the amide and the amine groups (both of which are necessary for
activity), and that in the more active isomer the methyl group
causes a more perfect combination to take place between the drug
and the receptor than would occur in its absence. In the less
active isomer, however, the methyl group would be directed away

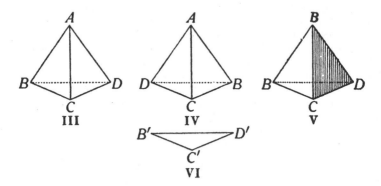

Biochemical Journal

Figure 1. Diagrammatic representation of "three-point contact" theory from 1933 paper of Easson and Stedman (33)

Biochemical Journal

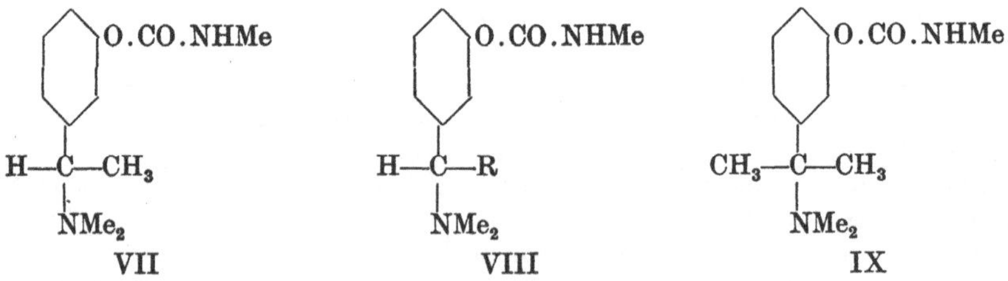

Figure 2. Chemical formulas from Easson and Stedman paper (33)

from the receptor and could not directly influence the fixation
of the drug. If this were the case, then one would expect, first
of all, that the less active isomer would have about the same
activity as VIII (where R is a hydrogen atom), since the methyl
group is not in a position to influence the fixation of the drug;
and, secondly, that if the hydrogen atom attached to the asymmetric carbon atom in VII were replaced by a methyl group, the
resulting product (IX) should have about the same miotic activity
as the active ℓ-isomer of VII, even though IX is optically inactive. Their own experimental studies on these compounds tended to
support their hypothesis, although the results were not clearly
definitive.

I should note that Easson and Stedman indicated that it was
not necessary for each of the three groups involved in fixing the
drug to actually combine chemically with the receptor, but that in
many cases one or more groups might merely cause a better "fit" of
the drug to the receptor (rather than being linked to the receptor
through "normal valencies") (33). H. R. Ing of Oxford, however,
criticized Easson and Stedman in 1937 for introducing the vague
notion of "fit," which he felt was unnecessary. Ing admitted that
the stereochemical configurations of the drug and the receptor are
important, but he felt that these factors could be included under
Cushny's explanation. The different physical and chemical properties of the diastereomeric drug-receptor compounds of Cushny's
theory, Ing noted, are presumably based upon the mutual spatial
arrangements of the drug and the receptor in the compound formed
by them (34). Ing's criticism of the concept of "fit" may seem at
first inconsistent with his own statement in 1935 that: "The conception of fit between drug molecules and the tissues on which
they act appears to the author to be fundamental to any general
theory of how drugs act." This statement, however, was followed
by the remark that "the hypothesis of fit between drugs and
tissues is at present infertile" because "nothing is known of the
nature of the receptors on which drugs are supposed to act" (35).
Presumably Ing's criticism of the Easson-Stedman hypothesis was
based on this feeling that such theories were at the time sterile,
and on the fact that Cushny's hypothesis could encompass "fit" if
one assumed that the physical properties of the drug-receptor compound depended upon the "fit" between the drug and the receptor.

A few years later, in 1943, Ing had to admit that Cushny's
view was hard to reconcile with the receptor theory as developed
by A. J. Clark in the 1930's. Under Cushny's view, both isomers
combined with equal facility with the receptor, but the two drug-
receptor compounds had different properties and therefore were not
equally effective pharmacologically. If this were the case, however, the less active isomer should antagonize the action of the
more active isomer, because it would compete on equal terms for
the available receptors but would form a less active compound.
The experimental evidence indicated, however, that optical isomers
generally did not antagonize each other but acted additively. If

one accepts the receptor theory, Ing noted, then the difference in activity of optical isomers must be presumed to depend upon the ease with which each isomer combines with the receptor, with both isomers forming equally effective drug-receptor compounds. In that case, one would not expect antagonism between the isomers.

He went on to add that this conclusion appears remarkable. Ing apparently found it hard to imagine, in spite of the fact that he knew of the Easson-Stedman theory (which he did not mention in the 1943 paper), that the receptor could differentiate between two molecules as identical in structure as optical isomers. In the case of stereoisomers which are not optical enantiomers, however, he felt that it was quite reasonable to expect that their ease of combination with the receptor is determined by their stereochemical configuration (36).

Ing's reaction may well typify the initial general response to the hypothesis of Easson and Stedman. It does not seem to have received widespread attention or acceptance until about 1950, when suddenly the "three-point contact theory" (essentially the Easson-Stedman model) found general favor in pharmacology and biochemistry. Some discussion of the theory, and evidence for or against it, did appear in the literature in the 1930's and 1940's (34,37, 38,39), but it apparently did not excite general interest or enthusiasm. In addition to conflicting evidence concerning the Easson-Stedman view, I would suspect that its slow acceptance was also partly due to a factor suggested by Colin Russell in his paper at this symposium with respect to the "puckered" ring model for cyclohexane. He suggested that the question of the conformation of the six-membered ring may have been largely irrelevant to what most organic chemists were doing in the first half of the twentieth century. In a similar way, I think that the Easson-Stedman model was in many ways "irrelevant" to the problems tackled by pharmacologists and medicinal chemists of the 1930's and 1940's. Their attention was focused on the synthesis of new drugs and on investigations to determine the site and general mode of action of both old and new drugs. There was still much to be done at the organism and organ level in terms of the understanding of drug action, and theories at the molecular level were rather speculative (and difficult to prove or disprove) and largely incapable of application to the practical problems faced by pharmacologists and medicinal chemists in that period (recall Ing's comment that the concept of fit was "infertile" in 1935).

It is interesting to note that beginning in 1935 Max Bergmann and his co-workers developed a similar theory for enzymes, postulating that for an enzyme to differentiate between two enantiomeric substrates it must contain three or more atoms or atomic groups, fixed in space with respect to one another, which enter into combination with a similar number of groups on the substrate (forcing the latter into a fixed spatial position) (40,41). They do not refer to Easson and Stedman in their work. The "polyaffinity theory" of Bergmann, however, also does not seem to have received

widespread attention at the time. It was not until A. G. Ogston
developed a similar theory in 1948, as we shall see, that the
"three-point contact" theory of enzyme action made a significant
impact on biochemistry, thus paralleling the situation in pharmacology.

In the late 1940's and early 1950's, the three-point contact
theory began to appear in a number of guises to explain the action
of certain enzymes, drugs, hormones, etc. It is not completely
clear as to why this hypothesis, which was essentially the view
suggested by Easson and Stedman in 1933, suddenly came into
prominence around 1950. No doubt an improved understanding of
chemical bonding and of stereochemistry played a significant role.

Certain work in biochemistry and pharmacology had also led to
a heightened concern with three-dimensional factors in drug action
by this time. The recognition in the early 1940's, for example,
that sulfanilamide competes with p-aminobenzoic acid, a natural
metabolite, because of their similar architecture helped to focus
attention on the importance of molecular size and shape in determining drug action (42,43). In 1946, F. W. Schueler demonstrated
the importance of the distance between the hydroxyl or keto groups
of estrogens in determining their relative activity (44). Two
years later, Carl Pfeiffer commented:

"Attempts to correlate structure-activity-relationships (SAR)
of chemical series of pharmacological importance have hitherto
mainly considered activity as variations in chain length of ali-
phatic series as drawn in two dimensions. Occasionally theories
have been centered around the well-known ring systems of organic
chemistry. Greater correlation and understanding of SAR might be
obtained by depicting formulas in three dimensions, with bond
distances calculated as accurately as our present knowledge will
allow" (45).

Pfeiffer then applied his suggestion to a study of muscarinic
drugs (drugs which simulate the effects of parasympathetic nerve
stimulation), calculating the distances between the three "pros-
thetic" chemical groups which he believed were responsible for
muscarinic activity, and relating these interprosthetic distances
to pharmacological activity (45).

In that same year, 1948, A. G. Ogston of Oxford University
introduced a hypothesis similar to that of Easson and Stedman in
an attempt to explain how an enzyme could produce an asymmetric
product from a symmetrical reactant. Ogston was apparently unaware of the Easson-Stedman theory, or at least he made no mention of it in his short paper. Nor did he mention the previously
noted "polyaffinity theory" of Max Bergmann and his colleagues.
His own concept developed out of a consideration of two metabolic
studies utilizing isotopic tracers in which the investigators had
concluded that certain compounds could not be intermediates because they were symmetrical molecules and the products formed were
asymmetric. Ogston pointed out, however, that it was entirely
possible that an enzyme could distinguish, for example, between

the two supposedly identical carboxyl groups in amino-malonic acid. If a three-point combination is involved between the enzyme and the substrate, he postulated, then it is conceivable that de-carboxylation might take place only at site a' (Figure 3) or only at site b', since they are catalytically different. The product produced would then be asymmetric (46).

The similarity of the Ogston hypothesis to the Easson-Stedman model is obvious. The Ogston hypothesis soon became widely accepted in biochemistry and probably helped to pave the way for the adoption of a similar view for drugs by pharmacologists (47,48,49).

The three-point contact theory was utilized shortly there-after (1950) by Ogston's colleague at Oxford, H. K. F. Blaschko, to explain the difference in activity between the two optical iso-mers of the hormone adrenaline (which had been demonstrated by Cushny). Blaschko, after describing the three-point contact theory of enzyme action (but without specifically mentioning Ogston), stated that:

"The adrenaline molecule has an asymmetric carbon atom; its laevorotatory isomer, which occurs in nature, is highly active. We shall therefore assume that three of the groups attached to the asymmetric carbon atom are essential in the reaction with the ex-citable tissue. We assume that these three groups are:

    (a) the catechol group,

    (b) the group $-CH_2 \cdot NH \cdot CH_3$, and

    (c) the hydroxyl group.

These three groups are assumed to be arranged in a fixed spatial relationship relative to the tissue receptors. We might say: the tissue receptors for adrenaline have three receptacles or anchorages, one for each of these groups.

The stereochemical specificity of the action of adrenaline differs from that of the enzyme discussed above; the specificity is not absolute: dextro-adrenaline has about 1/12 to 1/15 of the action of laevo-adrenaline on the arterial blood pressure. How can this be explained? It is obvious that dextro-adrenaline can-not attach itself in the same way to the receptors as laevo-adrenaline. We must assume that one of the three receptacles is not engaged: the dextro-adrenaline molecule is attached by the basic group and by the catechol group; the hydroxyl group is not engaged. The receptacle for the hydroxyl group is faced by the hydrogen atom attached to the asymmetric carbon atom. The dextro-adrenaline molecule is therefore held in two points; this attach-ment is less firm; the dextro-adrenaline molecule has a greater degree of freedom on the receptor and is therefore less active" (50).

Blaschko made no reference to the hypothesis of Easson and Stedman. At about this same time, the three-point contact theory was used by R. L. Wain and his associates to account for differences in activity between optical enantiomers of certain plant growth-regulating substances (51,52). Unlike Blaschko, Wain and his co-workers specifically refer to the earlier work of Easson and Stedman (51).

As one final example of the widespread interest in the three-point contact theory in the early 1950's, I will mention the application of the theory to explain differences in activity among optical isomers of various synthetic analgesics by A. H. Beckett of the School of Pharmacy of Chelsea College of Science and Technology. Beckett, who has contributed significantly to our knowledge of the stereochemistry of drug action in the past two decades, utilized the diagram shown in Figure 4 in a 1954 article on synthetic analgesics (coauthored by A. F. Casy). In all of these compounds the tertiary basic group and the aromatic ring seem to be essential for activity, so Beckett and Casy assumed that they are involved in the drug-receptor interaction. The third group (X), a hydrocarbon moiety, forms a third point of interaction with the receptor surface and hence helps to promote the formation of the drug-receptor complex. It can only be in the right position to become involved in the interaction, however, in one of the two enantiomers, in this case the (-)-isomer. Hence the (-)-isomer is more active than the (+)-isomer (53). In 1955, Beckett and Casy published a general review article on "Stereoisomerism and Biological Action," a paper in which they refer to the Easson and Stedman paper of 1933 for the first time (54).

By the mid-1950's, the three-point contact theory of drug action seems to have become well established as a mechanism of explaining differences in biological activity among optical enantiomers. By 1951, H. R. Ing (probably influenced by the work of his Oxford colleagues Ogston and Blaschko) had fully accepted this view (55).

There have, of course, been many advances in the understanding of the stereochemistry of drug action in the past twenty years. It is now clear, for example, that stereospecificity can be explained on the basis of a one-point or two-point contact theory as well as a three-point contact hypothesis (56,57). The influence of conformation on drug action has become a subject of investigation as stereochemical studies increase in sophistication. I shall leave the discussion of recent work, however, to the chemists. I have tried to provide some insight into the impact that stereochemistry has had on pharmacology over the past hundred years, but my paper has presented only a broad outline of this complex subject. There are many details which will have to be filled in by further research into the history of chemical pharmacology.

Literature Cited

1. Parascandola, John, Pharm. Hist. (1971) 13, 3-10.
2. Bynum, William, Bull. Hist. Med. (1970) 44, 518-538.
3. Crum Brown, Alexander and Fraser, Thomas, Proc. R. Soc. Edinburgh (1872) 7, 663-665.

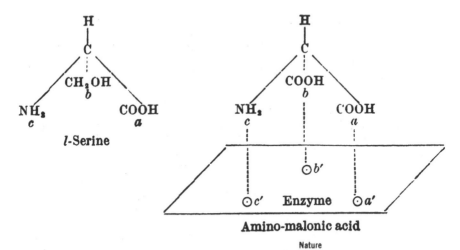

Figure 3. The Ogston hypothesis (46)

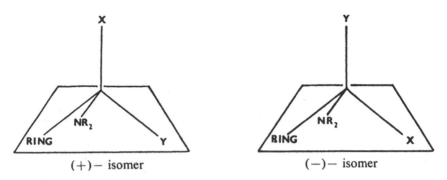

Journal of Pharmacy and Pharmacology

Figure 4. Diagram of Beckett and Casy representing the action of synthetic analgesics
(53)

4. Vulpian, A., Arch. physiol. normale pathol. (1868) 1, 472-473.
5. Rabuteau, A., C. R. Soc. Biol. (1882) 34, 127-137.
6. Rabuteau, A., C. R. Soc. Biol. (1882), 34, 195-200.
7. Kaufmann, George in "Werner Centennial," pp. 41-69, American Chemical Society, Washington, D. C., 1967.
8. Pope, William and Peachey, J., J. Chem. Soc. (1900) 77, 1072-1075.
9. Fränkel, Sigmund, "Die Arzneimittel-Synthese auf Grundlage der Beziehungen zwischen chemischen Aufbau und Wirkung," 2nd edition, pp. 126-131, Julius Springer, Berlin, 1906.
10. Francis, Francis and Fortesque-Brickdale, J. M., "The Chemical Basis of Pharmacology," pp. 53-54, Edward Arnold, London, 1908.
11. Stewart, A. W., Sci. Prog. (1908) 2, 449-481.
12. Ing, H. R., Physiol. Rev. (1936) 16, 527-544.
13. Foderà, A., Chem. Zentralbl. (1896) 67(I), 210-211.
14. Ishizuka, T., Bull. Coll. Agric., Tokyo Imp. Univ. (1897) 2, 484-486.
15. Kahlenberg, Louis and True, Rodney, Bot. Gaz. (1896) 22, 81-124.
16. Cooper, E. A. and Edgar, S. H., Biochem. J. (1926) 20, 1060-1070.
17. Butler, Thomas, J. Pharmacol. Exp. Ther. (1944) 81, 72-76.
18. Stewart, Alfred, "Stereochemistry," pp. 544-556, Longmans, Green and Co., London, 1907.
19. Cushny, A. R., "Biological Relations of Optically Isomeric Substances," pp. 18-29, Williams and Wilkins, Baltimore, 1926.
20. Parascandola, John, "Arthur Cushny, Optical Isomerism and the Mechanism of Drug Action," paper delivered before the Division of History of Chemistry, American Chemical Society, Chicago, August, 1973.
21. Cushny, A. R., J. Physiol. (1903) 30, 176-194.
22. Cushny, A. R., J. Physiol. (1905) 32, 501-510.
23. Cushny, A. R., J. Physiol. (1908) 37, 130-138.
24. Cushny, A. R., J. Physiol. (1909) 38, 259-262.
25. Parascandola, John, Pharm. Hist. (1974) 16, 54-63.
26. Parascandola, John and Jasensky, Ronald, Bull. Hist. Med. (1974) 48, in press.
27. Cushny, A. R., J. Pharmacol. Exp. Ther. (1921), 17, 41-61.
28. Cushny, A. R., "Biological Relations of Optically Isomeric Substances," pp. 54-55, Williams and Wilkins, Baltimore, 1926.
29. Cushny, A. R., J. Pharmacol. Exp. Ther. (1920) 15, 105-127. The quotation is from page 112.
30. Stewart, Alfred, "Chemistry and Its Borderland, pp. 129-130, Longmans, Green and Co., London, 1914.
31. Fränkel, Sigmund, Ergeb. Physiol. (1904) 3, 290-308.
32. Macht, David, Proc. Nat. Acad. Sci. USA (1929) 15, 63-70.
33. Easson, Leslie and Stedman, Edgar, Biochem. J. (1933) 27, 1257-1266.
34. Ing, H. R., Proc. R. Soc. London, Ser. B (1937) 121, 595-598.

35. Ing, H. R., Sci. Prog. (1935) 30, 252-267.
36. Ing, H. R., Trans. Faraday Soc. (1943) 39, 372-380.
37. Schaumann, Otto in "Medicine in its Chemical Aspects," pp. 361-369, Bayer, Leverkusen, Germany, 1938.
38. Alles, Gordon and Knoefel, Peter, Univ. Calif. Publ. Pharmacol. (1938) 1, 101-118.
39. Badger, G. M., letter to the editor (and reply by E. Stedman), Nature (1947) 159, 194-196.
40. Bergmann, Max, Zervas, Leonidas, Fruton, Joseph, Schneider, F. and Schleich, H., J. Biol. Chem. (1935) 109, 325-346.
41. Bergmann, Max, Zervas, Leonidas and Fruton, Joseph, J. Biol. Chem. (1936) 115, 593-611.
42. Woods, D. D., Br. J. Exp. Pathol. (1940) 21, 74-90.
43. Bell, P. and Roblin, R., J. Am. Chem. Soc. (1942) 64, 2905-2917.
44. Schueler, F. W., Science (1946) 103, 221-223.
45. Pfeiffer, Carl, Science (1948) 107, 94-96. The quotation is from page 94.
46. Ogston, A. G., Nature (1948) 162, 963.
47. Boyer, Paul, Lardy, Henry and Myrbäck, Karl, "The Enzymes," 2nd edition, volume 1, pp. 240-243, Academic Press, New York, 1959.
48. Bentley, Ronald, "Molecular Asymmetry in Biology," volume I, pp. 148-153, Academic Press, New York, 1969.
49. Alworth, William, "Stereochemistry and Its Application in Biochemistry," pp. 8-14, Wiley-Interscience, New York, 1969.
50. Blaschko, H. K. F., Proc. R. Soc. London, Ser. B (1950) 137, 307-317. The quotation is from page 310.
51. Smith, M. S. and Wain, R. L., Proc. R. Soc. London, Ser. B (1951) 139, 118-127.
52. Smith, M. S., Wain, R. L. and Wightman, F., Ann. Appl. Biol. (1952) 39, 295-307.
53. Beckett, A. H. and Casy, A. F., J. Pharm. Pharmacol. (1954) 6, 986-999.
54. Beckett, A. H. and Casy, A. F., J. Pharm. Pharmacol. (1955) 7, 433-455.
55. Ing, H. R., Chem. Ind. (1951), 926-928.
56. Mautner, Henry, Pharmacol. Rev. (1967) 19, 107-144.
57. Bentley, Ronald, "Molecular Asymmetry in Biology," volume I, pp. 154-155, Academic Press, New York, 1969.

Acknowledgment

I wish to thank the National Science Foundation for support of this research under grants GS-28549 and GS-41462.

V

Arthur Cushny, Optical Isomerism, and the Mechanism of Drug Action

INTRODUCTION

The fact that optical enantiomers (isomers which are nonsuperimposable mirror images of each other and rotate the plane of polarized light in opposite directions) may differ greatly in their pharmacological activity is often cited today as evidence that the shape of a drug molecule must be such that it fits a structure complementary to it on the surface of a receptor in the cell, and as an example of the close relationship between chemical structure and pharmacological activity. This view is neatly summarized, for example, in the following quotation from a 1964 review article on structure-activity relationships:

> To explain some of the types of structural specificity just referred to is difficult unless we infer that there are "drug receptors" which bear much the same relationship to certain drugs as do locks to the corresponding keys. Some of the best evidence for the existence of drug receptors has been obtained by comparing the effects of stereo-isomers. It has been found with morphine and numerous other drugs for which optical isomers exist that these isomers may differ strikingly in potency. Since optical isomers have identical properties except insofar as their molecules are mirror images, we are led to suppose that the shape of the drug molecule is important in these cases because part of the drug must fit a structure complementary to it.[1]

In light of the rather general acceptance of this view among contemporary pharmacologists and medicinal chemists, it is not surprising

---

1. F.N. Fastier, "Modern Concepts in Relationship between Structure and Activity," *Ann. Rev. Pharmacol., 4* (1964), 53. For other expressions of this view, see E.W. Gill, "Drug Receptor Interactions," *Prog. Med. Chem., 4* (1965), 39–40, and Andrejus Korolkovas, *Essentials of Molecular Pharmacology: Background for Drug Design* (New York: Wiley-Interscience, 1970), pp. 87–88, 97–101, 123–128.

that the work of Arthur Cushny, the pharmacologist who first demonstrated in a convincing manner the difference in pharmacological activity between certain optical isomers in the early twentieth century, has in recent years been interpreted historically by some scientists as supporting the receptor theory of Ehrlich and Langley and as favoring a chemical over a physical view of drug action. For example, one author has claimed that the discovery that pairs of optically active isomers can differ in pharmacological activity was an "early confirmation" for the existence of drug receptors. Cushny, according to this author, was the first to realize that differences in the biological activity of these isomers was caused by one enantiomer fitting the receptor surface much better than the other did.[2] Another account states that Cushny's work pointed to the correctness of the receptor theory and added the concept of "spatial arrangement" to this view, and that it favored a chemical over a physical theory of drug action.[3]

Upon examination of the historical evidence, however, it becomes apparent that Cushny himself interpreted the results of his work on optical isomerism in a different manner. While I have seen at least two articles by present-day scientists which recognize that Cushny's explanation of the difference in activity of optical isomers was not based upon the concept of one isomer "fitting" the receptor surface better that the other, these works make only brief passing reference to his views.[4] Cushny's studies on optical isomerism, his interpretation of the implications of his work for theories of drug action, and the relationship of his views about optical isomers to his more general concept of the mechanism of drug action have not been subjected to detailed historical analysis. This subject can provide us with historical insight into the understanding of the mechanism of drug action in the early twentieth century, and it would therefore seem worthwhile to explore it in further detail, which is the purpose of this paper.

---

2. Adrien Albert, "Relations between Molecular Structure and Biological Activity: Stages in the Evolution of Current Concepts," *Ann. Rev. Pharmacol., 11* (1971), 17; Adrien Albert, *Selective Toxicity*, 5th ed. (London: Methuen, 1973), p. 428.

3. William D.M. Paton, "The Significance of Stereoisomerism for the Growth of Pharmacology," *Actes XIe Cong. Int. Hist. Sci.* (1971), pp. 178–180.

4. Arnold H. Beckett, "Stereochemical Factors in Biological Activity," *Prog. Drug. Res., 1* (1959), 467–468; T.C. Daniels and E.C. Jorgensen, "Physiochemical Properties in Relation to Biologic Action," in Charles Wilson, Ole Grisvold, and Robert Doerge, ed., *Textbook of Organic and Medicinal Chemistry*, 5th ed. (Philadelphia: Lippincott, 1966), p. 27.

Arthur Cushny, Optical Isomerism and Drug Action

DISCOVERY OF DIFFERENCES IN PHARMACOLOGICAL ACTIVITY BETWEEN OPTICAL ISOMERS

The fact that living organisms have the ability to distinguish between optical enantiomers has been known since 1860, when Louis Pasteur demonstrated that certain microorganisms preferentially destroy dextrorotatory-tartrate over its enantiomer levorotatory-tartrate (dextrorotatory and levorotatory will be abbreviated as d and l, respectively, throughout the rest of the paper).[5] A number of similar observations were made later in the century with various microorganisms and certain ferments such as zymase, and it was also shown that the tissues of higher organisms sometimes oxidize one optical isomer more readily that another.[6] The fact that optical isomers may differ in taste (e.g., d-asparagine has a sweet taste, while l-asparagine is insipid) was also

5. Louis Pasteur, "Recherches sur la dissymétrie moléculaire des produits organiques naturels" (two lectures delivered before the Chemical Society of Paris, 1860; originally published in *Leçons de chimie professées en 1860*, Paris, 1861), in Pasteur Vallery-Radot, ed., *Oeuvres de Pasteur*, vol. I, *Dissymétrie moléculaire* (Paris: Masson, 1922), pp. 342–343. As indicated above, I shall use the symbols d and l, as Cushny ordinarily did, to designate direction of rotation (dextrorotatory and levrotatory, respectively). Unfortunately, there is some confusion in the literature of the period on the use of the d and l designations since Emil Fischer used these same symbols to denote configuration in the sugars (with respect to the two enantiomers of glyceraldehyde). Sugars which could be chemically derived from dextrorotatory-glyceraldehyde were designated d-sugars (regardless of their sign of rotation), while sugars which could be derived from levorotatory-glyceraldehyde were designated l-sugars. In Fischer's system a d-compound could thus be either dextrorotatory or levorotatory, and the same was true of an l-compound. For compounds other than the sugars, however, the terms d and l generally referred to direction of rotation, rather than configuration, throughout Cushny's lifetime. See, for example, M.A. Rosanoff, "On Fischer's Classification of Stereo-Isomers," *J. Amer. Chem. Soc.*, 28 (1906), 114–121; H.T. Clarke, *An Introduction to the Study of Organic Chemistry* (London: Longmans, Green, 1920), p. 124; and J.B. Conant, *Organic Chemistry: A Brief Introductory Course* (New York: Macmillan, 1928), p. 146. Eventually the symbols D and L replaced d and l in denoting configuration (R and S are also frequently used today), and the symbols (+) and (−) have largely supplanted d and l in designating dextrorotatory and levorotatory, respectively.

6. See, for example, Emil Fischer, "Bedeutung der Stereochemie für die Physiologie," *Z. Physiol. Chem.*, 26 (1898), 60–87, and Albert Brion, "Ueber die Oxydation der stereoisomeren Weinsäuren in thierischen Organismus," *Z. Physiol. Chem.*, 25 (1898), 283–295.

observed.[7] A number of attempts were made in the late nineteenth and early twentieth century to compare the pharmacological and toxicological properties of pairs of optical isomers,[8] but the first convincing examples of differences in pharmacological activity between two optical isomers were provided by the work of the Scottish pharmacologist Arthur Cushny.

Arthur Robertson Cushny (1866–1926) was one of the most prominent pharmacologists of the early twentieth century.[9] He studied at the University of Aberdeen, where he graduated with an M.A. in 1886 and degrees as Bachelor of Medicine and Master of Surgery in 1889. One of his teachers, John Theodore Cash, had aroused his interest in pharmacology, and Cushny then spent several years studying physiology and pharmacology in Germany (including a year as assistant to the noted pharmacologist Oswald Schmiedeberg at Strasbourg). In 1893, he was appointed to the chair of materia medica and therapuetics at the University of Michigan, a position which had been vacated when John J. Abel moved to Johns Hopkins University.

It was in Ann Arbor that Cushny began his work on optical isomers, a study that he was to continue during his tenure at University College, London (1905–1918), and the University of Edinburgh (1918–1926). Cushny obtained pure samples of *l*-hyoscyamine and atropine (a racemic, i.e., optically inactive, mixture of *d*- and *l*-hyoscyamine) from his colleagues Albert Prescott and Julius Otto Schlotterbeck of the College of Pharmacy at Michigan. He compared their pharmacological action on frogs and various mammals and found that while the two substances were equivalent in their action on some tissues (e.g., the central nervous system in mammals), they exhibited markedly different

7. M.A. Piutti, "Sur une nouvelle espèce d'asparagine," *C.R. Acad. Sci., 103* (1886), 134–137. Pasteur, who presented the paper on behalf of Piutti, commented in his observations (p. 138) that this difference in taste could be explained by assuming that the two optical isomers combine with an optically active substance in the nervous system to give two disymmetric compounds with different properties (compare this view with Cushny's explanation with respect to pharmacological activity, which is discussed below).

8. For discussions of these early efforts, see Alfred Stewart, *Stereochemistry* (London: Longmans, Green: 1907), pp. 544–556, and Arthur R. Cushny, *Biological Relations of Optically Isomeric Substances*, (Baltimore: Williams and Wilkins, 1926), pp. 18–29.

9. For biographical information on Cushny, see John J. Abel, "Arthur Robertson Cushny and Pharmacology," *J. Pharmacol. Exp. Ther., 27* (1926), 265–286; Henry H. Dale, "Arthur Robertson Cushny, 1866–1926," *Proc. Roy. Soc., 100B* (1926), pp. xix–xxvii; Helen MacGillivray, "A Personal Biography of Arthur Robertson Cushny, 1866–1926," *Ann. Rev. Pharmacol., 8* (1968), 1–24.

Arthur Cushny, Optical Isomerism and Drug Action

activities in their action on certain other tissues. For example, *l*-hyoscyamine proved to have twice the activity of atropine, the racemic mixture, on the motor nerve endings in the heart, in the salivary glands, and in the pupil of the eye. He concluded that the *d*-isomer is almost devoid of activity on these nerve endings, and that the activity of atropine on these nerves is due to the presence of the *l*-isomer. One could readily explain the experimentally observed fact that *l*-hyoscyamine is twice as active as atropine (which consists of equal quantities of *d*- and *l*-hyoscyamine) on the motor nerve endings on the assumption that the *d*-isomer has no appreciable activity on these nerves. On the other hand, atropine seemed to possess a more powerful stimulant action on the reflexes of the spinal cord in the frog than hyoscyamine (suggesting that the *d*-isomer is responsible for the action on the spinal cord).[10]

A small amount of pure *d*-hyoscyamine was then made available to Cushny so that he was able to directly compare the activities of the *d*- and *l*-isomers to a certain extent. He found that *d*-hyoscyamine was not completely inactive with regard to the motor nerve endings, but that it had only about one-twelfth to one-fourteenth of the activity of the *l*-compound.[11] Years later, on the basis of experiments with purer compounds, he revised this ratio to one to twenty.[12]

In the five years following his first publication on atropine and hyoscyamine, Cushny was able to demonstrate a similar difference in activity with two other pairs of optical isomers. In 1905, he demonstrated that *l*-hyoscine and racemic hyoscine differ markedly in certain pharmacological actions (e.g., the *l*-isomer is about twice as powerful as the racemic form in antagonizing the salivary secretion caused by

10. Arthur R. Cushny, "Atropine and the Hyoscyamines: A Study of the Action of Optical Isomers," *J. Physiol., 30* (1903), 176–194.

11. Ibid., pp. 188–192.

12. Arthur R. Cushny, "On Optical Isomers. V. The Tropeines," *J. Pharmacol. Exp. Ther., 13* (1919), 71–93. This article was reprinted in ibid., *15* (1920), 105–127, because the original version contained a large number of mistakes which were missed in proofreading. Cushny did not have an opportunity to proofread the article himself and wrote to John Abel, the editor of the journal and his friend, complaining about the large number of errors, whereupon Abel decided to reprint the paper (letter of August 17, 1919, John J. Abel papers, Welch Medical Library, Johns Hopkins University). I am grateful to the Johns Hopkins Institute of the History of Medicine for permission to use the Abel papers. The errors do not involve any of the passages quoted or discussed here, and they do not affect Cushny's main arguments, so I have cited the original version throughout my paper.

V

pilocarpine).[13] These studies were extended to adrenaline in 1908, and once again differences in activity were noted between *l*-adrenaline and racemic adrenaline (e.g., the natural *l*-adrenaline caused about twice as great an increase in blood pressure as the synthetic racemic adrenaline).[14] As with hyoscyamine, Cushny concluded that *d*-hyoscyine and *d*-adrenaline were essentially devoid of action on the tissues mentioned. Later experiments with the pure *d*-isomers, when these became available, showed that *l*-hyoscine was actually about fifteen to eighteen times as active as the *d*-isomer, and *l*-adrenaline about twelve to fifteen times as active as the *d*-isomer with respect to these tissues.[15]

Later in his career, Cushny returned again to the study of optical isomers and investigated the pharmacological activity of various tropeine compounds. Once again he was able to demonstrate significant differences in the activity of certain optical isomers.[16]

CUSHNY'S EXPLANATION OF THE MECHANISM OF DIFFERENTIATION

How did Cushny interpret the results of his researches on optical isomers with respect to theories of the mechanism of drug action? In his original 1903 paper on hyoscyamine, he did not speculate on the mechanism by which the cell might distinguish between optical isomers. He did make it clear, however, that he did not view his work as an illustration of a close relationship between structure and activity. On the contrary, he emphasized that his results illustrated the *independence* of pharmacological action and chemical structure, "for nothing can be more nearly related chemically than the two hyoscyamines, yet some of the most characteristic features in the action of the one are almost entirely wanting in the other."[17]

In the same year (1903), he did speculate about this difference in activity in a paper entitled "The Pharmacologic Action of Drugs; Is It

13. Arthur R. Cushny and A.R. Peebles, "The Action of Optical Isomers, II. Hyoscines," *J. Physiol., 32* (1905), 501–510.

14. Arthur R. Cushny, "The Action of Optical Isomers. III. Adrenalin," *J. Physiol., 37* (1908), 130–138.

15. Arthur R. Cushny, "Further Note on Adrenalin Isomers," *J. Physiol., 38* (1909), 259–262; Arthur R. Cushny, "Optical Isomers. VII. Hyoscines and Hyoscyamines," *J. Pharmacol. Exp. Ther., 17* (1921), 41–61.

16. See, for example, Arthur R. Cushny, "Optical Isomers. V. The Tropeines;" Arthur R. Cushny, "On Optical Isomers. VIII. The Influence of Configuration on the Activity of Tropeines," *J. Pharmacol. Exp. Ther., 29* (1926), 5–16.

17. Cushny, "Atropine and the Hyoscyamines," p. 194.

Arthur Cushny, Optical Isomerism and Drug Action

Determined by Chemical Structure or by Physical Characters?"[18] Optical isomers, he argued, could not be differentiated by "ordinary chemical means" and would be regarded as identical if it were not for the fact that they rotate the plane of polarized light in opposite directions. It seemed likely to him that this "physical characteristic," rather than the difference in configuration, was the direct determining cause of differences in pharmacological activity, although he admitted that "the physical factor undoubtedly rests on a structural difference ultimately."[19]

It should be noted that the emphasis of this paper was on the importance of physicochemical properties in determining drug action. In many cases, Cushny claimed, the facts could be more satisfactorily explained by assuming that physical properties, rather than chemical properties, were the immediate determinants of the action of a drug (although these properties ultimately depended upon the structure of the molecule).[20] Since the pharmacological action of many drugs, he felt, did not involve their entering into chemical combinations, the chemical structure of these drugs was of much less interest to the pharmacologist than physical properties such as solubility and volatility (which played a crucial role in determining their action).

Since optical isomers have essentially identical physical properties, however, Cushny was not able to explain how the cell could distinguish between them solely on the basis of these properties. By 1905, in his paper on the action of hyoscyines, he had admitted the likelihood that a chemical reaction was involved in the cell's ability to differentiate between enantiomers. He noted that certain substances which are themselves optically active show a greater "elective affinity" for one member of a pair of optical isomers than for the other. For example, d-tartaric acid crystallizes more readily with d-coniine than with l-coniine. Analogy would suggest, he stated, that the motor nerve endings, which have an ability to distinguish between d- and l-hyoscine, may possess an optically active acid which exhibits a preference for levorotatory bases, or which perhaps "deposits" dextrorotatory bases in a nonpoisonous form.[21] By his 1908 paper on adrenaline, he had begun to speak of optically active "receptive substances" in the cell which entered into

18. Arthur R. Cushny, "The Pharmacologic Action of Drugs; Is It Determined by Chemical Structure or by Physical Characters?," *J. Amer. Med. Assoc., 41* (1903), 1252–1255.

19. Ibid., p. 1254.

20. Ibid., p. 1255.

21. Cushny and Peebles, "Optical Isomers. II. Hyoscines," p. 505.

V

combinations with *l*-isomers that were somehow different from those formed with *d*-isomers.[22] The term "receptive substance" had been introduced by Langley in 1905 (I have discussed elsewhere the development of the receptor concept of drug action by Ehrlich and Langley in the period 1905–1908).[23]

Before assuming that Cushny had in mind a view of the *d*- and *l*-isomers competing for the same site on the receptor surface, with one isomer fitting better than the other, however, one must ask what he meant by "elective affinity" and how he viewed the "somewhat different" compounds formed by combination of the *d*- and *l*-isomers with the receptive substances. These questions cannot be answered as clearly as we might like on the basis of these early papers, although it seems likely that he had in mind the analogy he later utilized in explaining his views, that is, the reaction of both isomers with an optically active acid or base to form two diastereoisomers (stereoisomers which are dissymmetric, at least in part, and hence are not mirror images of each other) with different properties (such as solubility). Note the example mentined above, where *d*-tartaric acid forms a compound with d-coniine which is less soluble (and hence crystallizes more readily) than the compound it forms with *l*-coniine.

An expanded and clearer treatment of these views was presented by Cushny during the course of his renewed investigations on optical isomerism beginning about 1919. The fifth paper of his series of articles on optical isomers was published in 1919, after a gap of ten years since his previous paper on the subject, and it dealt with tropeines. Cushny was able to demonstrate that there were significant differences in activity between the optical isomers of various tropeine compounds. He returned again to the question of what was the underlying cause of these differences in activity. Optical isomers differ, he noted, in the direction in which they rotate the plane of polarized light, in their crystalline form, in the solubilities of the compounds they form on reacting with other optically active substances, and, of course, in their pharmacological effects on certain tissues. It did not seem promising to Cushny to attempt to relate the first two qualities (rotation of light and crystalline form) to the effects of the compounds on living tissues. He preferred to retain and expand the explanation which I believe is implied in his earlier work, that is, that the pharmacological effects were

22. Cushny, "Optical Isomers. III. Adrenalin," p. 136.
23. John Parascandola and Ronald Jasensky, "Origins of the Receptor Theory of Drug Action," *Bull. Hist. Med., 48* (1974), 199–220.

related to the different properties of the compounds formed by combination of the two isomers of the drug with an optically active receptor (similar to Pasteur's view, mentioned in note 7, concerning differences in taste between optical isomers): "Living matter is itself optically active, that is, contains asymmetric carbon atoms, and the difference in the action of the two hyoscyamines in living organisms may plausibly be explained by their forming compounds with the molecule containing asymmetric carbon, these compounds differing in solubility or other physical characters."[24]

Note that while Cushny admitted the involvement of a chemical reaction, he emphasized that it was the difference in physical properties (especially solubility) of the compounds formed by this reaction (diastereoisomers) which determined the difference in pharmacological activity. In an entry made in one of his research notebooks in 1917, he emphasized that it is not the presence of the asymmetric carbon atom itself which confers activity on a compound such as hyoscyamine (since one isomer may be active and the other relatively inactive), but the "physical characters" which arise from the presence of the asymmetric carbon atom.[25] He certainly did not suggest that the difference in activity between optical isomers was due to one enantiomer fitting the receptor surface better than the other. In fact, he specifically denied that the facility with which the two isomers combined with the receptor played any part in this process of differentiation. Aware that his views might be misinterpreted to favor a chemical theory of drug action (as they have been by some), he wrote:

At first sight this may seem to suggest that the reaction of these bases with the receptor is a purely chemical one and that their pharmacological action depends on this, which would run counter to the tendency of pharmacological thought at present, and would be in direct opposition to previous work in which I showed that the activity of atropine depends upon the law of mass action and not on that of chemical affinity; but this would be an erroneous deduction. It is true that I assume some chemical reaction to occur between the receptor and the alkaloid, but this follows whether the *l* or the

24. Cushny, "Optical Isomers. V. Tropeines," p. 77.
25. Arthur R. Cushny, Research Notebooks, vol. VII (June 1916–January 1918), MS, Manuscripts Division, Edinburgh University Library, Edinburgh, Scotland. The entry is not dated, but was apparently made between September 25 and October 2, 1917, the dates of the preceeding and succeeding entries. I am grateful to the Library for permission to use the Cushny manuscripts.

d form is present, just as in their reaction with *d* camphorsulphonic acid, which combines with either *d* or *l*-hyoscyamine indifferently. The difference in action lies not in the facility with which the chemical combination is formed, but in the physical characters of the resultant compound. In the case of camphorsulphonic acid these compounds differ in solubility, and some similar difference in the compound of the living receptor and the alkaloid may explain the marked change in pharmacological activity which accompanies the change in sign.[26]

In this statement, Cushny not only rejected the concept of the drug and the isomer fitting each other like a "lock and key," but also emphasized his belief that physical properties were more important than chemical affinities in determining pharmacological action. It should be noted that he suggested that in cases where two optical isomers exerted identical pharmacological effects on a tissue, the physical properties of the uncombined drug molecules were probably responsible for the action.[27] Cushny can thus hardly be considered a defender of the chemical over the physical view of drug action. An example of his advocacy of a physical or physicochemical approach was given earlier in this paper. Since I have discussed the subject elsewhere in some detail,[28] I will here offer only two further pieces of evidence on this point. The first of these is a quotation from Cushny's influential *Textbook of Pharmacology and Therapeutics:*

> As a matter of fact the physical properties of drugs appear to have a more direct bearing upon their action than the chemical structure; that is, the properties of the molecule as a whole determine its effects more than any of its constituent parts. For such properties as solubility in the fluids of the tissues, volatility, and diffusibility in colloid solutions determine whether a drug can be absorbed and come into contact with the living cells; thus, if two drugs differ in solubility in water their effects may be very different, although they

26. Cushny, "Optical Isomers. V. Tropeines," pp. 77–78.
27. Cushny, "Optical Isomers. VII. Hyoscines and Hyoscyamines," p. 60. Cushny once referred to his view as "a special case of Fischer's lock and key reactions" (Cushny, "Optical Isomers. V. Tropeines," p. 92), but this seems to me to be stretching the analogy too far. Cushny, for example, did not favor Ehrlich's "lock and key" theory of drug action (as discussed below).
28. John Parascandola, "The Controversy over Structure-Activity Relationships in the Early Twentieth Century," *Pharmacy in History, 16* (1974), 54–63.

Arthur Cushny, Optical Isomerism and Drug Action

are nearly related chemically. These physical characters depend ulti-mately upon the chemical structure, but as yet little has been done to correlate them with it and it is impossible to deduce them from the structural formulae.[29]

The second piece of evidence is from Cushny's manuscript notes for his pharmacology lectures at the University of Edinburgh. In these notes, he states that the group of substances which are supposed to act by chemical combination is being slowly reduced and that "it seems likely that it may finally *disappear*" (italics mine). Apparently he felt that this wording was too strong, even for a speculation in a lecture (although it is interesting to note that he entertained the thought), and he crossed out the word "disappear." He replaced it (at the top of the next page) with the phrase: "to embrace very few molecules as far as true chemical combinations are concerned. Probably many of [the] supposed cases are really of the nature of adsorption phenomena."[30]

It is also incorrect to portray Cushny as a supporter of the receptor theory of Ehrlich and Langley, which was developed in the first decade of the twentieth century. Paul Ehrlich conceived of the cell as a giant protoplasmic molecule with a chemical nucleus to which various chemical side chains were attached. For a drug to act on the cell, he envisioned, it first had to be anchored chemically to one of the cell's side chains, or "chemoreceptors." An atom group on the drug ("hapto-phore" group) had to possess a specific chemical affinity for a particu-lar atom group on the side chain in order for this "chemical union" to take place. Once the drug was thus anchored to the cell, its "pharmaco-phore" or "toxophore" group (the chemical moiety of the molecule which endowed it with its specific pharmacological or toxicological properties) could then exert its action on the cell. John Newport Langley also postulated that many drugs and poisons act by combining with specific "receptive substances" in the cell, and he suggested that these "receptive substances" might be radicals or side chains of the protoplasmic molecule.[31]

Many pharmacologists and chemists of the early twentieth century,

29. Arthur Cushny, *A Textbook of Pharmacology and Therapeutics*, 5th ed. (London: Churchill, 1910), p. 25.
30. Arthur R. Cushny, "Notes for Lectures on Materia Medica at the Univer-sity of Edinburgh (1918–1926)," Lecture 1, pp. 4–5, MS, Manuscripts Division, Edinburgh University Library, Edinburgh, Scotland.
31. For a discussion of the origins of the receptor theory, see Parascandola and Jasensky, "Origins of the Receptor Theory."

however, were skeptical of the receptor theory. A controversy developed over whether physical properties (such as solubility) or chemical reactivity played a greater part in determining pharmacological action. In a period when little was known of the biochemistry of the cell, and when the concept of the electronic nature of chemical bonding was only just emerging, it is understandable that a distinction developed between physical and chemical factors which today seems too rigid and artificial. Cushny tended to support the view that drugs very often acted through their physical properties as "uncombined foreign bodies" rather than through chemical combination (which was thought of at that times essentially in terms of firm linkages of the type that we would now refer to as covalent and ionic bonds). The structure of the molecule as a whole determined these physical properties, he felt, rather than the presence or absence of specific chemical groups.[32] While he used the concept of receptive substances in dealing with optically active drugs, he did not support the Ehrlich-Langley receptor concept as a general theory of drug action. It should be pointed out that while Cushny did not specifically identify what he thought the optically active receptive substances in the cell were, he never referred to them as "side chains" of the protoplasmic molecule. Instead, he frequently compared the reaction of optical isomers with the cell to their reaction with organic acids and bases, such as camphorsulfonic acid and cinchonidine,[33] although he admitted that the reaction in the living cell was probably more complicated.[34]

Cushny criticized or challenged the receptor theory on a number of occasions. In discussing Ehrlich's view, for example, that Salvarsan is effective against certain parasites because the "anchoring group" of the drug has a greater chemical affinity for the chemoreceptors of the

32. Cushny, "Pharmacologic Action of Drugs;" Cushny, *Textbook of Pharmacology*, 5th ed., p. 25. On physical versus chemical theories of drug action in this period, see Parascandola, "Controversy over Structure-Activity Relationships."

33. See, e.g., Cushny, "Optical Isomers. V. Tropeines," p. 78; Cushny, *Biological Relations*, pp. 56–57.

34. Cushny, *Biological Relations*, p. 58. It seems unlikely that Cushny would have accepted Ehrlich's "side chain" theory of cellular function, since supporters of the physiocochemical view of drug action tended to be critical of the concept of the cell as a giant protoplasmic molecule, a concept which was under attack from various quarters in the early twentieth century. They generally argued that the cell is a heterogeneous physicochemical system consisting of various components and phases. See, e.g., Carl Alsberg, "Chemical Structure and Physiological Action," *J. Wash. Acad. Sci., 11* (1921), 321–341, and William Bayliss, *Principles of General Physiology* (London: Longmans, Green, 1915), pp. 17–20.

parasite than for those of the mammalian cell, he remarked that it was simpler to assume that the drug permeates the cell of the parasite more readily than it does the mammalian cell.[35] In discussing the selective action of drugs of known structure on tissues, he stated that he felt it only led to confusion to attempt to explain this action in terms of Ehrlich's "haptophore" and "toxophore" groups. In many cases, he argued, the difference in the effects of drugs on different tissues appears to arise more from "differences in the behavior of the molecule as a whole" than from "differences in the affinities of the special parts" — that is, more from physical properties than from chemical structure. In addition, the fact that certain tissues exhibit a common reaction to certain chemicals may arise from "community of physical relationship," from "a common arrangement of the aggregate molecules," rather than from the presence of some chemical substance in common.[36]

In one of his papers on optical isomers, Cushny specifically rejected an opportunity to use the receptor theory to explain drug specificity. He noted that in the tropeine series the highest activity is attained when an asymmetric carbon atom is associated with a hydroxyl group. It is tempting to assume, he pointed out, that the asymmetric carbon atom is the anchoring or haptophore group and that the hydroxyl is the pharmacophore group (in Ehrlich's terminology). The fact that tropeines which contain neither asymmetric carbon atoms nor hydroxyl groups still have some pharmacological activity, however, indicates that such molecules must still be able to act on the "receptor." Cushny concluded that perhaps the activating power of the hydroxyl group might be due to some physical property with which it endows the whole molecule. For example, he pointed out the change in physical and pharmacological properties which is produced in ethane by the introduction of a hydroxyl group to form ehtyl alcohol.[37]

Cushny summarized his work on optical isomers in his Dohme Lectures in 1925 (published in 1926 as *Biological Relations of Optically Isomeric Substances*). In that monograph he makes a statement which is frequently quoted or referred to in discussions of his work. With regard to optical isomers, he says: "In pharmacological effects there can

35. Cushny, *Textbook of Pharmacology*, 7th ed. (1918), p. 605.

36. Arthur R. Cushny, "On the Analysis of Living Matter through Its Reactions to Poisons," *Science, 44* (1916), 487.

37. Cushny, "Optical Isomers, V. Tropeines," p. 91.

hardly be any question that the action is on a single receptor, which embraces both isomers, though with unequal warmth."[38]

This statement could perhaps be interpreted to mean that the receptor combines more readily with one isomer than the other; that is their structures are compementary. If this interpretation is correct, then Cushny would have been contradicting his 1919 statement that the difference in activity of two enantiomers is not due to the facility with which they combine with the receptor. Did Cushny change his mind in the six years between 1919 and 1925? This explanation seems unlikely to me, because throughout his 1925 lectures he continued to emphasize, as he has earlier, that it is the difference in physical properties of the two diastereoisomers formed by the combination of the *d*- and *l*-isomers with the receptor which is responsible for the difference in pharmalogical activity. In discussing the differences observed between the reactions of two optical isomers with optically active chemicals, with enzymes, or with receptors, he stated:

> There can, I think, be no question that in all these conditions the differences observed between the reactions of two isomers arise from the same fundamental cause and that for example *l*-adrenaline contracts the vessels of the conjunctiva more strongly than *d*-adrenaline from the same principle that makes *d*-tartrate more readily oxidised by penicillium and less easily precipitated by cinchonine than the *l*-tartrate, that is because in the tissues, as in the test-tube, the isomers form compounds with some optically active substance and these compounds are no longer mirror images and no longer identical in their physical characteristics. For example, it may be supposed that *l*-adrenaline may cause a precipitate readily in the myoneural junction, while *d*-adrenaline does so only when it is present in much higher concentration, just as they differ in their reaction with camphor-sulphonic acid.[39]

Nowhere in his lectures on optical isomerism, or in his other writings of this period, does he suggest that the difference in activity between

38. Cushny, *Biological Relations*, p. 67.
39. Ibid., p. 55. Cushny rejected other possible explanations in his 1925 lectures (although he did not even mention any views based on ease of combination with the receptor). For example, he argued that the stronger action of *d*-hyoscyamine on the brain could not be explained by assuming that *l*-hyoscyamine is more rapidly destroyed by body tissues because *l*-hyoscyamine has a stronger action on the nerve endings.

Arthur Cushny, Optical Isomerism and Drug Action

enantiomers depends upon their structure relative to that of the receptor. His 1925 statement that the receptor "embraces both isomers, though with unequal warmth," is a vague phrase which need not imply any consideration of structural "fit" or complementarity. I believe that when Cushny spoke of the receptor "embracing" one enantiomer more "warmly," he meant that the receptor has a greater affinity for this isomer and thus forms a compound which is more tightly bound, hence more insoluble (less likely to be broken apart by solvent molecules) and perhaps more stable in other ways. If he were pressed as to the cause of the different properties of the two compounds formed upon combination of the receptor with the enantiomers, I suspect that he would have admitted that these properties probably depended ultimately upon the chemical structures of the compounds. But this was a problem for the chemist rather than for the pharmacologist, and Cushny did not foresee any immediate success in relating physical properties to chemical structure.[40]

This statement about the receptor embracing the isomers with unequal warmth must also be considered in its proper context. It appeared in a discussion of the question of whether the slight activity of *d*-hyoscyamine on the nerve endings, for example, might be due to partial racemization to form some *l*-hyoscyamine. In other words, perhaps the *d*-isomer is not one-twentieth as active as the *l*-isomer, perhaps it is not active at all. Cushny went on to say that a similar question had been discussed with regard to enzymes which digest enantiomers at unequal rates. It was suggested that two enzymes were present, one of which acted on the *d*-isomer and the other on the *l*-isomer, but this view was later abandoned. He then added that in pharmacological effects there could be little doubt that both isomers act on a single receptor (though with unequal warmth).[41] The point he was emphasiz-

40. Examples were given earlier in this paper of Cushny's willingness to admit that physical properties ultimately depend on chemical structure, and his doubts that the two would soon be correlated. In 1903, he wrote: "if no true chemical combinations are formed, the structure is of less immediate interest to the pharmacologist, and the physical characters ought to receive his chief attention, while the connection between the structure and the physical properties scarcely comes within his sphere of action." See Cushny, "Pharmacologic Action of Drugs," p. 1253. Compare this statement with one by Carl Alsberg, another supporter of the physicochemical view: "Of course, in the last analysis the physical state is but an extension of the chemical constitution and vice versa, but these are problems for the chemist, not the pharmacologist." See Alsberg, "Chemical Structure," p. 324.

41. Cushny, *Biological Relations*, pp. 66–67.

ing, in other words, was that the *d*- and *l*-forms both act on the same receptor, and not on different receptors. The phrase "though with unequal warmth" was added to indicate that he recognized, of course, that the enantiomers did not produce the same quantitative effect on combining with the receptor.

In his 1925 lectures, Cushny also attempted to evaluate the various factors contributing to the specific activity of a drug such as hyoscyamine.[42] He listed three factors which had to be taken into account:

(1) the general structure of the molecule (a tropeine ester, preferably of an aromatic acid), which gives a slight activity as a general rule;

(2) the presence of an alcoholic hydroxyl group in the side chain of the acid, which greatly intensifies the activity;

(3) the presence of an asymmetric carbon atom (which gives optical rotation to the molecule), which may vary the activity 15 to 20 times in certain situations.

The first of these, the general structure or configuration of the molecule, is a necessary preliminary to the onset of action. Cushny argued, however, that since the configuration of the whole molecule rather than the presence of individual radicals seems to be the determining factor, the influence of this feature may be physical rather than chemical (though he admitted that it may not be possible to distinguish physical from chemical influences).

The presence of the hydroxyl group, he felt, might possibly affect pharmacological activity by giving to the molecule certain physical properties (such as solubility) which promote its reaction with the receptors of the tissues.

The effect of the third factor, direction of rotation, he believed was almost certainly due to a chemical combination between the receptor and the drug, forming two diastereoisomers with different properties (as he had explained earlier).

Note that Cushny continued to emphasize the physical factors involved in drug action. In addition, we can see that he clearly separated out the influence of the asymmetric carbon atom from that of the general configuration or structure of the molecule. Whenever he explained the effect of asymmetry on pharmacological action, he tended to speak of the difference in the direction of optical rotation of the isomers rather than their different configurations (although he was aware that two substances which have the same configuration could have opposite signs

42. Ibid., pp. 74–75.

Arthur Cushny, Optical Isomerism and Drug Action

of rotation).[43] In 1932, in fact, his explanation of the differences in activity between optical isomers was criticized by Leopold Rosenthaler because of its emphasis on the direction of rotation rather than on the configuration of an optical isomer.[44] Cushny's discussions of the pharmacological action of optical isomers did not explicitly consider the spatial arrangement around the asymmetric carbon atom, and he did not even use structural formulas to any significant extent in his treatment of the subject.

I should point out, however, that in his 1925 lectures Cushny does seem to have been willing to grant more importance to chemical factors in drug action than in his earlier works. He noted, for example, that

43. Cushny did recognize, for example, that the compounds designated by Emil Fischer as *d*-glucose (now D-glucose) and *d*-fructose (now D-fructose) had a similar configuration, although the former was dextrorotatory and the latter was levorotatory (see Cushny, *Biological Relations*, pp. 28–29). Fischer, of course, used the symbols *d* and *l* to refer to configuration, rather than direction of rotation, in the sugars (see n. 5). When explaining the pharmacological activity of optical isomers, Cushny generally spoke in terms of direction of rotation (e.g., ibid., pp. 74–75; Cushny and Peebles, "Optical Isomers. II. Hyoscines," p. 505; Cushny, "Optical Isomers. V. Tropeines," pp. 78, 90–92). It is interesting to note that although he listed the three factors influencing the action of a drug such as hyoscyamine (discussed above) under the general heading of "Influence of Configuration on Pharmacological Action," he separated out the effect of the asymmetric carbon atom from that of the general structure or configuration of the molecule, and related it to direction of rotation (Cushny, *Biological Relations*, pp. 74–75). In another publication he used the word "configuration" in the title, but it never appeared in the text of the article, nor did he utilize the concept of configuration in this paper. See Cushny, "Optical Isomers. VIII. Influence of Configuration." It may be that by 1926 (the year in which both of these works were published, and the year in which he died) he was at least becoming more aware of the need to attempt to speak in terms of configuration. The question of the configuration (as opposed to the optical rotation) of compounds other than the sugars and a few organic acids (such as lactic and tartaric acids) does not seem to have received much attention in the scientific literature during Cushny's lifetime.

44. Leopold Rosenthaler, "Ueber die Beziehungen zwischen pharmakologischer Wirkung and optischer Drehung," *Schweiz. Med. Wochenschr.*, *13* (1932), 305–306. Cushny did not, however, claim (as Rosenthaler suggests) that only levorotatory compounds are pharmacologically active. One year later, Cushny was criticized for separating out optical activity as a factor distinct from general structure by Easson and Stedman, who offered an alternative theory for explaining the differences of activities between optical isomers (see below). See Leslie Easson and Edgar Stedman, "Studies on the Relationship between Chemical Constitution and Physiological Action. V. Molecular Dissymmetry and Physiological Activity," *Biochem. J.*, *27* (1933), 1257–1266.

V

while there was at the time a general tendency to attribute pharmacological action almost exclusively to physical changes produced in the
cells by drugs, chemical factors also sometimes play a part (as clearly
demonstrated by the reaction of optical isomers with receptors). He
suggested that the relation between the living cell and the drug is probably seldom purely chemical or physical, and that the proportion of
these forces varies from time to time. He particularly emphasized the
fact that one cannot always differentiate clearly between physical and
chemical processes ("the frontiers of physics and chemistry can no
longer be drawn with the precision that was formerly supposed to be
possible"). In addition, he emphasized that where a drug has a similar
action on different tissues, this fact suggests that these tissues may have
certain common chemical features.[45] As a result of developments such
as the theories of chemical bonding proposed by Irving Langmuir,
Walther Kossel, and G.N. Lewis, Langmuir's studies on adsorption, and
the work of W.H. and W.L. Bragg on X-ray crystallography, Cushny
(like most of his contemporaries) was becoming more aware by 1925 of
the difficulty of attempting to distinguish between chemical and physical
forces.[46]

THE VIEWS OF SOME OF CUSHNY'S CONTEMPORARIES

While I have not made a systematic and comprehensive search of the
pharmacological literature for reactions to Cushny's work on optical
isomers, it can readily be shown that Cushny's contemporaries did not

45. Cushny, *Biological Relations*, pp. 58–59, 77–78. The quotation is from
p. 59.
46. For a discussion of some of these developments, see Aaron J. Ihde, *The
Development of Modern Chemistry* (New York: Harper & Row, 1964),
pp. 536–541, 550–552, and 555–557. Langmuir's work seems to have been
particularly influential in breaking down the barriers between chemical and
physical forces. See Irving Langmuir, "The Constitution and Fundamental Properties of Solids and Liquids," in C. Guy Suits, ed., *The Collected Works of Irving
Langmuir*, vol. VIII, *Properties of Matter* (New York: Pergammon Press, 1961),
pp. 1–130 (reprinted from *J. Amer. Chem. Soc., 38*, 1916). See also Henry
Eyring, "Introduction to Volume 8," *Properties of Matter*, pp. xvii–xxix; Albert
Rosenfeld, "The Quintessence of Irving Langmuir: A Biography," *The Collected
Works of Irving Langmuir*, vol. XII, *Langmuir, the Man and the Scientist* (1962),
pp. 152–161; Eric Rideal, "Some of the Chemical Aspects of the Work of
Langmuir," ibid., pp. 419–432; P.W. Bridgman, "Some of the Physical Aspects of
the Work of Langmuir," ibid., pp. 433–457. See also Robert Kohler, Jr., "Irving
Langmuir and the 'Octet' Theory of Valence," *Hist. Stud. Phys. Sci., 4* (1974),
39–67.

V

Arthur Cushny, Optical Isomerism and Drug Action

necessarily interpret his work as supporting the receptor theory of Ehrlich and Langley or the view that drug action depends directly on the chemical structure of a drug. The physiologist William Bayliss, for example, referred to Cushny's work in criticizing the concept that drug action involves the fitting of a drug to a receptor like a "lock and key." If this analogy were correct, he argued, one would expect that one member of a pair of optical isomers would have no activity at all, instead of some fraction of the activity of its enantiomer (as shown by Cushny).[47] The pharmacologist Walter Dixon, in discussing the fact that drug action cannot always be related to chemical structure, used optical isomers as an example of the limits of the chemical view: "No two bodies can be more closely related chemically than the two hyoscyamines (optical isomers), yet some of the most characteristic features in the action of the one are almost entirely wanting in the other."[48]

Some scientists in the early twentieth century, however, did attempt to explain the difference in activity between enantiomers in terms of the stereochemical configurations of the drug and the receptor. For example, Alfred Stewart, a chemist and the author of a 1907 book on *Stereochemistry*, argued that spatial or three-dimensional factors play a part in many chemical reactions involved in vital processes. He suggested that the speed of reaction of an optically active drug with an asymmetric receptive substance sometimes depends upon the spatial arrangement of the atoms.[49] Stewart noted that it was probable that the tissues, which are themselves asymmetric, select those substances whose "stereochemical configurations best fit in with their own"[50] (similar to Emil Fischer's well-known "lock and key" analogy for the reaction between an enzyme and its substrate, first expressed in 1894).

These early attempts at stereochemical explanations were rather vague "lock and key" or "hand and glove" analogies, and no satisfactory three-dimensional explanation of how a receptive substance could distinguish between optical isomers seems to have been offered until 1933. In that year Leslie Easson and Edgar Stedman of Edinburgh University expounded an alternative to Cushny's view based on the

47. Bayliss, *Principles of General Physiology*, p. 728. Bayliss held a similar view with respect to enzyme action (ibid., p. 726).

48. Walter Dixon, *Manual of Pharmacology* (London: Edward Arnold, 1906), p. 19. Note the similarity of his statement to that quoted above from Cushny's 1903 paper (n. 17).

49. Alfred Stewart, *Chemistry and Its Borderland* (London: Longmans, Green, 1914), pp. 129–130.

50. Stewart, *Stereochemistry*, p. 545.

molecular arrangement of the drug relative to the receptor.[51] While the hypothesis of Easson and Stedman was not immediately adopted, this type of "three-point contact" model eventually received widespread use in biochemistry and pharmacology, beginning about 1950, as I have discussed elsewhere.[52]

CONCLUSION

While contemporary scientists tend to point to differences in the pharmacological behavior of optical isomers as evidence of the structural complementarity that must exist between a drug and its receptor, it seems clear that Arthur Cushny did not hold such a view. His own explanation for the differences in activity between optical enantiomers, based on differences in the physical properties of the different drug-receptor compounds formed by the two isomers, was in harmony with his general view of the mechanism of drug action, which tended to give preference to physical over chemical factors. Some of his contemporaries also declined to view the results of his work as evidence for a close relationship between structure and activity. However, there were some early attempts to explain the difference in activity between optical isomers in terms of the stereochemical configurations of the drug and the receptor, but it was not until 1933 that a satisfactory explanation of this type was offered by Easson and Stedman (and it was many years before their theory was widely adopted).

Current views of the action of optical isomers based on structural complementarity therefore derive more from the tradition of Stewart, Easson and Stedman, and others than from Cushny's hypothesis. This fact does not detract from the importance of Cushny's work, which demonstrated the existence of these differences in activity and measured their magnitude, in addition to offering a plausible theory to explain them. Indeed, views about the mechanism of action of optical enantiomers are constantly being refined and modified, and may evolve in the future in directions which are now unforeseen. Perhaps this study can serve to remind us again (if historians of science need any further reminders on this point) of the care that must be taken to avoid the interpretation of past concepts in terms of current views.

51. Easson and Stedman, "Molecular Dissymmetry and Physiological Action."
52. John Parascandola, "The Evolution of Stereochemical Concepts in Pharmacology," in O. Bertrand Ramsay, ed., van 't Hoff – Le Bel Centennial Symposium, American Chemical Society Symposium Series Number 12, 1975, pp. 143–158.

Arthur Cushny, Optical Isomerism and Drug Action

Acknowledgments

This paper is part of a study on "The History of Chemical Pharmacology" funded by the National Science Foundation (under grants GS–28549 and GS–41462). Some of the research for this paper was also carried out under a grant from the Wisconsin Alumni Research Foundation University of Wisconsin Graduate School. A preliminary and abbreviated version of this paper was presented to the Division of the History of Chemistry, American Chemical Society, in August 1973. I wish to thank John Edsall of Harvard University and Aaron Ihde of the University of Wisconsin for helpful suggestions concerning certain points in the paper, and my colleague Phillip Hart for informative discussions on the stereochemical aspects of drug action.

VI

Carl Voegtlin and the 'Arsenic Receptor' in Chemotherapy

T HE birth of modern chemotherapy is generally associated with the work of Paul Ehrlich in the early twentieth century, and particularly with his introduction in 1910 of the drug 'salvarsan' (606) for the treatment of syphilis and trypanosomiasis. Ehrlich explained the chemotherapeutic action of salvarsan on the basis of his receptor theory, postulating that the arsenic-containing drug exerted its toxic effect by combining with an 'arsenoreceptor' in the cell of the microorganism. He speculated that the chemical group involved in reacting with arsenic might be a hydroxyl or sulfhydryl group.

In the 1920s Carl Voegtlin and his colleagues in the Hygienic Laboratory of the United States Public Health Service provided convincing evidence that arsenical drugs combined with essential sulfhydryl-containing compounds in the cell, thereby interfering with normal metabolism. It would thus seem reasonable to view Voegtlin's work as providing experimental confirmation of Ehrlich's suggestion that sulfhydryl groups might act as receptors for arsenic, and as supporting his receptor theory. While there is some justification for such a view, it represents an oversimplification of the actual historical situation. For one thing it does not recognize adequately the significance and the originality of Voegtlin's contribution. More importantly, however, it overlooks the facts that one of the motivating forces behind Voegtlin's chemotherapeutic researches appears to have been a dissatisfaction with Ehrlich's receptor theory, that Voegtlin rejected some of

The author wishes gratefully to acknowledge the support of the National Science Foundation under Grant GS-41462. A preliminary and abbreviated version of this paper was presented at the International Congress of the History of Pharmacy, Bremen, West Germany, October 1975. Part of the research was carried out while I was a visiting worker at the National Institute for Medical Research in London, England, and I wish to thank the Director, A. S. V. Burgen, for the use of the institute's facilities, and the Librarian, R. J. Moore, for his assistance in the use of library materials. I also appreciate my being granted permission to use the Wellcome Institute for the History of Medicine Library and the Library of the University College London.

the fundamental concepts of Ehrlich's theory, and that Voegtlin's own explanation of the action of arsenical drugs differed significantly from that of Ehrlich.

Carl Voegtlin (1879–1960) has not received much attention from historians, but the importance for chemotherapy and pharmacology of his research on arsenicals has been discussed by a number of scientists.[1] He was born in Switzerland, received his doctoral training in organic chemistry in Germany in the early years of this century, and in 1904 came to the United States to serve as an instructor in chemistry at the University of Wisconsin for one year.[2] He was to remain in the United States for the rest of his life, eventually becoming a naturalized citizen. In 1905 he moved to Johns Hopkins University where he established a biochemical or metabolic research laboratory in the Department of Medicine, but he later shifted to the Department of Pharmacology under the influence of Prof. John J. Abel.

John Abel is often considered to be the father of American pharmacology. After receiving his undergraduate training at the University of Michigan and pursuing further studies at Johns Hopkins, Abel made the pilgrimage to Europe so customary for ambitious young Americans in the late nineteenth century. His European apprenticeship is one of the longest on record, as he spent six and one-half years working in various laboratories in Germany and Switzerland, including two years at Strassburg where he received his M.D. degree in 1888. Here he came into contact with the distinguished pharmacologist Oswald Schmiedeberg and worked in his laboratory. Abel brought with him to his first university position at Michigan the German tradition of experimental pharmacology as molded by such pioneers of the discipline as Rudolph Buchheim and Oswald Schmiedeberg. Pharmacology in their view was an experimental biological science closely related to physiology, and distinct from traditional ma-

1. Historian of pharmacy Glenn Sonnedecker delivered a brief but informative paper on 'Carl Voegtlin and chemotherapy' at the 1960 annual meeting of the American Institute of the History of Pharmacy in Washington, D.C. (unpublished; copy in Kremers Reference Files, University of Wisconsin School of Pharmacy Library, Madison). Scientists who have commented on the significance of Voegtlin's work include Thomas S. Work and Elizabeth Work, *The basis of chemotherapy* (New York, 1948), pp. 27–28; Adrien Albert, *Selective toxicity*, 5th ed. (London, 1973), pp. 139, 393–395; and B. Holmstedt and G. Liljestrand, eds., *Readings in pharmacology* (Oxford, 1963), pp. 292–294.

2. Biographical information concerning Voegtlin is relatively meager, especially considering his significant contributions to chemotherapy and his role as first head of the National Cancer Institute. See 'Carl Voegtlin (1879–1960), first Director of Cancer Research of the Public Health Service and first Chief of the National Cancer Institute,' *J. Nat. Cancer Instit.*, 1960, *25*, v–xv (includes a bibliography of Voegtlin's papers); K. K. Chen, ed., *The American Society for Pharmacology and Experimental Therapeutics: the first sixty years, 1908–1969* (n.p., 1969), pp. 29–30; Hans Ritter, 'Carl Voegtlin,' *Schweiz. med. Wochen.*, 1961, *91*, 216–217; and H. Fischer, 'Carl Voegtlin,' *Bull. Schweiz. Akad. med. Wiss.*, 1960, *16*, 323–326.

teria medica, which had concerned itself largely with questions of the origins and constituents of drugs, their preparation, etc. In 1893 Abel moved to Johns Hopkins University to join the faculty of the newly created medical school, occupying what was apparently the first chair in this country to bear the title of 'pharmacology.' His laboratory became a mecca for young Americans interested in pursuing pharmacological researches.

Abel was firmly convinced of the importance of chemistry for the medical sciences, and had himself acquired a strong training in physiological chemistry. Most of his pharmacological researches had a biochemical bent, and he played a significant role in the establishment of biochemistry as a discipline in the United States. Because of his interest in chemistry, he was no doubt especially alert to the value of Voegtlin's particular training and skill. In 1908 Voegtlin accepted a position in Abel's department, thus determining, as he later said, the course of his future life.[3]

Carl Voegtlin taught pharmacology and engaged in research in Abel's laboratory until 1913 when he became Chief of the Division of Pharmacology of the Hygienic Laboratory of the United States Public Health Service at Washington. At the Hygienic Laboratory Voegtlin began the studies on the chemotherapy of arsenic compounds as a result of a practical problem facing the Hygienic Laboratory. Before the First World War, the United States depended upon Germany for its supply of arsenicals such as salvarsan. With the outbreak of the war in Europe in 1914 the German supply was almost completely cut off. Imports of these drugs into the United States had reached such a low level by 1917, when the United States entered the war, that the Federal Trade Commission had abrogated foreign patent rights to allow selected American manufacturers to produce salvarsan (given the generic name 'arsphenamine' in the United States) and its derivatives. In Germany, because of difficulties in obtaining uniform preparations of the drug, Ehrlich's laboratory had been testing each batch of salvarsan produced by the original manufacturer, Hoechst. In the United States, under the 1902 Biologics Control Act, the Hygienic Laboratory had already assumed responsibility for testing biologic products (serums, vaccines, etc.) sold in interstate commerce. It was thus a logical step to bring the testing and control of arsenicals under its jurisdiction. Manufacturers

3. Carl Voegtlin, 'John Jacob Abel, decade, 1903–1913,' *Bull. Johns Hopkins Hosp.*, 1957, *101*, 303–305, p. 303. For biographical information on Abel see *Dictionary of scientific biography*, s.v. 'Abel, John Jacob'; Carl Voegtlin, 'John Jacob Abel, 1857–1938,' *J. Pharmacol. exp. Ther.*, 1939, *67*, 373–406; and idem, *John Jacob Abel, M.D., investigator, teacher, prophet, 1857–1938* (Baltimore, 1957).

were required to test for toxicity and arsenic content in each lot of arsenicals produced, and to submit samples of each lot to the Public Health Service for possible testing by this agency. Voegtlin's laboratory was responsible for developing the chemical and pharmacological tests used.[4]

Voegtlin then moved beyond the immediate problem of developing toxicity tests to an investigation of the fundamental mechanism of biological action of arsenic compounds. In 1920 he published the first two papers, in what would become a series of chemotherapeutic studies from the Hygienic Laboratory, on the trypanocidal effect of arsenic and antimony compounds. In the first paper Voegtlin and his co-worker Homer Smith noted that the development of new chemotherapeutic agents was essentially empirical, consisting of the testing of hundreds of chemicals. Progress in chemotherapy was retarded by ignorance of the fundamental mechanism by which the drug killed the parasite. They had therefore decided to investigate the mechanism of action of certain known chemotherapeutic drugs rather than synthesize and study new compounds.[5]

Attempts to understand the action of chemicals on living cells go back to the nineteenth century. Pharmacologists such as Thomas Fraser and T. Lauder Brunton, for example, postulated in the 1870s that physiological action was probably usually due to a chemical reaction between the drug and some constituent of the cell or tissue. Not until the first decade of the twentieth century, however, was the concept of *receptors* in the cell, that is, substances which were thought to combine with drug molecules, clearly developed into a systematic theory by Paul Ehrlich in Germany and by John Newport Langley in England.[6]

Paul Ehrlich conceived of the cell as a giant protoplasmic molecule consisting of a chemical nucleus to which were attached various chemical side

4. Ralph C. Williams, *The United States Public Health Service, 1798–1950* (Washington, D.C., 1951), pp. 182–183, 592–594; 'Carl Voegtlin, . . . first Director of Cancer Research' (n. 2), p. vi; 'Arsphenamine (salvarsan), licenses ordered and rules and standards prescribed for its manufacture,' *Pub. Hlth. Rep.*, 1917, *32*, 2071–2072; and Carl Voegtlin and D. W. Miller, 'The relative parasiticidal value of arsphenamine and neoarsphenamine, with a description of the trypanocidal test,' *Pub. Hlth. Rep.*, 1922, *37*, 1627–1641. A similar situation arose in Great Britain where Henry Dale's Department of Biochemistry and Pharmacology at the National Institute of Medical Research was called upon to test the salvarsan manufactured in that country. See W. S. Feldberg, 'Henry Hallett Dale, 1875–1968,' *Biog. Mem. Fellows Roy. Soc.*, 1970, *16*, 77–174, p. 106; and *Reports of the special committee upon the manufacture, biological testing and clinical administration of Salvarsan and of its substitutes. No. 1*, Medical Research Committee special report no. 44 (London, 1919), pp. 23–24.

5. Carl Voegtlin and Homer Smith, 'Quantitative studies in chemotherapy. I. The trypanocidal action of antimony compounds,' *J. Pharmacol. exp. Ther.*, 1920, *15*, 453–473, p. 453.

6. For a discussion of the theories of Ehrlich and Langley, and for references to the views of Fraser, Brunton, and others, see John Parascandola and Ronald Jasensky, 'Origins of the receptor theory of drug action,' *Bull. Hist. Med.*, 1974, *48*, 199–220.

chains which were involved in such vital processes of the cell as oxidation. This was a concept similar to Edward Pflüger's view of protoplasm and a forerunner of Max Verworn's *biogen* hypothesis. Ehrlich utilized the giant molecule concept of the cell in 1897 to explain the process of immunization. He postulated that bacterial toxins poisoned the cell by combining with specific side chains on the protoplasmic molecule, hence rendering them incapable of performing their normal physiological function. He thought that the combination was very specific and that it depended upon the possession by the toxin of an atom group (the *haptophore* group) which had a specific tendency to combine with a particular atom group on a side chain. Antibodies against a toxin were formed by the production of more side chains by the cell to replace those incapacitated by the toxin. Overcompensation resulted in the production of excess side chains which were released into the bloodstream. Such excess side chains formed the antibodies or antitoxins in the serum and served to neutralize the toxin by combining with it in the blood and thus preventing it from injuring the cell. Ehrlich's side chain theory exerted an important influence on immunology at the turn of the twentieth century, although it soon began to lose support in favor of a more physical view of the toxin-antitoxin reaction based upon the principles of colloid science.[7]

Ehrlich hesitated at first to apply his side chain or receptor concept to explain the action of drugs on the cell, but in 1907, as a result of researches in his laboratory on the phenomenon of drug resistance, together with an awareness of John Newport Langley's theory (first expounded in 1905–06) that drugs and poisons act by combining with 'receptive substances' in the cell, he adopted a modified version of his side chain theory of immunity to explain the action of various chemotherapeutic agents then being studied in his laboratory.[8]

About 1903 Ehrlich and his co-workers began in earnest an investigation of the effects of various chemicals on trypanosome infections, trypanosomes being the microorganisms responsible for sleeping sickness. In 1907 Ehrlich postulated that in order for a chemical to be effective against trypanosomes, the trypanosomes must possess side chains or *chemoreceptors* which are capable of combining with the poison, as in the case of bacterial toxins. Ehrlich also thought that the chemoreceptors of the trypanosomes

7. Pauline Mazumdar, 'The antigen-antibody reaction and the physics and chemistry of life,' *Bull. Hist. Med.*, 1974, *48*, 1–21.

8. For a discussion of the reasons why Ehrlich did not at first apply his side chain theory to drugs, see Parascandola and Jasensky (n. 6), pp. 205–209.

156

must possess a greater avidity for the drug than did the chemoreceptors of the host cells, otherwise the drug would be more toxic for the human host than for the parasite. Trypanosomes which acquired a resistance to an arsenic-containing chemical, such as atoxyl, also tended to exhibit increased resistance toward other arsenicals, but not toward compounds of different chemical natures, such as the azo dyes. The specificity of drug resistance acquired by the trypanosomes indicated to Ehrlich that different types of drugs attack different receptors in the cell, and that the reaction between drug and receptor is of a rather specific nature, similar to the reaction between toxin and antitoxin.

In the case of arsenical drugs, Ehrlich suggested that the arsenical radical was the specific chemical group that was bound by the chemoreceptors. In 1909 he even hazarded a guess about the chemical nature of the receptor for arsenic, suggesting that it might be a hydroxyl or sulfhydryl group. Since Ehrlich believed that sulfhydryl and/or hydroxyl groups were probably involved in oxidation-reduction processes in the cell, he may have thought that arsenic compounds could poison the cell by combining with such hydroxyl or sulfhydryl groups, thus interfering with normal oxidation-reduction reactions. The possibility that the toxic action of arsenic might involve an effect on cellular oxidation had already been suggested by other investigators.[9]

In 1913 Ehrlich elaborated further on this concept of the mechanism of action of arsenicals to explain the action of salvarsan.[10] He noted that for

9. For Ehrlich's discussion of the possible chemical nature of the arsenic receptor, see Paul Ehrlich, 'Über den jetzigen Stand der Chemotherapie,' in The collected papers of Paul Ehrlich, ed. F. Himmelweit, 3 vols. (London, 1956–60), III, 150–170, pp. 166–167 (reprinted from Ber. dt. chem. Ges., 1909). Binz and Schulz theorized as early as 1879 that arsenic compounds interfered with cellular oxidation by alternately supplying and withdrawing oxygen through the interconversion of arsenious acid and arsenic acid by an oxidation-reduction process. See C. Binz and H. Schulz, 'Die Arsengiftwirkungen von chemischen Standpunkt betrachtet,' Arch. exp. Path. Pharmak., 1879, 11, 200–230. Although this particular theory was criticized on the grounds that arsenious and arsenic acids should be equally toxic, which they were not, if they were readily interconvertible, the more general concept that arsenic in some way inhibited oxidation was entertained by a number of pharmacologists in the early twentieth century. Arthur Cushny, for example, in his Textbook of pharmacology and therapeutics, 4th ed. (London, 1906), p. 612, stated that many of the metabolic changes produced by arsenic could be explained on the assumption that it 'lessens the oxidation of the tissues and causes fatty degeneration of the cells of various organs.' Hans Meyer and R. Gottlieb claimed in Die Experimentelle Pharmakologie als Grundlage der Arzneibehandlung, 2nd ed. (Berlin, 1911), p. 366, that arsenic in small doses inhibits oxidation.

10. For Ehrlich's views on the mechanism of action of salvarsan, see Paul Ehrlich, 'Chemotherapeutics: scientific principles, methods and results,' Lancet, 1913, ii, 445–451, pp. 445–446. This same address, delivered before the Seventeenth International Congress of Medicine in 1913 and published in the Proceedings of the Congress (1914), was also reprinted (with slight amendments by the editor) under the title of 'Chemotherapy' in Collected papers (n. 9), III, 505–518.

more complicated synthetic medicaments the haptophore group, which anchors the molecule to the cell so that the drug can exert its action, is generally different from the toxophore group, which actually injures the cell. The two groups will often be residues attached, like side chains, to a chemical molecule. In the case of salvarsan, the *ortho*-aminophenol group (i.e., the hydroxyl and amino group next to one another on the benzene ring) primarily anchors the drug to the parasite. As a result of this anchorage the trivalent arsenic radical can combine chemically with the arsenoreceptor of the cell, thereby exerting its toxic action.

$$HCl.H_2N \qquad\qquad NH_2.HCl$$

$$HO \qquad As = As \qquad OH$$

Salvarsan
(Arsphenamine)

Thus in Ehrlich's view there were two receptors for the salvarsan molecule, the *ortho*-aminophenolreceptor and the arsenoreceptor. He compared the drug to a poison arrow, with the benzene nucleus of the molecule corresponding to the shaft, the *ortho*-aminophenol group (haptophore group) to the tip, and the trivalent arsenic radical (toxophore group) to the poison on the tip. This dualistic theory enabled him to explain how the substitution of sulfonic acid and amine groups in phenylarsonic acid (the mother substance of salvarsan), a substitution which did not affect the arsenic radical, might modify its activity several hundred times. The substitution changed the nature of the haptophore group, thereby altering the affinity of the drug for the chemoreceptors that attached it to the cell, thus making it easier or more difficult for the arsenic radical to exert its toxic effect.[11]

Ehrlich's discovery of salvarsan generated great enthusiasm for chemotherapy and his chemoreceptor hypothesis stimulated discussion and controversy concerning the nature of interactions between drug and cell. But Carl Voegtlin was not satisfied with the explanation of drug action offered by Ehrlich's theory. In 1924, in an article on drug resistance, Voegtlin and his co-workers argued that the experimental evidence was insufficient to

11. *Ibid.*, p. 447 (in *Collected papers* (n. 9), III, 510).

158

provide a firm foundation for Ehrlich's theory, and they agreed with the criticisms of the theory expressed by the British pharmacologist Henry Dale the year before.[12] They added that it was their realization of the inadequacy of Ehrlich's theory that led them to take up the study of chemotherapeutic action.[13]

Early in their studies, Voegtlin and his co-workers concluded that salvarsan, an arsenobenzene compound of the type $R' - As = As - R$, did not itself possess any trypanocidal activity, but that it must be converted to the active oxide derivative, $R - As = O$, before it could attack the parasites. Ehrlich had already shown that pentavalent arsenic compounds (such as atoxyl) of the type

$$
\begin{array}{c}
\text{OH} \\
| \\
R - As = O \\
| \\
\text{OH}
\end{array}
$$

had to be reduced to the trivalent form in order to act on the parasites, since pentavalent compounds did not exhibit any toxicity toward microorganisms in vitro. He argued that the toxicity of these pentavalent compounds for animals, and their in vivo activity against trypanosomal infections, was due to their conversion to the trivalent state in the body.[14] The trivalent arsenic atom, present in compounds such as salvarsan, was thus, in Ehrlich's view, the active toxic portion of the molecule.

Voegtlin's group compared the toxic effect of various arsenicals on trypanosomes in in vitro samples of the blood of infected rats and on rats. Their results confirmed the fact that trivalent arsenicals are much more toxic than the pentavalent compounds, and also indicated that compounds of the arsenoxide type $(R - As = O)$ began to produce their toxic effects within a few minutes after administration whereas trivalent arsenobenzene compounds, such as salvarsan, exhibited a significant latent period before signs of intoxication appeared. If, however, a solution of salvarsan was incubated for about three hours at $37°c$, the latent period was abolished and the solution possessed a much greater trypanocidal effect than a freshly prepared solution. Therefore, Voegtlin's group concluded that salvarsan

12. Carl Voegtlin, Helen Dyer, and D. Wright Miller, 'On drug resistance of trypanosomes with particular reference to arsenic,' *J. Pharmacol. exp. Ther.*, 1924, *23*, 55–86, pp. 57, 80. The review article referred to is Henry Dale, 'Chemotherapy,' *Physiol. Rev.*, 1923, *3*, 359–393.

13. Voegtlin, Dyer, and Miller (n. 12), p. 57. The authors further emphasized their dissatisfaction with Ehrlich's theory by repeating this point later in the article (p. 80).

14. Ehrlich (n. 9), III, 155–159.

must be oxidized in the air or in the animal body to arsenoxide $(R - As = O)$ before it can exert its toxic effects.[15] The active toxic group of arsenicals was not, as Ehrlich believed, the trivalent arsenic atom itself, but the trivalent arsenic oxide group.

Ehrlich had himself observed that the toxicity of a solution of salvarsan increased when it was kept in contact with air, and he assumed that this increased toxicity was due to oxidation of the drug to produce the much more toxic arsenoxide.[16] He did not recognize, however, that arsenoxide, rather than salvarsan, was the active therapeutic agent. The oxidation of salvarsan was seen as a problem leading to undesirable toxic reactions, and Ehrlich developed procedures to avoid oxidation during the various processes of manufacture of the drug.[17]

It is interesting to note that while Voegtlin and his colleagues correctly concluded that salvarsan must be converted in the animal body to arsenoxide before it can affect trypanosomes, they did not recommend the use of the latter substance as a chemotherapeutic agent. Their experimental studies suggested that the physical properties of the arsenicals, especially their solubility in water, played a significant role in determining their therapeutic efficacy through the regulation of their distribution in the body and of their rate and pathway of excretion. Pentavalent arsenicals, which exhibited a relatively low trypanocidal effect, were apparently excreted rapidly in the urine and hence much of the drug was removed from the body before it could be reduced to the active trivalent oxide. Arsenoxide, on the other hand, was excreted relatively slowly and was very toxic. They believed that the great advantage of salvarsan was that it was itself nontoxic and was retained in the tissues for a much longer time than the pentavalent arsenicals, although, probably because of differences of distribution in the body, it was excreted more rapidly than arsenoxide. The drug was deposited in the tissues where it was gradually oxidized into arsenoxide, thus providing a slow but steady supply of the active agent over a prolonged period of time, leading to the destruction of the parasites.

15. Carl Voegtlin, Helen Dyer, and C. S. Leonard, 'On the mechanism of action of arsenic upon protoplasm,' *Pub. Hlth. Rep.*, 1923, *38*, 1882–1912.

16. Paul Ehrlich and A. Bertheim, 'Über das salzsäure 3,3'-Diamino-4,4'-dioxy-arsenobenzol und seine nachsten Verwandten,' in *Collected papers* (n. 9), III, 405–411 (reprinted from *Ber. dt. chem. Ges.*, 1912); Paul Ehrlich, 'Über den jetzigen Stand der Salvarsantherapie mit besonderer Berücksichtigung der Nebenwirkung und deren Vermeidung,' in *Collected papers* (n. 9), III, 393–404, esp. p. 399 (reprinted from *Z. Chemother.*, 1912); and Paul Ehrlich, 'Chemotherapie,' in *Collected papers* (n. 9), III, 443–455, esp. pp. 448–449 (reprinted from *Soziale Kultur und Volkswohlfahrt während der ersten 25 Regierungsjahre Kaiser Wilhelms II*, Berlin, 1913).

17. For a discussion of this point, see Martha Marquardt, *Paul Ehrlich* (London, 1949), pp. 189–191.

The arsenoxide was eventually eliminated, probably by conversion to the rapidly excreted pentavalent state by further oxidation, thus preventing prolonged toxic action on the tissues after the parasites had been killed.[18]

Voegtlin thus felt that it was safer and more effective to administer salvarsan, because of its slow conversion to arsenoxide, so that the amount of arsenoxide in the tissues would not be too great at any given time. Not until 1934 did A. Tatum and G. Cooper show that arsenoxide was actually a safer drug than salvarsan because it was relatively more toxic for the parasite than for the host, so that smaller doses were required for treatment.[19]

Voegtlin and his co-workers amassed a significant amount of experimental evidence to support their hypothesis that the arsenoxide group was the active portion of the arsenical drugs. In itself, however, this evidence only indicated that Ehrlich had been incorrect in assuming that the trivalent arsenic atom itself was directly responsible for trypanocidal properties. It did not challenge the more general chemoreceptor hypothesis, because one might readily postulate the presence in the cell of arsenoreceptors which could combine only with an arsenoxide group rather than with an arsenic radical. But Voegtlin drew upon their experimental results to make a number of objections to Ehrlich's theory, which he felt was 'rather speculative' and 'not well supported by experimental evidence,'[20] and to offer alternative explanations for the observed phenomena.

Voegtlin's group, for example, criticized Ehrlich for adopting 'a purely chemical theory of drug action,' whereas their evidence indicated that 'purely physical factors' were of great importance in determining chemotherapeutic action. While they agreed with Ehrlich that the chemical constitution of the drug was a key factor in its activity, they believed that the importance of constitution was indirectly mediated through physical properties. Chemical structure was important insofar as it determined the retention and distribution of the drug in the body through physical properties

18. Carl Voegtlin and J. W. Thompson, 'Quantitative studies in chemotherapy. VI. Rate of excretion of arsenicals, a factor governing toxicity and parasiticidal action,' *J. Pharmacol. exp. Ther.*, 1922, *20*, 85–105; and Carl Voegtlin, Helen Dyer, and Dorothy Miller, 'Quantitative studies in chemotherapy. VII. Effects of ligation of the ureters or bile duct upon the toxicity and trypanocidal action of arsenicals,' *J. Pharmacol. exp. Ther.*, 1922, *20*, 129–151.

19. A. L. Tatum and G. A. Cooper, 'An experimental study of mapharsen (meta-amino parahydroxy phenyl arsine oxide) as an antisyphilitic agent,' *J. Pharmacol. exp. Ther.*, 1934, *50*, 198–215. Tatum and Cooper pointed out that the term 'arsenoxide' was frequently employed to designate that specific trivalent arsenic derivative of salvarsan obtained by controlled partial oxidation (as I have used it in this paper). They introduced the name 'mapharsen,' a shortening of the long chemical name given in the title of their paper, to distinguish this specific oxide from other oxides which might logically be included under the generic title 'arsenoxide.' *Ibid.*, p. 198.

20. Voegtlin, Dyer, and Miller (n. 18), p. 129.

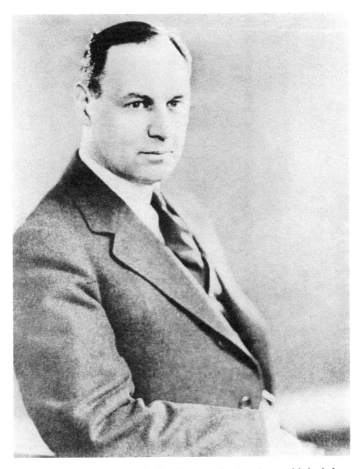

Carl Voegtlin (1879–1960), the pharmacologist who established that arsenical drugs react with sulfhydryl-containing substances in the cell. Photograph courtesy of the National Library of Medicine.

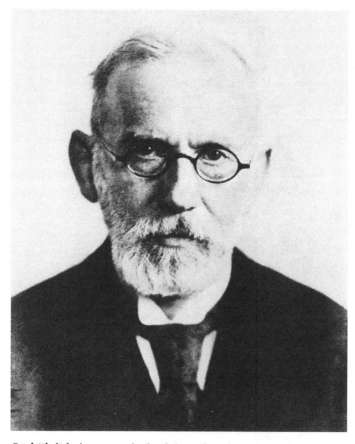

Paul Ehrlich (1854–1915), the father of modern chemotherapy, towards the end of his life. Photograph courtesy of the National Library
of Medicine.

such as solubility.[21] Their work had indicated, as previously mentioned, that the rate of excretion of arsenicals had a potent influence on their toxicity and parasiticidal influence.

To Ehrlich the structure of the molecule was important because, in order for the arsenic residue to exert its toxic effect, the drug had to possess a specific haptophore group capable of combining with a chemoreceptor of the cell. In salvarsan and related compounds, the haptophore group was the *ortho*-aminophenol group. Voegtlin and his colleagues showed, however, that in some cases the nature of substituent groups might be modified significantly without altering the trypanocidal activity of the compound. For example, the trypanocidal activity of the compound C_6H_5AsO was not altered at all by the addition of an amino group or an amino and a hydroxyl group as substituents on the benzene ring. They thought that such observations were evidence against Ehrlich's hypothesis in which the substituent groups were thought to be involved in the attachment of the drug to the cell through the chemoreceptors.[22] Where changes in the chemical structure did produce an alteration of therapeutic activity, the Voegtlin group explained the modification of activity, as previously noted, on the basis of the changes in physical properties which accompanied the structural modifications.

Voegtlin's emphasis on the importance of physical factors in determining the activity of drugs harmonized with the views of many of his contemporaries. The rise of physical chemistry as a distinct discipline at the end of the nineteenth century had eventually led to a greater interest in the influence of physical factors, such as solubility, upon drug action. In the first quarter of the twentieth century, many pharmacologists leaned toward the view that drugs often induce their effects through their physical properties, by altering the surface tension, electrolytic balance, osmotic pressure, etc. of cells, rather than through the formation of chemical bonds with protoplasmic constituents. Supporters of the physical view generally argued that chemical structure was important largely insofar as it determined physical properties, and opposed the Ehrlich-Langley receptor hypothesis as a general theory of drug action. The controversy in pharmacology was a part of a broader discussion in various biological sciences (e.g., biochemistry, immunology) concerning physicochemical, especially colloidal chemical, as

---

21. *Ibid.*, pp. 129–130; and Voegtlin and Thompson (n. 18), pp. 99–100.
22. Carl Voegtlin and Homer Smith, 'Quantitative studies in chemotherapy. IV. The relative therapeutic value of arsphenamine and neoarsphenamine of different manufacture,' *J. Pharmacol. exp. Ther.*, 1921, *16*, 449–461, see esp. p. 460.

162

opposed to organic chemical approaches. Robert Kohler has argued that the 1920s was the heyday of the 'colloidal school' in biochemistry, and no doubt Voegtlin was influenced by such currents of thought, although his later view of the mechanism of action of arsenicals explained the toxic action of these compounds, if not their distribution, on the basis of a specific chemical reaction.[23]

Voegtlin also challenged Ehrlich's assumption that a drug, in order to be of therapeutic value, must show very little or no affinity for the host tissues.[24] The research of Voegtlin's group had indicated that a sufficiently prolonged retention of the drug by the host tissues appeared to be an essential requirement for the chemotherapeutic action of arsenicals. Arsenicals, such as the pentavalent compounds, which were too quickly eliminated from the host had relatively little therapeutic value. Instead of accounting for the greater toxicity of salvarsan to parasites than to the host tissues by its greater affinity for trypanosome cells than for host cells, as Ehrlich had done, Voegtlin suggested that animal tissues might be capable of detoxifying arsenoxide by oxidizing it to the nontoxic pentavalent compound, whereas trypanosomes either did not possess this ability or possessed it only to a slight degree.[25]

Another piece of evidence advanced against the chemoreceptor theory was the observation that half of the minimum effective dose of antimony lactate and half of the minimum effective dose of arsenoxide when administered together proved therapeutically effective, although neither was effective alone. The fact that antimony and arsenic were trypanocidally complementary, Voegtlin argued, contradicted Ehrlich's hypothesis of chemoreceptor specificity.[26] Voegtlin was obviously making the assumption that both drugs had to act on the same receptor in order for their toxic effects to be additive. Ehrlich, however, would have disagreed with this assumption as he had observed that drugs such as parafuchsin and salvarsan, which he felt sure attacked different chemoreceptors—on the basis of evidence derived from the specificity of drug resistance—acted addi-

23. For a discussion of the controversy over physical versus chemical theories of drug action in the first quarter of the twentieth century, see John Parascandola, 'The controversy over structure-activity relationships in the early twentieth century,' *Pharmacy in History*, 1974, *16*, 54–63. For discussions of the similar controversies in biochemistry and immunology, see Robert Kohler, 'The history of biochemistry: a survey,' *J. Hist. Biol.*, 1975, *8*, 275–318, pp. 288–294, 306–308; Mazumdar (n. 7); and Joseph Fruton, 'The emergence of biochemistry,' *Science*, 1976, *192*, 327–334.

24. Voegtlin, Dyer, and Miller (n. 18), p. 148.

25. *Ibid.*, pp. 149–150.

26. Carl Voegtlin and Homer Smith, 'Quantitative studies in chemotherapy. II. The trypanocidal effect of arsenic compounds,' *J. Pharmacol. exp. Ther.*, 1920, *15*, 475–493, p. 492.

tively when given in combination. In fact, Ehrlich argued that the two drugs may even potentiate each other so that their combined effect was more than a summation of the individual actions.[27] One might assume, as Ehrlich apparently did, that the poisoning of x number of arsenic receptors and x number of parafuchsin receptors in a trypanosome cell produced a toxic effect that was equal to or even greater than that produced by the poisoning of $2x$ arsenic receptors.

On the other hand, evidence had already accumulated in Ehrlich's own laboratory by 1908 that antimony and arsenic probably did react with the same receptor, as Voegtlin was later to argue. Ehrlich and his co-workers had produced a trypanosome strain that was resistant to tartar emetic (an antimony compound) by exposing it to arsenious acid. Ehrlich pointed out, however, that arsenic and antimony were very closely related chemically.[28] He thus saw no need to abandon the idea of chemoreceptor specificity. In fact, he held firm to the idea of receptor specificity even in the face of more serious problems. Ehrlich and his associates produced a strain of trypanosomes resistant to *ortho*-quinoid dyes, organic chemicals which contain no metallic element, and found that this strain had also simultaneously acquired resistance to arsenicals. These experiments forced him to conclude that the arsenoreceptor also has the ability to combine with the purely organic *ortho*-quinones. Ehrlich's attempt to salvage the concept of highly specific chemoreceptors was attacked by the British pharmacologist Henry Dale in his 1923 review article on chemotherapy. To state that the chemoreceptor for the chemically unrelated arsenicals and *ortho*-quinoid dyes is identical, argued Dale, 'is to offer no explanation for a wholly mysterious phenomenon; it is merely to state the fact of reciprocal action in producing resistance in other words.'[29]

In their early studies, Voegtlin and his colleagues did not suggest a biochemical mechanism by which the arsenicals poisoned the cell. They had shown that arsenicals such as salvarsan were oxidized in the host tissues to arsenoxide compounds, which were the active therapeutic agents, and that physical properties, such as solubility, played a role in determining chemo-

27. Ehrlich (n. 10), p. 450 (in *Collected papers* [n. 9], III, 514–515).

28. Paul Ehrlich, 'On partial functions of the cell,' in *Collected papers* (n. 9), III, 183–194, pp. 192–193. This publication was Ehrlich's Nobel Prize Lecture, delivered in Stockholm on 11 December 1908 and originally published in *Les Prix Nobel* (Stockholm, 1909).

29. For Ehrlich's discussion of the development of simultaneous resistance to *ortho*-quinoid dyes and arsenicals, see Paul Ehrlich, 'Über die neuesten Ergebnisse auf dem Gebiete der Trypanosomenforschung,' in *Collected papers* (n. 9), III, 195–212, esp. pp. 206–207 (reprinted from *Verh. dt. tropenmed. Ges.*, 1909). For Dale's criticism, see Dale (n. 12), p. 381.

164

therapeutic activity through their influence on the retention and distribution of the drug in the body. They had challenged Ehrlich's chemoreceptor hypothesis, but had not yet developed a specific alternative mechanism to explain the toxic action of arsenic on the cell.

Not much was known at the time about the specific chemical interactions between drugs and the living cell. There had been some speculation about the possible nature of the chemical groups in the cell involved in binding drugs, such as Oscar Loew's hypothesis[30] in 1893 that the aldehyde or amino groups in protoplasm were important in this respect or Ehrlich's suggestion that a hydroxyl or sulfhydryl group was responsible for fixing arsenic. But carbon monoxide was a rare example of a drug or poison whose mode of action was understood in terms of a biochemical mechanism, in this case, the displacement of oxygen from its combination with hemoglobin.[31] A major problem was that relatively little was known about the biochemistry of the cell in the early part of the century. Of attempts to elucidate the changes produced in the cell by chemical substances, Voegtlin and his co-workers wrote in 1923: 'The investigator who has the temerity to attack such problems is naturally confronted by great difficulties on account of the heterogeneous system which constitutes protoplasm, and for this reason very little or no information is available concerning the cellular action of most chemicals.'[32]

In the 1920s rapid advances in biochemistry began to open up the possibility of elucidating the biochemical mechanisms involved in the action of drugs. Biochemists such as F. Gowland Hopkins, Otto Warburg, and Otto Meyerhof began to provide information about the enzyme systems and metabolic reactions of the cell, information that was essential to an understanding of the reaction between drugs and cellular constituents.[33] The iso-

30. For Loew's views, see Oscar Loew, *Ein natürliches System der Giftwirkungen* (Munich, 1893).

31. The mode of action of carbon monoxide was elucidated by Claude Bernard in 1856. See J. M. D. Olmsted and E. H. Olmsted, *Claude Bernard and the experimental method in medicine* (New York, 1952), p. 96; and Claude Bernard, *An introduction to the study of experimental medicine*, trans. H. C. Greene (New York, 1927), pp. 159–162. John Edsall has pointed out, however, that there was still a controversy in the early twentieth century over whether the reaction between oxygen and hemoglobin involved a nonspecific adsorption or a specific chemical combination. See John Edsall, 'Blood and hemoglobin: the evolution of knowledge of functional adaptation in a biochemical system. Part I: the adaptation of chemical structure to function in hemoglobin,' *J. Hist. Biol.*, 1972, 5, 205–257, pp. 229–235.

32. Voegtlin, Dyer, and Leonard (n. 15), p. 1882.

33. For information on relevant biochemical developments in this period see Joseph Fruton, *Molecules and life: historical essays on the interplay of chemistry and biology* (New York, 1972); and Marcel Florkin, *A history of biochemistry, parts I and II* (Amsterdam, 1972); and idem, *A history of biochemistry, part III* (Amsterdam, 1975). See also Kohler (n. 23) for references to Robert Kohler's recent articles on the history of biochemistry and to other useful works on the subject.

lation and study of glutathione by Frederick Gowland Hopkins in the early 1920s provided the Voegtlin group with the clue that they needed to postulate a specific mechanism of action for arsenicals, a mechanism that preserved at least certain features of Ehrlich's theory. In 1921 Hopkins isolated from yeast cells and animal tissues a compound of cysteine and glutamic acid which he named glutathione. The reduced form of the compound, containing a sulfhydryl (–SH) group, was readily oxidized so that two molecules of glutathione were joined by an –S–S– bridge, and the oxidized form could also be converted relatively easily back to the reduced form. The substance thus acted as a hydrogen acceptor or as an oxygen acceptor (hydrogen donor) and Hopkins suggested that it might play a role in the dynamics of the cell. In the following year, he and Malcolm Dixon offered further evidence that glutathione was involved in the oxidation–reduction system of the cell.[34]

Arsenious oxides (including arsenoxide) were known to combine readily with hydrogen sulfide or with sulfhydryl compounds to give the following reaction:

$$R - As = O + 2R'SH \rightarrow R - As{\overset{\displaystyle R'}{\underset{\displaystyle R'}{\big\langle}}} + H_2O$$

Since glutathione, on the basis of the evidence provided by Hopkins, seemed to play an important role in the oxidative and reductive processes of the cell, it seemed reasonable to Voegtlin to assume that arsenoxide might exert its toxic effect by combining with the sulfhydryl group of this compound (or some closely related sulfhydryl compound) according to the above reaction. If this hypothesis were correct, he reasoned, then it should be possible to overcome the toxic effects of arsenic, at least temporarily, by supplying the cell with an extra amount of glutathione.[35] It is not clear whether or not Voegtlin knew of Ehrlich's suggestion that a hydroxyl or sulfhydryl group might be the arsenoreceptor, but there is little doubt that it was Hopkins's work on glutathione which attracted Voegtlin's attention to sulfhydryl compounds.

Experiments carried out in the Hygienic Laboratory and published in 1923 revealed that glutathione in the reduced form and certain other sulfhydryl compounds (such as glycylcysteine and thioglycollic acid) did coun-

34. F. G. Hopkins, 'On an autoxidisable constituent of the cell,' *Biochem. J.*, 1921, *15*, 286–305; and F. G. Hopkins and M. Dixon, 'On glutathione. II. A thermostable oxidation–reduction system,' *J. biol. Chem.*, 1922, *54*, 527–563.

35. Voegtlin, Dyer, and Leonard (n. 15), pp. 1885–1886.

teract the toxic effect produced by arsenoxide on trypanosomes in rat blood (in vitro and in vivo) and on rats. The corresponding disulfide compounds (R′ – S – S – R) and various amino acids and other substances without sulfhydryl groups were, on the other hand, without effect. Voegtlin concluded, therefore, that arsenoxide most likely exerted its effect by reacting chemically with the sulfhydryl group of glutathione and perhaps also with that of other sulfhydryl compounds that might occur in protoplasm. The death of the cell by arsenic poisoning was probably due to an interference with the oxidative processes governed by glutathione.[36] As previously mentioned, the idea that arsenic compounds might somehow inhibit oxidation had already been suggested.

The work of Voegtlin and his co-workers in one sense supported Ehrlich's view that arsenicals acted by combining chemically with a cellular constituent, and thereby interfering with the metabolism of the cell. It provided evidence for the view that many drugs exert their action by virtue of their chemical properties rather than their physical properties. Perhaps their suggested mechanism of action for these drugs was closer to the chemoreceptor hypothesis than they had anticipated at the beginning of their chemotherapeutic researches. Voegtlin and his associates stated in a 1925 paper that their studies provided strong experimental evidence for 'a somewhat modified conception of Ehrlich's chemoreceptor theory,' and referred to the sulfhydryl group of glutathione as the 'arseno-receptor' of the cell.[37] They qualified the latter term in the title of their paper, however, by referring to the 'so-called arsenic receptor,' and in another paper Voegtlin noted that the sulfhydryl group could only be considered the arsenic receptor with certain obvious reservations.[38] Since Voegtlin's theory differed significantly from Ehrlich's in many respects, it would be misleading to consider the work of his group as a confirmation of Ehrlich's chemoreceptor hypothesis.

In 1924 Voegtlin and his colleagues referred to Ehrlich's theory as being 'far too simple to explain the intricate mechanism of chemotherapeutic action and the cause of drug resistance.'[39] They criticized his interpretation of drug resistance, which had provided the original evidence for his chemoreceptor theory. Ehrlich had explained the development of resistance

---

36. *Ibid.*, pp. 1905–1910.

37. Carl Voegtlin, Helen Dyer, and C. S. Leonard, 'On the specificity of the so-called arsenic receptor in the higher animals,' *J. Pharmacol. exp. Ther.*, 1925, *25*, 297–307, p. 305.

38. *Ibid.*, p. 297; and Carl Voegtlin, 'Arsphenamine and related arsenicals,' *Physiol. Rev.*, 1925, *5*, 63–94, p. 89.

39. Voegtlin, Dyer, and Miller (n. 12), p. 80.

to arsenicals in a trypanosome strain by postulating that the chemoreceptors of the resistant strain had somehow developed a reduced affinity for arsenic. Voegtlin's group offered the alternative suggestion that the drug resistant trypanosomes perhaps contained a sufficient excess of sulfhydryl compounds above the physiological requirements, and hence were more likely to survive treatment with arsenicals than the ordinary trypanosomes. Prolonged exposure to arsenic might cause trypanosome cells to respond by producing more sulfhydryl compounds or converting more of their oxidized sulfur compounds to the reduced sulfhydryl form.[40]

Voegtlin and his colleagues also criticized Ehrlich's theory for its failure to recognize the active role of the host cells in producing the active therapeutic agent (arsenoxide), the necessity that the drug possess considerable 'organotropic' properties (i.e., be retained in the host for a considerable period of time), and the importance of physicochemical properties such as solubility in determining the chemotherapeutic action of the drug.[41] It was also in this same paper that Voegtlin's group acknowledged their agreement with Henry Dale's criticism of the chemoreceptor theory and indicated that their dissatisfaction with the theory had stimulated their work in this area.

In 1925 Voegtlin remained critical of Ehrlich's theory, although complimenting him for his attempts to provide a theoretical foundation for chemotherapy. After summarizing Ehrlich's views, Voegtlin noted that Ehrlich's theory was no longer tenable in its original form. Ehrlich's view of the cell as a giant protoplasmic molecule (biogen) with chemical side chains—a view that Langley also tended to support—was, Voegtlin argued, no longer acceptable. In 1925, said Voegtlin, the cell was conceived of as 'a complex physicochemical system made up of a great variety of chemical substances, undergoing constant change but being adjusted to a certain (dynamic) equilibrium with regard to the various components.'[42] Ehrlich's theory had already been criticized on these grounds by others because the biogen concept had fallen into disrepute early in the twentieth century.[43] Voegtlin thus rejected one of the central features of Ehrlich's

40. *Ibid.*, pp. 83–84. Voegtlin and his co-workers also suggested that the ability of *ortho*-quinoid dyes to produce arsenic resistance in trypanosomes might be due to the reversible oxidation-reduction properties of these compounds allowing them to affect the sulfhydryl compounds of protoplasm in the same manner that arsenic does.

41. *Ibid.*, p. 80.

42. Voegtlin (n. 38), p. 89.

43. See, for example, William Bayliss, *Principles of general physiology* (London, 1915), pp. 17–20, 723–726; Carl Alsberg, 'Chemical structure and physiological action,' *J. Washington Acad. Sci.*, 1921, *11*, 321–341, pp. 322–323; and F. G. Hopkins, 'The dynamic side of biochemistry,' *Nature*, 1913, *92*, 213–223, pp. 220–221.

view of such physiological processes as biological oxidation, immunological reactions, and drug action, namely the side chain concept of cellular function. Arsenicals, in Voegtlin's opinion, did not attack side chains on a hypothetical protoplasmic molecule, but instead they attacked specific individual molecules within the cell such as glutathione. The sulfhydryl group of a glutathione molecule was not the 'arseno-receptor' as envisioned by Ehrlich, that is, a chemical group attached to a side chain of the cellular molecule.

Voegtlin also did not adopt Ehrlich's concept of haptophore and toxophore groups. While he identified the arsenic oxide radical as the active portion of the arsenoxide molecule, what one might call the toxophore group, he did not accept Ehrlich's view that certain substituent groups (haptophore groups) on the benzene nucleus of salvarsan are chemically bound to chemoreceptors, thus anchoring the drug in the cell. He tended to view the distribution of the drug in the body as determined by physicochemical properties such as solubility and degree of dissociation. Changing the substituent groups on the benzene nucleus probably altered the chemotherapeutic properties of aromatic arsenicals, Voegtlin believed, by modifying their physicochemical properties.[44]

Ehrlich had explained the fact that salvarsan was more toxic for the parasites than for the host by assuming that the arsenic receptors of trypanosomes possessed a greater affinity for the drug than did the arsenic receptors of mammalian tissues. In Voegtlin's view, however, the arsenic receptor was clearly the same (the sulfhydryl group of glutathione) in trypanosomes and mammals, so it was difficult to conceive of a difference in affinity for the drug. Voegtlin tentatively suggested that the difference in toxicity might be due to a greater oxidation potential of the host's tissues for arsenoxide, permitting a ready conversion of arsenoxide into the nontoxic and easily excreted pentavalent arsenic compound and thereby resulting in a better protection for the host.[45]

Voegtlin stated that the experimental evidence obtained in his laboratory showed that there was 'a kernel of truth in Ehrlich's theory.'[46] But Voegtlin's conception of cellular processes, including the mechanism of

44. Voegtlin reaffirmed his earlier views on the subject, already mentioned in this paper, in Voegtlin (n. 38), pp. 90–91.

45. *Ibid.*, p. 90. Voegtlin had earlier suggested that the difference in toxicity might be based on the different amounts of SH compounds in the cells of trypanosomes and rats, with other factors, such as the permeability of the cells to the arsenic, also probably playing a role. See Voegtlin, Dyer, and Leonard (n. 15), p. 1909.

46. Voegtlin (n. 38), p. 89.

action of salvarsan, was quite different from that of Ehrlich. It was based upon the biochemical picture, as developed by F. G. Hopkins and others, of the cell as a complex, heterogeneous physicochemical system in dynamic equilibrium, its reactions being carried out by a host of enzymes, coenzymes, and related substances. Glutathione appeared to be one of the important constituents of the cell, playing a significant role in biological oxidations and reductions.

While glutathione was originally the major focus of Voegtlin's attention, he did admit the possibility that other sulfhydryl compounds in the cell might also be involved in reactions with arsenicals. In 1930 Carl Voegtlin and Sanford Rosenthal indicated their tentative belief that arsenic might also react with 'the so-called fixed SH groups of tissue proteins.' This hypothesis might explain, they noted, why subsequent, as opposed to prior or simultaneous, treatment of arsenic-poisoned trypanosomes and rats with reduced glutathione did not remove the toxic effect of the arsenic (i.e., glutathione was more of a preventive than a cure for arsenic poisoning). It was conceivable that the hypothetical compound of arsenic with the sulfhydryl group of a protein could not be dissociated by treatment with glutathione, presumably because the arsenic-protein compound was exceptionally stable.[47] Two years later Sanford Rosenthal, working in Voegtlin's laboratory, was able to demonstrate that arsenoxide did combine chemically with proteins containing sulfhydryl groups.[48]

Further work by other investigators led to the conclusion that the toxic effects of arsenicals were due to their ability to combine with the sulfhydryl groups of certain enzymes. Even before Voegtlin's group had carried out their studies with sulfhydryl compounds, some evidence had appeared in the literature to suggest that arsenicals might inhibit the action of certain enzymes.[49] Among the chemical warfare agents studied by Rudolf Peters under the direction of Joseph Barcroft during the First World War were arsenical vesicants such as Lewisite, and Peters continued to investigate these compounds at Oxford during the 1920s. Peters and his colleague Ernest Walker concluded that the toxicity of Lewisite and of mustard gas involved a combination with sulfhydryl groups of cellular constituents.

---

47. Sanford Rosenthal and Carl Voegtlin, 'Biological and chemical studies of the relationship between arsenic and crystalline glutathione,' *J. Pharmacol. exp. Ther.*, 1930, *39*, 347–367, p. 365.

48. Sanford Rosenthal, 'Action of arsenic upon the fixed sulphhydryl groups of proteins,' *Pub. Hlth. Rep.*, 1932, *47*, 241–256.

49. In 1920, for example, Rona and Bach studied the inhibition of the action of the enzyme serum lipase by atoxyl. See P. Rona and E. Bach, 'Beitrage zum Studium der Giftwirkung. Über die Wirkung des Atoxyls auf Serumlipase,' *Biochem. Z.*, 1920, *111*, 166–188.

170

At about the same time, Voegtlin had reached a similar conclusion for the therapeutic arsenicals. In the early part of the Second World War, the study of vesicants was again taken up in Peters's laboratory. Peters and his co-workers found that the pyruvate-oxidase enzyme system was particularly sensitive to Lewisite and arsenite, and they obtained evidence of the involvement of a sulfhydryl group. These studies led to the development of British Anti-Lewisite (BAL), a compound containing two sulfhydryl groups, as an antidote for arsenical vesicants.[50] Work in other laboratories in the 1930s and 1940s further established the inhibiting effect of arsenicals on a number of enzyme systems.[51]

While Ehrlich had made the speculative suggestion that arsenic might combine with a hydroxyl group or a sulfhydryl group (attached to a chemical side chain) in the cell, Voegtlin and his co-workers clearly identified the arsenic receptor as a sulfhydryl group and provided substantial evidence that arsenic (in the form of the trivalent oxide) combined chemically with the sulfhydryl group. Their work was part of the growing effort in the 1920s and 1930s to understand the biochemical reactions that took place in the cell and the effects of drugs and poisons on such reactions.

Ehrlich's chemoreceptor hypothesis, coupled with the practical therapeutic success of salvarsan, undoubtedly helped to stimulate research on the intimate mechanisms by which drugs act. The receptor theory advanced by Ehrlich and Langley provided a general theoretical framework within which one could view the action of many drugs, a framework that basically still exists today although in a greatly modified form. This original theory, however, was based on a concept of the cell that was already losing favor amongst biological scientists when the theory was being developed. In 1924 Henry Dale argued that Ehrlich's chemoreceptors could no longer satisfy pharmacologists, but regretted that there was nothing equally definite to replace them. He pointed to Voegtlin's interpretation of the action of arsenoxide as a hopeful sign of contact between biochemistry and pharmacology that showed promise for the future.[52] Two decades later, in

50. On the work in Peters's laboratory, see Ernest Walker, 'Chemical constitution and toxicity,' *Biochem. J.*, 1928, *22*, 292–305; Rudolph Peters, 'Development and theoretical significance of British Anti-Lewisite (BAL),' *Brit. med. Bull.*, 1948, *5*, 313–319; idem, *Biochemical lesions and lethal synthesis* (Oxford, 1963), pp. 40–46; L. A. Stocken and R. H. S. Thompson, 'Reactions of British Anti-Lewisite with arsenic and other metals in living systems,' *Physiol. Rev.*, 1949, *29*, 168–194; and R. H. S. Thompson, 'The reactions of arsenicals in living tissues,' *Biochem. Soc. Sym.*, 1948, *2*, 28–38.

51. For further information on these later developments, see George Doak and Harry Eagle, 'The biological activity of arsenobenzenes in relation to their structure,' *Pharmacol. Rev.*, 1951, *3*, 107–143; and Albert, *Selective toxicity* (n. 1), pp. 392–397.

52. Henry Dale, 'Progress and prospects in chemotherapy,' *Science*, 1924, *60*, 185–191, pp. 190–191.

1943, Dale, heartened by such developments as the explanation of the mechanism of action of arsenicals and of sulfanilamide in biochemical terms,[53] wrote: 'But now, in place of vaguely conceived chemoreceptors, labels for observed but unexplained affinities, it begins to be possible to think in terms of interference with activities of vital enzyme systems, or supplanting essential substrate molecules on the specific surfaces of enzymes.'[54]

Pharmacologists and biochemists still have not elucidated the biochemical mechanism of action of most drugs. The receptors for many drugs appear to be complex macromolecular structures whose nature is only beginning to be understood. In most cases, the reaction between the drug and the cell would appear to be more complex than that between an arsenic group and a sulfhydryl group. But significant progress has been made along these lines in the past half-century, and the work of Carl Voegtlin and his colleagues on arsenicals represents one of the pioneering efforts in the development of biochemical pharmacology.

53. On sulfanilamide see D. D. Woods, 'The relation of *p*-aminobenzoic acid to the mechanism of action of sulfanilamide,' *Brit. J. exp. Path.*, 1940, *21*, 74–90; and Paul Fildes, 'A rational approach to chemotherapy,' *Lancet*, 1940, *i*, 955–957.

54. Henry Dale, 'Modes of drug action: a general discussion,' *Trans. Faraday Soc.*, 1943, *39*, 319–322, p. 321.

VII

The Theoretical Basis
of Paul Ehrlich's Chemotherapy

N spite of all that has been written about Paul Ehrlich (1854–1915), especially with respect to his work in chemotherapy, an understanding of his ideas and contributions is far from satisfactory.[1] My aim in this paper is to analyze in detail one important aspect of Ehrlich's thought, the theoretical basis of his chemotherapy.

Paul Ehrlich is generally acknowledged to be the founder of modern chemotherapy. What did Ehrlich mean by the term *chemotherapy*, which was introduced into medicine through his work?[2] Chemical substances

1. The bibliography of secondary sources in the article on Paul Ehrlich by Claude Dolman in the *Dictionary of scientific biography*, which makes no claim to completeness, contains some sixty-five references. Ehrlich's contributions have received a significant amount of attention in the popular literature (and even in a Hollywood motion picture), but such accounts are generally superficial and often inaccurate. Even more serious studies of Ehrlich, however, have failed to provide an in-depth historical analysis of the development of his scientific work. The article by Dolman is useful, but provides only a relatively brief overview of Ehrlich's life and work. The few existing book-length biographies are undocumented and inadequate. The biography by his secretary, Martha Marquardt, *Paul Ehrlich* (London, 1949), gives a vivid picture of Ehrlich's personality, but treats his scientific work in a disjointed and superficial manner. Professor James Hirsch of the Rockefeller University is studying the Ehrlich manuscript materials with the goal of providing a biographical study emphasizing Ehrlich's scientific contributions.

2. Ehrlich is generally credited with having coined the term *chemotherapy*. See H. A. Skinner, *The origin of medical terms*, 2nd ed. (Baltimore, 1961), p. 103; and Henry Wain, *The story behind the word: some interesting origins of medical terms* (Springfield, Ill., 1958), p. 65. The term certainly is associated with Ehrlich's name in the literature of the early twentieth century, and there can be little doubt that it entered the medical vocabulary through his work, but it is possible that someone may have used the word earlier. Ehrlich's earliest use of the word *chemotherapy* (*Chemotherapie*), as far as I know, was in his 'Address delivered at the dedication of the Georg-Speyer Haus' on 6 September 1906, but not published until 1960 in *The collected papers of Paul Ehrlich*, ed. F. Himmelweit, 3 vols. (London, 1956–60), III, 53–63. His earliest published use of the term appears to have been in 1907 in his 'Chemotherapeutische Trypanosomen-Studien,' *ibid.*, pp. 81–105 (*Berl. klin. Wschr.*, 1907, 44, 233–236, 280–282, 310–314, 341–344).

A preliminary version of this paper was delivered at a symposium on the history of chemotherapy at the American Chemical Society meeting in Chicago on 29 August 1977. The research was supported by grants from the National Science Foundation (GS-41462) and the University of Wisconsin Graduate School. I am grateful to Mr. Gunther Schwerin and to the Wellcome Institute for the History of Medicine, London, for permission to use the Ehrlich manuscript materials housed in the Wellcome Institute at the time of my research. The Ehrlich manuscripts are currently on loan to the Rockefeller University, New York.

had been used in therapeutics long before Ehrlich's time. Sometimes Ehrlich appears to have used the term in a general sense to refer simply to the use of chemicals in therapy, as when he stated that '. . . from the very origin of the art of healing, chemotherapy has been in existence, since almost all of the medicaments that we employ are chemical.'[3] Usually, however, he had a much more specific and limited use in mind, and he often qualified the term with the adjectives *specific* or *experimental*. Pharmacologist Hans Herken has recently argued: 'The term "chemotherapy" introduced by Paul Ehrlich is incomplete without the adjective "specifica" which was also added by him.'[4] Chemotherapy in this sense meant to Ehrlich the use of chemical substances, especially those produced synthetically, to destroy pathogenic microorganisms within the body. Ehrlich expressed the task of his institute of chemotherapy at the Georg-Speyer-Haus in Frankfort as follows:

Here we shall . . . be concerned with the problem of curing organisms infected by certain parasites in such a way that the parasites are exterminated within the living organism, so that the organism is disinfected . . . by the use of substances which have had their origin in the chemist's retort. Thus, the task of the new institute will be a *specific chemotherapy of infectious diseases*.[5]

Ehrlich generally used the term *chemotherapy* in this sense. Chemotherapy, as he saw it, was a part of the broader field of experimental therapeutics, a field he differentiated clearly from pharmacology. The science of pharmacology had emerged as a separate discipline in the nineteenth century under the guidance of such men as Rudolf Buchheim and especially Oswald Schmiedeberg, a contemporary of Ehrlich's and the most prominent and influential pharmacologist of his time. While admitting that pharmacology had contributed significantly to our knowledge of physiology and had led to the introduction of a number of drugs that were valuable for symptomatic treatment (analgesics, antipyretics,

3. Paul Ehrlich, 'Chemotherapy,' *Collected papers* (n. 2), III, 505–518, p. 505 (International medical congress, 17th, London, 1913, *Proceedings* [London, 1914], pp. 94–111). Ehrlich went on to add that 'on the other hand, experimental chemotherapy could only develop in a fruitful manner in modern times.'

4. Hans Herkin, *Paul Ehrlich: pioneer of chemotherapy* (Berlin, n.d.), p. 8. Address delivered at the Weizmann Institute of Science, Rehovat, Israel, 25 March 1976.

5. Ehrlich, 'Address' (n. 2), p. 60. For similar expressions of this definition of specific or experimental chemotherapy see Ehrlich, 'Chemotherapeutische' (n. 2), p. 81; and Paul Ehrlich and R. Gonder, 'Experimentelle Chemotherapie,' in S. von Prowazek, ed., *Handbuch der pathogenen Protozoen*, 3 vols. (Leipzig 1912–31) II, 752–780 (*Collected papers* [n. 2], III, 559–582, p. 559). For a discussion of the problem of agreeing upon a single definition of chemotherapy since Ehrlich's time, see Glenn Sonnedecker, 'The concept of chemotherapy,' *Am. J. pharm. Ed.*, 1962, *26*, 1–3.

hypnotics, etc.), Ehrlich argued that the discipline had contributed little to the discovery of 'specific (that is, truly curative) drugs.' Pharmacology had concentrated on the effects of drugs upon healthy animals, and therefore could not solve the problem of curing disease.[6]

Experimental therapeutics, Ehrlich explained, involved producing diseases experimentally in animals and then studying the action of drugs against these diseases. The infectious diseases were the easiest to reproduce in laboratory animals, and experimental therapeutics had already achieved significant progress in the development of immunological agents to control or treat certain of these diseases.[7] Ehrlich divided experimental therapeutics into three categories: organotherapy (the use of organ extracts, or what we would call hormones), bacteriotherapy (the use of immunological agents such as antitoxins), and experimental chemotherapy, the newest and perhaps the most difficult of these fields.[8]

Ehrlich's chemotherapy was based upon the concept of selective affinity. In order for a drug to exert its effect on a pathogenic microorganism, or on any cell for that matter, it must first be fixed within the cell. In an address on chemotherapy, Ehrlich stated:

The whole field is governed by a simple, I might even say natural, principle. If the law is true in chemistry that *corpora non agunt nisi liquida*, then for chemotherapy the principle is true that *corpora non agunt nisi fixata*. When applied to the special case in point, this means that parasites are killed only by those substances for which they have a certain affinity, by virtue of which these are fixed by the parasites. I call such substances *parasitotropic*.[9]

The problem is, however, that chemicals that have an affinity for the cells of parasites are likely also to have an affinity for human cells, or in Ehrlich's terminology to be *organotropic*. Therefore one must search for therapeutic agents that are selective and that possess a relatively high affinity, and toxicity, for the parasite in relation to the animal body, so that it is possible to kill the parasites without serious damage to the body.[10] The most ideal agents in this sense are the immunological products of the body because these antitoxins and antibodies exert an extremely specific action on the parasites evoking their production, and having no effect

6. Paul Ehrlich, 'Über der jetzigen Stand der Chemotherapie,' *Collected papers* (n. 2), III, 150–170, pp. 150–151 (*Ber. dt. chem. Ges.*, 1909, 42, 17–47).

7. *Ibid.*, p. 151.

8. Letter from Paul Ehrlich to A. von Rosthorm, 18 January 1907, Paul Ehrlich copybooks, Rockefeller University, New York, Ser. v, No. XXI, pp. 138–140.

9. Ehrlich (n. 3), p. 507.

10. Ehrlich (n. 6), p. 153.

22

on the cells of the host. These immune substances are like 'magic bullets' which seek out and destroy the enemy without harming the body. But many infectious diseases are not amenable to treatment by serum therapy; hence we must turn to chemotherapy.

In general, Ehrlich noted, chemotherapy is a more complicated task than serum therapy because chemical agents, in contrast to antibodies, are likely to be harmful to the body. It was not easy to score direct hits as with the antibodies. We must learn, Ehrlich added, to aim in a chemical sense. Ehrlich thus recognized the difficulty of obtaining perfect chemotherapeutic drugs which attacked only the microorganism and not the host.[11] He did not claim that Salvarsan, the most important chemotherapeutic agent that he developed, was a 'magic bullet' for therapeutic purposes in the same sense that the antitoxins were. He did hold out the hope, however, that it might be possible someday to synthesize such an ideal chemical medicament,[12] and he probably thought that Salvarsan was closer to that ideal than it actually was.[13]

Ehrlich developed an interest in the selective action of drugs and chemicals while he was still a student. The idea that drugs have a selective action was not original to Ehrlich. The fact that drugs may exert their effects on specific organs had long been recognized empirically and expressed vaguely in the traditional designation of certain remedies as cordials, hepatics, etc.[14] In the late eighteenth and early nineteenth centuries, the belief that most drugs exerted their effects by acting directly on the nerves at the site of action came to dominate pharmacological thought. The theory of the action of drugs on nerves argued that selective action was more apparent than real. The theory supposed that the drug produced a generalized reaction in the body with each organ responding in its own peculiar manner. Some body responses, however, were more dominant than others, thus giving rise to an erroneous impression that the drug acted selectively only on certain organs.[15]

11. *Ibid.*, pp. 152–153; Paul Ehrlich, 'Über moderne Chemotherapie,' *Collected papers* (n. 2), III, 140–149, pp. 140–141 (*Verh. Kongr. dt. derm. Ges.*, 1908, *10*, 52–70).

12. Ehrlich (n. 3), p. 510.

13. See, for example, his overly optimistic statements about Salvarsan in 'Closing notes to the experimental chemotherapy of spirilloses,' *Collected papers* (n. 2), III, 282–309, especially pp. 308–309 (*Die experimentelle Chemotherapie der Spirillosen* [Berlin, 1910], pp. 114–164).

14. M. P. Earles, 'Early theories of the mode of action of drugs and poisons,' *Ann. Sci.*, 1961, *17*, 97–110, p. 98.

15. M. P. Earles, 'The action of medicines: problems of explanation in the eighteenth and early nineteenth centuries,' International Congress of the History of Medicine, 13th, London, 1972, *Proceedings*, 2 vols. (London, 1974), II, 1177–1181, pp. 1177–1178.

By 1850 the pharmacological studies of François Magendie, James Blake, and others in the first half of the nineteenth century had largely discredited the theory of action through the nerves. Most pharmacologists and physiologists had by mid-century come to accept the concept that drugs are absorbed into the bloodstream at the site of administration and must be transported by the blood to the specific organ or organs on which they act. The absorption theory emphasized the selective action of a drug at a specific site distant from the site of administration. Magendie, for example, was able to demonstrate that strychnine-containing arrow poisons acted specifically on the spinal cord.

The absorption theory raised the question of how drugs or poisons, present in the blood and in contact with all organs, might act only on one organ, leaving the others unaffected. One might attempt to offer a physicochemical explanation for this fact or one might fall back upon a vitalistic approach by assuming, as Anthony Todd Thomson did in the 1830s, that specific medicines possess 'peculiar energies' to excite an organ.[16]

The question of the selective action of drugs and poisons attracted Ehrlich's attention early in his career. Ehrlich recalled that while still a medical student in the early 1870s he read a work on lead poisoning by Emil Heubel which greatly impressed him.

In order to elucidate the nature of this poisoning, the author had estimated quantitatively the lead content of the liver, the kidney, and the heart and had discovered that there were remarkable differences in the amount of lead to be found in various organs. When he immersed organs of normal animals in dilute lead-solutions and subsequently subjected the organs to chemical analysis, he believed that he obtained exactly the same difference. This experiment seemed to me, at that time, a revelation. The possibility emerged that this technique might be used also to ascertain the site of action of poisons.[17]

That lead was to be found in certain organs, for example, the brain, was for Ehrlich only the starting point for an investigation. The brain was a complex structure made up of various tissues. Ehrlich wanted to know within which cells of the organ the poison was concentrated, but his attempts to determine the location of the poison with the aid of a microscope resulted in failure.

He became fascinated by the distribution of substances among the cells

16. *Ibid.*, pp. 1178–1179.
17. Ehrlich, 'Address' (n. 2), p. 54. The publication that Ehrlich referred to is undoubtedly Emil Huebel's *Pathogenese und Symptome der chronischen Bleivergiftung Experimentelle Untersuchungen* (Berlin, 1871).

of the body. The concept that drugs act only upon those organs that take them up was an old one, but Ehrlich felt that it had not been given sufficient emphasis in pharmacology and that it had remained only a general theoretical principle because the laws governing distribution were so little understood. He decided to investigate this *storage-axiom*, as he termed the principle.

Ehrlich began by studying the distribution of dyes in living tissues because only here could he easily determine the distribution of the substance by its color.[18] His interest in dyes may well have been aroused by his cousin Carl Weigert, a pioneer in the field of histological staining. The thesis that Ehrlich presented for his graduation in medicine at the University of Leipzig in 1878 dealt with the theory and practice of histological staining. It is of interest to us here because it clearly demonstrates Ehrlich's early concern with the question of selective affinity, in this case the affinity of particular dyes for certain types of tissues, and also his commitment to a chemical viewpoint. He rejected the idea that the process of staining involved only a physical adhesion of the dye to the tissue, but believed that the interaction was of a chemical nature (probably similar to that involved in the formation of so-called *double salts*, that is, the linking together of two apparently saturated compounds such as silver chloride and mercurous oxide). Ehrlich also noted in this dissertation that he believed there were colorless substances that had similar 'sticking' properties to those of dyes.[19]

Ehrlich's interest in dyes continued, and his *Habilitationschrift* for his appointment as *Privatdocent* in the University of Berlin in 1885 was an investigation of the ability of various tissues to reduce certain dyestuffs. This work is important in the present context largely because it concerns the first indication of his side-chain theory of cellular action, a concept that played a very significant role in his later thinking about immunology and chemotherapy. Ehrlich adopted Eduard Pflüger's view that protoplasm may be envisioned as a giant molecule consisting of a chemical nucleus of special structure which is responsible for the specific functions of a particular cell (for example, a liver cell or a kidney cell), with attached chemical side chains. These side chains are more involved in the vital processes common to all cells, such as cellular oxidation. Some side chains, Ehrlich believed, possess the ability to fix oxygen or, more accurately, to give up hydrogen to oxygen and thus become oxidizing agents themselves. Other

18. Ehrlich, 'Address' (n. 2), pp. 54–55.
19. Paul Ehrlich, 'Contributions to the theory and practice of histological staining,' *Collected papers* (n. 2), I, 65–98, pp. 67–76 (M.D. diss., University of Leipzig, 1878).

side chains were involved in nutrition, and probably consisted of 'combustible molecule-groups' that were consumed during the process of oxidation and then regenerated.[20]

At about this same time (1885), Ehrlich was also becoming involved in his first significant pharmacotherapeutic investigations. In the period 1885 to 1894 he published studies on the properties of various drugs, including iodine, thalline, methylene blue, and cocaine.[21] An examination of these studies reveals that Ehrlich was continuing to develop some of the methods and concepts that were to play a part in his later work on the chemotherapy of trypanosomal diseases and syphilis. Once again we see Ehrlich's concern with selective affinity and distribution in this work.

Let us consider, for example, his investigation of methylene blue. In the course of his work on histological staining, Ehrlich reported in 1886 that methylene blue selectively stained living nerve tissue.[22] The dye thus exhibited a selective affinity towards nerve tissue, or, in Ehrlich's words, it was 'neurotropic.' Ehrlich's conviction, already developing at that time, that a drug must first become fixed or stored in a cell in order to act on it led him in 1890 to try methylene blue in the clinical treatment of pain in neuralgia because of its affinity towards nerve cells.[23] The following year, stimulated by the knowledge that methylene blue is an excellent stain for plasmodia, the causative agent of malaria, Ehrlich tried the dye in the treatment of two cases of malaria in humans.[24] The results were promising, but since Ehrlich was working in Berlin where cases of malaria were rare, and since at that time the disease could not be reproduced experimentally in laboratory animals, he had little opportunity to follow up on this work. This study marks Ehrlich's first real foray into the chemotherapy of infectious disease and the beginning of his search for parasitotropic substances.

These early therapeutic studies also reveal Ehrlich's interest in understanding the relationship of the pharmacological activity of a drug to its chemical structure and in attempting to modify that structure to produce

20. Paul Ehrlich, 'The requirement of the organism for oxygen: an analytical study with the aid of dyes,' *Collected papers* (n. 2), I, 433–496 (*Das Sauerstoffbedürfnis des Organismus: eine farbenanalytische Studie* [Berlin, 1885]).

21. See, for example, Paul Ehrlich, 'Über Wesen und Behandlung des Jodismus,' *Collected papers* (n. 2), I, 530–534 (*Charité-Ann.*, 1885, *10*, 129–135); and idem, 'Experimentelles und Klinisches über Thallin,' *Collected papers* (n. 2), I, 542–551 (*Dt. med. Wschr.*, 1886, *12*, 849–851).

22. Paul Ehrlich, 'Über die Methylenblaureaction der lebenden Newensubstanz,' *Collected papers* (n. 2), I, 500–508 (*Dt. med. Wschr.*, 1886, *12*, 49–52).

23. Paul Ehrlich and A. Leppman, 'Über schmerzstillende Wirkung des Methylenblau,' *Collected papers* (n. 2), I, 555–558 (*Dt. med. Wschr.*, 1890, *16*, 493–494).

24. P. Guttmann and Paul Ehrlich, 'On the action of methylene blue on malaria,' *Collected papers* (n. 2), III, 15–20 (*Berl. klin. Wschr.*, 1891, *28*, 953–956).

26

desired changes in activity, again foreshadowing his later chemotherapeutic work with azo dyes and arsenicals. Ehrlich was by no means the first to study the relationship between structure and activity, a subject that had been pioneered by British scientists such as James Blake, Benjamin Ward Richardson, Alexander Crum Brown, and Thomas Fraser in the period from about 1840 to 1870.[25] But Ehrlich was eventually to utilize structure-activity considerations in a sustained and systematic way in the first successful synthesis of a significantly effective chemotherapeutic agent, namely, Salvarsan.

Working with Alfred Einhorn in the early 1890s, Ehrlich investigated the properties of cocaine and various related compounds and determined that the benzoic acid radical was the portion of the molecule responsible for anesthetic action or, as Ehrlich phrased it, was the 'anesthesiophore group' of the molecule.[26] The chemical constitution of the drug molecule was also important in determining the distribution of the substance in the body. Ehrlich tended to attribute the specific therapeutic action of a drug (such as anesthetic properties) to the presence of a particular functional group, whereas he felt that the distribution of the drug depended upon the entire constitution or structure. In 1898 he expressed his conception of the best approach to the synthesis of pharmacologically active agents: 'If one is desirous of studying organ therapy in this sense, it is first of all necessary to seek for substances which possess a particular affinity for a certain organ. Having found such substances, one could then use them, so to speak, as a vehicle, with which to bring therapeutically active groups to the organ in question.'[27] Ehrlich's later conception of the search for chemotherapeutic agents was basically similar, except that the emphasis was on finding substances that had a particular affinity for a pathogenic microorganism rather than for a specific organ within the human body.

In the 1890s, however, Ehrlich's attention was largely diverted from synthetic chemical drugs to the newly emerging field of immunological therapy. In 1890 he was provided with laboratory space in Robert Koch's newly founded Institute for Infectious Diseases at Berlin and became actively involved in immunological work. Emil von Behring's discovery of

25. See John Parascandola, 'Structure-activity relationships: the early mirage,' *Pharm. Hist.*, 1971, *13*, 3–10. Cf. William F. Bynum, 'Chemical structure and pharmacological action: a chapter in the history of 19th century molecular pharmacology,' *Bull. Hist. Med.*, 1970, *44*, 518–538.

26. Paul Ehrlich and A. Einhorn, 'Über die physiologische Wirkung der Verbindungen der Cocain-reihe,' *Collected papers* (n. 2), I, 567–569 (*Ber. dt. chem. Ges.*, 1894, *27*, 1870–1873).

27. Paul Ehrlich, 'The relations existing between chemical constitution, distribution and pharmacological action,' *Collected papers* (n. 2), I, 596–618, p. 618 (*Ernst von Leyden Festchrift* [Berlin, 1902], pp. 647–679).

diphtheria antitoxin at Koch's institute in late 1890, with Ehrlich's later important role in helping to develop a sufficiently potent and standardized preparation for therapeutic use, stimulated great interest in serum therapy.[28] Although Ehrlich's contributions to immunology, which were significant enough to merit the Nobel Prize in 1909, are beyond the scope of this paper, we must consider at least briefly his famous side-chain theory of immunity because of its later influence on his concept of chemotherapy.

In 1897, to explain the process of immunization, Ehrlich called upon the side-chain theory which he had used earlier to explain cellular oxidation. Assume, he postulated, that one of the side chains (or *receptors*, as he later also referred to them) of the cell possesses an atom group with a specific combining property for a particular toxin, such as tetanus toxin. This side chain is normally involved in ordinary physiological processes, such as nutrition, and it is merely coincidental that it has the ability to combine with tetanus toxin. Combination with the toxin, however, renders the side chain incapable of performing its normal physiological function. The cell then produced more of these side chains to make up for the deficiency, but it overcompensates so that excess side chains are produced, break away from the cell, and are released into the bloodstream. These excess side chains in the blood are what we call antibodies or antitoxins. They neutralize the toxin by combining with it, thus preventing it from anchoring itself to the cell and exerting its poisonous effects.[29]

Ehrlich went on to distinguish between what he called the *toxophore* and the *haptophore* groups of the toxin. The haptophore group is the atom group involved in binding the toxin to the side chain. Once the toxin is thus anchored to the cell, the cell comes under the influence of the toxophore group, which is responsible for the poisonous properties of the toxin.[30] He may well have derived this concept from an analogy with

28. On Ehrlich's role in the development of the diphtheria antitoxin see Dolman (n. 1) and Marquardt, *Ehrlich* (n. 1), pp. 29–40.

29. Paul Ehrlich, 'The assay of the activity of diphtheria-curative serum and its theoretical basis,' *Collected papers* (n. 2), II, 107–125, pp. 113–115 (*Klin. Jb.*, 1897, *6*, 299–326). He referred in this paper (p. 115) to 'receptive side chains,' but did not use the term *receptor* until 1900. See Paul Ehrlich, 'On haemolysins: third communication,' *ibid.*, pp. 205–212, especially p. 205 (*Berl. klin. Wschr.*, 1900, *37*, 453–458). For more detailed discussions of Ehrlich's immunological theory, see Pauline Mazumdar, 'The antigen-antibody reaction and the physics and chemistry of life,' *Bull. Hist. Med.*, 1974, *48*, 1–21; and Lewis P. Rubin, 'Styles in scientific explanation: Paul Ehrlich and Svante Arrhenius on immuno-chemistry,' *J. Hist. Med.*, 1980, *35*, 397–425.

30. In his first paper on the side-chain theory Ehrlich differentiated between the binding group and the toxic group of the toxin, using the terms *combining group* and *toxophore group*, respectively. See his 'Diphtheria-curative serum' (n. 29), pp. 113–117. He introduced the term *haptophore* for the combining group the very next year. See Paul Ehrlich, 'Über die Constitution des Diphtheriegiftes,' *Collected papers* (n. 2), II, 126–133, p. 131 (*Dt. med. Wschr.*, 1898, *24*, 597–600). For a more elaborate

28

dyes, in which the chemical grouping responsible for color is different from that responsible for fixing the dye to the fabric or tissue.

Ehrlich's theory became more elaborate as he struggled to explain various immunological phenomena, but we need not consider these modifications for our present purposes. I have outlined Ehrlich's side-chain theory of immunity because this concept was later to play a key role in his theory of chemotherapy. It must be stressed, however, that Ehrlich did not immediately apply the side-chain theory to the question of drug action. In fact, he did not do so for some ten years, and at first he specifically denied that drugs were bound to the cell in a manner similar to the binding of toxins, a fact that is generally overlooked in accounts of Ehrlich's work.

The reason for Ehrlich's reluctance to apply the side-chain concept to drugs derived from the observations that many drugs can be easily extracted from tissues by solvents and that the action of many drugs is of a transitory character. Therefore, chemical drugs could not be bound firmly by the cell in the manner of toxins because they were not incorporated into the protoplasmic molecule by a chemical union. They did not possess haptophore groups and were not capable of evoking the production of antibodies.

Yet Ehrlich was well aware that drugs exhibit a selectivity for certain tissues. How then did he explain this specificity if not on the basis of his side-chain or receptor concept? It is not surprising that Ehrlich again drew upon his experience with dyes in explaining the specificity of drug action. As noted earlier, he believed that the fixing of dyes was not simply a physical or mechanical process involving surface attraction and adsorption. He discussed two current theories of the mechanism of action of dyeing or staining, each of which he felt might be correct in certain cases. The first of these involved the combination of the dye with a constituent of the fabric to form an insoluble, salt-like compound called a *lake*. A similar process might occur, he believed, in the tissues of the organism in the case of drugs, with a drug combining with a free substance (such as an acid) in the cell to form an insoluble compound that precipitates out of solution and is thus fixed in the cell. Cells that possessed constituents capable of forming a lake with a particular drug could thus localize that drug. The second theory of dyeing discussed by Ehrlich involved the formation of

summary of his theory of immunity, see Paul Ehrlich, 'On immunity with special reference to cell life,' *Collected papers* (n. 2), II, 178–195 (*Proc. roy. Soc. Lond.*, 1900, *66*, 424–448).

solid solutions in which the dye forms a homogeneous mixture with the substance of the fabric. He suggested that some drugs might be fixed in cells through a similar process, by being dissolved in the fat-like substances of certain tissues. Note that both of these mechanisms are different from the side-chain theory and do not involve combination of the drug with a receptor in the cell, although Ehrlich did note that they both involved 'chemical affinities in the widest meaning of the term.'[31]

Ehrlich's doubt about the probability of a true chemical combination taking place between the drug and the cell were shared by many of his contemporaries. Chemical combination was generally thought of at the time essentially in terms of what we would call covalent or ionic bonds, which are not easily broken. Such concepts as hydrogen bonds and Van der Waals bonds had not yet been developed. It was thus hard to reconcile phenomena such as the ease with which many drugs could be washed out of tissues by solvents with the contemporary concepts of chemical bonding. Many pharmacologists leaned towards the view that drugs often induce their effects through their physical properties, by altering the surface tension, electrolytic balance, osmotic pressure, etc., of the cell, rather than through the formation of chemical bonds with protoplasmic constituents.[32]

Ehrlich was to change his mind about the mechanism of action of drugs, however, as he became deeply involved in chemotherapeutic studies, and the receptor or side-chain theory was to come to form the theoretical basis of his chemotherapy. By 1898 Ehrlich was once again involved with therapeutic researches with dyes, and by 1903 he and his coworkers had begun an extensive series of chemotherapeutic investigations at the Institute for Experimental Therapy in Frankfort.[33] In 1906 Ehrlich was provided with additional space and funds for these studies when the Georg-Speyer-Haus for Chemotherapy, financed by Frau Franziska Speyer in memory of her late husband, was built adjoining the Institute for Experimental Therapy. From that time on, he turned his attention more and more away from immunology and towards chemotherapy. At the time that the Speyer-Haus was being planned, he wrote to a friend that he felt he had exhausted the

31. See John Parascandola and Ronald Jasensky, 'Origins of the receptor theory of drug action.' *Bull. Hist. Med.*, 1974, *48*, 199–220, pp. 205–209. See also Ehrlich (n. 27), pp. 608–616.

32. See John Parascandola, 'The controversy over structure-activity relationships in the early 20th century,' *Pharm. Hist.*, 1974, *16*, 54–63.

33. James G. Hirsch, 'The conquest of bacterial infectious diseases in the twentieth century: the greatest success story in the history of medical sciences,' Ms. Professor Hirsch notes that the Ehrlich copybooks provide evidence that by 1898 Ehrlich had set out to find a derivative of methylene blue that would have a better therapeutic index.

30

field of immunity and was pleased to have the opportunity to cultivate chemical therapy, which had always been his favorite field, in the proper way.[34]

In 1900 only a few drugs were available that actually combatted the causes of infectious diseases, that is, pathogenic microorganisms, and these had largely been discovered empirically. Quinine was perhaps the most prominent example of such a curative drug. The many new synthetic drugs developed in the late nineteenth century (such as phenacetin and aspirin) all tended to treat symptoms rather than causes of disease. They were antipyretics, analgesics, sedatives, etc. A number of chemical disinfectants such as carbolic acid did exist, but they were too toxic for use within the body. Efforts were made to find disinfectants that might be used internally, but the results were discouraging.[35] Little progress had been made in the nineteenth century towards developing the specific antimicrobial drugs that Ehrlich had in mind.

A rational, systematic search for specific chemotherapeutic agents against various infectious diseases could not have been carried out before the germ theory of disease was established in the latter part of the nineteenth century, and before methods had been developed for the identification, isolation, and culture of pathogenic microorganisms. Research in experimental therapeutics, as Ehrlich called it, was hampered also by the difficulty of reproducing certain human diseases in experimental animals (as in malaria).

Ehrlich and his coworkers began investigating the effects of various chemicals in the treatment of trypanosome infections in experimental animals, and, not surprisingly, their attention at first was concentrated on dyes. Many of the compounds tested were received through Dr. Arthur Weinberg, director of the Cassella and Company Dye Works near Frankfort.[36] Ehrlich found that dyes in the benzopurpurin series seemed the most promising of the compounds then under investigation, and by the addition of a sulfonic acid group to one of these dyes, to increase solubility, trypan red was prepared. This red dye seemed to cure mice with trypanosome infections completely, but unfortunately it was ineffective in rats and larger animals.[37]

34. Letter from Paul Ehrlich to Leopold Landau, 8 February 1905, Ehrlich copybooks (n. 8), Ser. V, No. XVI, pp. 26–28.

35. For a discussion of efforts to find 'internal disinfectants' in the nineteenth century, see John Crellin, 'Internal antisepsis or the dawn of chemotherapy?' *J. Hist. Med.*, 1981, *36*, 9–18.

36. Marquardt, *Ehrlich* (n. 1), p. 121. See also the correspondence between Ehrlich and Weinberg in the Ehrlich copybooks (n. 8) from this period.

37. Paul Ehrlich and K. Shiga, 'Farbentherapeutische Versuche bei Trypanosomenekrankung,' *Collected papers* (n. 2), III, 24–29 (*Berl. klin. Wschr.*, 1904); Ehrlich, 'Address' (n. 2), pp. 61–63.

Arsenic compounds also attracted the attention of Ehrlich's group. Arsenic had been used to some extent therapeutically in the treatment of certain trypanosomal diseases even before the microorganism had been identified as the cause.[38] It was thus natural that Ehrlich should exhibit an interest in arsenic, and he apparently tried atoxyl, a synthetic organic arsenic compound, in 1903 but rejected it because it did not exert a lethal action on the parasites in the test tube.[39] In 1902 Laveran and Mesnil had administered arsenious acid to experimental animals infected with trypanosomes, but they had been unable to effect a complete cure. After the publication of Ehrlich's results on trypan red in 1902, Laveran tried a combination of this dye with arsenious acid and found that in rats and mice it cured certain trypanosome infections that neither substance alone could treat successfully. These results were confirmed in Ehrlich's laboratory.[40]

In 1905 Thomas and Breinl of the Liverpool School of Tropical Medicine reported that atoxyl, which Ehrlich had earlier abandoned on the basis of *in vitro* tests, could eliminate trypanosomes from the blood of infected animals.[41] This discovery stimulated further interest in arsenicals on the part of Ehrlich and others, but it was soon found with respect to atoxyl that relapses commonly occur and that the large therapeutic doses required could damage the optic nerve and produce blindness in man.[42] Even before this discovery of its effect on sight, however, Ehrlich was attempting to modify the structure of atoxyl to produce a less toxic and more potent trypanocidal drug.

Atoxyl had been synthesized in the 1860s by Béchamp, and was believed to be an anilide with little potential for modification to produce active derivatives. Ehrlich and Bertheim found that atoxyl was a chemically stable compound and possessed a free amine group which could be reacted with various substances to produce a host of related derivatives. The chem-

38. David Livingstone tried arsenic as early as 1858 as a remedy for a horse afflicted with *nagana*, a disease later found to be caused by a trypanosome. See David Livingstone, 'Arsenic as a remedy for the tsetse bite,' *Br. med. J.*, 1858, *i*, 360–361. Arsenic preparations were also tried by David Bruce in the 1890s in an effort to cure trypanosomal diseases. See John J. McKelvey, Jr., *Man against tsetse: struggle for Africa* (Ithaca, N.Y., 1973), pp. 27–28, 66, 84–85.

39. Ehrlich (n. 13), p. 283.

40. A. Laveran and F. Mesnil, 'Recherches sur le traitement et la prévention du Ngana,' *Annls. Inst. Pasteur*, 1902, *16*, 785–817; A. Laveran, 'Le trypanroth dans le traitement de quelques Trypanosomiases,' *C. r. Séanc. Acad. Sci., Paris*, 1904, *39*, 19–22; Ehrlich, 'Chemotherapeutische' (n. 2), p. 85; letter from Ehrlich to A. Laveran, 13 February 1905, Ehrlich copybooks (n. 8), Ser. v, No. xvi, pp. 69–70.

41. H. W. Thomas and A. Breinl, *Report on trypanosomes, trypanosomiases and sleeping sickness* (Liverpool, 1905); H. W. Thomas, 'Some experiments in the treatment of trypanosomiases,' *Br. med. J.*, 1905, *i*, 1140–1141.

42. 'A danger of atoxyl,' *J. Am. med. Ass.*, 1907, *49*, 1149.

32

ists at the Georg-Speyer-Haus found that the toxicity of atoxyl could be increased or decreased by suitable modifications of the molecule.[43]

As is well known, several hundred organic arsenic compounds were prepared and tested in Ehrlich's laboratory. This work was carefully directed by Ehrlich himself. Each morning he would provide the various researchers in his laboratory with written instructions for their day's work, and he expected these instructions to be obeyed exactly.[44] Sometimes such detailed supervision led to resentment on the part of experienced coworkers who felt that they should have more independence.[45] When he was in the process of searching for skilled chemists to work in his new institute for experimental chemotherapy, Ehrlich described to a colleague the difficulty of finding suitable candidates from his point of view. He noted: 'they must be on the one hand entirely skilled and independent scientific workers, and, on the other hand, also disposed to acquiesce in my ideas and develop them therapeutically.' Ehrlich admitted that the task of preparing the compounds that he desired might not always be of great interest from a purely chemical point of view.[46]

In the course of the work on organic arsenic compounds it was found that only trivalent arsenic compounds killed trypanosomes *in vitro*, and Ehrlich postulated that the pentavalent atoxyl was converted to the trivalent state in the body. Particularly encouraging results were obtained with compounds of the arsenobenzene type R-As-As-R'. For example, compound number 418, arsenophenylglycine, yielded encouraging results in laboratory and clinical trials, but the search still continued in Ehrlich's institute for a better chemotherapeutic agent.[47]

After the *Spirochaeta pallida* had been isolated as the causal agent of syphilis in 1905, several investigators tried arsenical drugs such as atoxyl in the treatment of syphilis and other spirochaetal diseases because of the

43. Paul Ehrlich and A. Bertheim, 'Über p-Aminophenylarsinsäure,' *Collected papers* (n. 2), III, 135–139 (*Ber. dt. chem. Ges.*, 1907); Ehrlich (n. 13), pp. 283–284; Ehrlich, 'Moderne Chemotherapie' (n. 11), pp. 141–142. See also letter from Paul Ehrlich to L. Darmstädter, 25 November 1905, Ehrlich copybooks (n. 8), Ser. v, No. XVIII, pp. 303–305, on the structure of atoxyl.

44. Marquardt, *Ehrlich* (n. 1), pp. 53, 63, 130, 133–134. Reid Hunt, working in Ehrlich's laboratory in 1902, noted that in his supervision of coworkers such as Mogenroth and Sacks, 'Ehrlich writes down what they are to do and will never hear a word of suggestion from any of them.' Letter from Reid Hunt to John Abel, 10 November 1902, Abel Papers, Johns Hopkins University. Hunt may have exaggerated somewhat, but Ehrlich did not want his coworkers to become too independent. I am grateful to the Johns Hopkins University Institute of the History of Medicine for permission to use the Abel papers.

45. See Marquardt, *Ehrlich* (n. 1), pp. 141–144, 154–156.

46. Letter from Paul Ehrlich to A. Wohl, 9 May 1905, Ehrlich copybooks (n. 8), Ser. v, No. XVII, pp. 100–105.

47. Ehrlich (n. 6), pp. 154–165; Ehrlich, 'Moderne Chemotherapie' (n. 11), pp. 141–149.

apparent similarity between trypanosomes and spirochaetes.[48] As in the case of trypanosomal infections, arsenic preparations had been used to some extent in the treatment of syphilis long before the cause of the disease was known.[49] Ehrlich's laboratory did not carry out experiments on syphilis-infected animals before 1909, but Ehrlich was interested in spirochaetes and did arrange for his friend Albert Neisser to test the most promising arsenicals on syphilis in monkeys and apes.[50]

In 1909 Sahachiro Hata, who had carried out experimental studies on syphilis in rabbits at the Kitsano Institute of Infectious Diseases in Tokyo, came to work in Ehrlich's laboratory. Ehrlich set him to work testing the effects of numerous compounds on relapsing fever and on syphilis. When Hata tested compound number 606, he found it to be an effective anti-syphilitic agent. The compound had actually been synthesized in 1907, but the assistant who tested it at the time did not report any significant therapeutic activity. It is not clear why the effectiveness of 606 was missed at first, since the compound is, as was soon shown, useful in the treatment of certain trypanosomal diseases as well as syphilis.[51]

After extensive animal tests, limited supplies of 606 were distributed to selected specialists for clinical trials. In April 1910 Ehrlich was ready to announce the discovery of 606 at the Congress for Internal Medicine in Wiesbaden.[52] The announcement was greeted with great enthusiasm, and the demand for the drug soon outgrew the ability of the Georg-Speyer-Haus chemists to produce it. Ehrlich then arranged with the Höchst Chemical Works to manufacture 606, which was patented under the trade-

48. See P. Uhlenhuth, E. Hoffmann, and K. Roscher, 'Untersuchungen über die Wirkung des Atoxyls auf die Syphilis,' *Dt. med. Wschr.*, 1907, *33*, 873–876.

49. See John S. Haller, Jr., 'Therapeutic mule: the use of arsenic in the nineteenth century materia medica,' *Pharm. Hist.*, 1975, *17*, 87–100; and Alfred Fournier, *Traitement de la syphilis* (Paris, 1893), pp. 100–104.

50. Ehrlich (n. 13), pp. 294–295. References to spirochaetes in Ehrlich's letters and notes in the Ehrlich copybooks (n. 8) before 1909 indicate his interest in these microorganisms and the diseases they cause. As an example of Neisser's studies, see Albert Neisser, 'Ueber die Verwendung des Arsacetins (Ehrlich) bei der Syphilisbehandlung,' *Dt. med. Wschr.*, 1908, *34*, 1500–1504. See also Ehrlich's letter to Neisser, 12 April 1907, Ehrlich copybooks (n. 8), Ser. v, No. xxi, pp. 315–318.

51. Marquardt, *Ehrlich* (n. 1), pp. 163–175; Ehrlich (n. 13).

52. Paul Ehrlich, 'Allgemeines über Chemotherapie,' *Collected papers* (n. 2), III, 235–239 (*Verh. Kongr. inn. Med.*, 1910, *27*, 226–234). The Ehrlich copybooks (n. 8) for 1909–10 provide information on the distribution of 606 for clinical trials. See also Marquardt, *Ehrlich* (n. 1), pp. 172–177. Some results of animal studies with 606, along with other compounds, were briefly noted in a lecture by Ehrlich on 1 December 1909, but 606 was not singled out for special attention. See Paul Ehrlich, 'Chemotherapie von Infektionskrankheit,' *Collected papers* (n. 2), III, 213–227, pp. 220–221, 226 (*Z. ärztl. Fortbild.*, 1909 *6*, 721–733).

34

name *Salvarsan*.[53] Salvarsan represented the first practical success for Ehrlich's concept of chemotherapy, and the only truly significant one during his lifetime.

Ehrlich, as we have seen, was very much interested in understanding the mechanism of action of drugs, for he believed that a rational therapeutics must be based on such an understanding. He emphasized that in a chemotherapeutic institute one must search for the scientific foundations of drug action rather than carry out a purely empirical search for new drugs.[54] The first duty of experimental pharmacology, according to Ehrlich, was to clarify not only the questions 'What?' and 'How?' but also 'Why?' Therefore, he had decided to investigate the cause of the action of arsenic.[55] His chemotherapeutic researches led him to reject his earlier conception of the view of drug action and to apply a modified form of the side-chain theory which he had used to explain immune reactions to the question of drug action. Particularly instrumental in this regard was the discovery in his laboratory of the phenomenon of drug resistance.

In the period from 1905 to 1907, experiments carried out by Franke, Röhl, and Browning in Ehrlich's laboratory demonstrated that a strain of trypanosomes that is susceptible to treatment with a particular drug, such as atoxyl, may, on continued exposure to that drug, develop a resistance to such treatment. In other words, a trypanosome strain may be produced that no longer responds to treatment with the drug. Resistance was found to be not limited to the compound used to develop it, but to extend also to other compounds within the same chemical class. For example, the atoxyl-resistant strain exhibited a significant degree of resistance towards other arsenical compounds, such as acetyl-atoxyl, and the trypan-red-resistant strain exhibited some resistance towards other azo dyes, such as trypan blue and trypan violet. The development of resistance towards one group of compounds (for example, the arsenicals), however, did not

53. Marquardt, *Ehrlich* (n. 1), pp. 176–180. For an example of the enthusiasm with which Salvarsan was greeted, see 'Doctors in Congress,' London *Times*, 12 August 1913 (a report on the International Congress of Medicine in London, where Ehrlich spoke). On the reception of Salvarsan in this country, see Patricia Spain Ward, 'The American reception of Salvarsan,' *J. Hist. Med.*, 1981, *36*, 44–62. Salvarsan was not received enthusiastically by all. For discussions of opposition to the drug, which had potentially dangerous side effects, see Marquardt, *Ehrlich* (n. 1), pp. 234–238; and Harry Dowling, 'Comparisons and contrasts between the early arsphenamine and early antibiotic periods,' *Bull. Hist. Med.*, 1973, *47*, 236–249, p. 245.

54. In referring to the tasks of a chemotherapeutic institute, Ehrlich wrote that one should not grab blindly like a bear in the soup bowl if one wanted a good piece. See his notes dated 7 September 1909, Ehrlich copybooks (n. 8), Ser. IV, No. V, pp. 19–20.

55. Ehrlich, 'Moderne Chemotherapie' (n. 11), p. 145.

increase resistance towards compounds of other classes (for example, azo dyes).[56]

In order to explain the specificity of resistance, Ehrlich adopted the concept of *chemoreceptors* for drugs. In his Harben Lectures of 1907 in London, he revealed that he had come to believe that at least some drugs are bound to protoplasm by certain atom groupings ('side chains' or 'receptors'). The chemoreceptors for drugs are somewhat analogous to the toxin receptors, but are simpler in structure and less independent (that is, they cannot be separated from the cell to form antibodies). A given drug or poison, such as an arsenic compound, will only attack an organism, for example, a trypanosome, if that organism possesses chemoreceptors capable of combining with it. Like the *nutrireceptors* that are attacked by microbial toxins, however, chemoreceptors are ordinarily engaged with the normal substances of nutrition or metabolism, and hence are present in all cells. Hence, Ehrlich explained, any chemical drug is likely to have an affinity for the cells of the host organism as well as for the parasite. In order for a drug to be an effective chemotherapeutic agent, it must have a greater affinity for the chemoreceptors of the parasite cells than for those of the host cells, or its 'trypanotropic' force must be greater than its 'organotropic' force. In other words, one must be able to produce a curative effect with a dose that is not injurious to the host.

The studies on drug resistance, Ehrlich argued, supported the concept of chemoreceptors. The atoxyl-resistant strain, for example, was resistant to a number of arsenic compounds which otherwise possessed significant differences in their chemical characteristics. The arsenic acid radical, however, represented a common point of attack in this series. It was bound to the cell by chemoreceptors. The trypanosome cell possessed other chemoreceptors which represented the points of attack for other poisons.

The development of resistance could be readily explained by Ehrlich in terms of the receptor concept. The chemoreceptors of resistant trypanosome strains had somehow developed a reduced affinity for the drug, so that the distribution of the drug between the microorganisms and the host animal is shifted in the direction of the latter.[57] Ehrlich felt that the phe-

56. Ehrlich, 'Chemotherapeutische' (n. 2). See also Parascandola and Jasensky (n. 31), pp. 216–220, for a fuller discussion of the studies on drug resistance.

57. Paul Ehrlich, 'Experimental researches on specific therapy,' *Collected papers* (n. 2), III, 106–134, pp. 120–122, 132–133 (*The Harben Lectures for 1907 of the Royal Institute of Public Health* [London, 1908]). In his notes, Ehrlich wrote that chemical poisons are like wild birds that become captured and destroy the surroundings. See his notes of 28 March 1909, Ehrlich copybooks (n. 8), Ser. IV, No. IV, p. 380.

nomenon of drug resistance would play an important role in the development of 'therapeutic biology' and would help to bring order and light to the chaos of drug action.[58] Ehrlich's decision to apply the receptor concept to drugs was also influenced, as he himself admitted, by the development in 1905 of a similar theory of 'receptive substances' by John Newport Langley in England to explain the action of alkaloidal drugs such as nicotine and curare.[59]

In his early discussions of the mode of action of arsenicals, Ehrlich emphasized the binding of the arsenic radical to a chemoreceptor in the cell. He even speculated about the chemical nature of the 'arsenoreceptor,' suggesting that it might be a hydroxyl or sulfhydryl group, a remarkably accurate prediction, because Carl Voegtlin later showed that the chemical grouping involved in reacting with arsenic is indeed a sulfhydryl group.[60] But Ehrlich soon developed a more complex explanation of drug action involving more than one receptor for a given drug.

As Ehrlich noted in 1909, if aromatic arsenic compounds were anchored to the cell exclusively through the trivalent arsenic atom bound on the phenyl residue and this anchorage was the determining factor in the action of this class of drugs, then one would expect that the simplest compounds (such as phenylarsenic acid and arsenobenzene) would be the best substances for treatment. But such was not the case. In fact, the introduction of substituents in the *para*-position of the benzene ring in phenylarsenic acid greatly influenced toxicity and therapeutic action. For example, the introduction of an amino group in this position promotes the action of the drug.[61]

In order to explain the fact that substitutions in the benzene ring, which do not affect the arsenic radical itself, modify the action of the drug, Ehrlich postulated that for complicated drugs other groupings in the molecule besides the arsenic residue are also involved in binding the drug to the cell. The addition, removal, or modification of such groups therefore affects the fixation of the compound to the cell and consequently its pharmacological action. The drug becomes successively fastened by its various groupings to the specific 'fangs' or 'snares' (*Fangen*), that is, the chemoreceptors, of the protoplasm. Ehrlich, in his usual graphic way, compared the process to the mounting of a butterfly which is fixed first by the torso and then succes-

58. See Ehrlich's notes of 13 May 1908. Ehrlich copybooks (n. 8), Ser. VI, No. IV, p. 422.
59. For a discussion of Langley's views, see Parascandola and Jasensky (n. 31).
60. See John Parascandola, 'Carl Voegtlin and the "arsenic receptor" in chemotherapy,' *J. Hist. Med.*, 1977, *32*, 151–171.
61. Ehrlich (n. 6), pp. 164–165.

sively by the wings with pins. He noted, however, that one can frequently determine experimentally a grouping that brings about the primary anchoring, and that this grouping can be designated the *primary haptophore*. In the drug arsenophenylglycine (compound number 418), for example, Ehrlich felt that the acetic acid radical was the group that primarily anchored the drug to the cell.[62]

Ehrlich was essentially applying the haptophore-toxophore concept, which he utilized in immunology, to the problem of drug action. Originally, before he adopted the receptor concept for drugs, Ehrlich had denied that drugs possessed haptophore groups. He had argued that the entire constitution of the drug was involved in its distribution rather than specific atom groupings. Even before he published his first account of his chemoreceptor theory, however, he had come to accept the idea that drugs possess a 'selective group,' which governs distribution, and a 'pharmacophore group,' which evokes the specific activity.[63] With the development of the drug-receptor theory, Ehrlich came explicitly to adopt the haptophore-toxophore terminology of his immunological theory (with the stipulation that there could be more than one haptophore group involved in binding a drug).

This fact is perhaps seen most clearly in Ehrlich's discussion of the mode of action of Salvarsan. Ehrlich expressed the point best at the International Congress of Medicine in 1913:

Now, if we are to look for specific medicaments, the first condition is that they must possess a certain definite group which is chemically allied to one of the chemoreceptors of the parasites. This is only one of the prerequisites necessary for the medicament to be effective, but generally it is not sufficient in itself. Hundreds of substances may fix themselves to a parasite but only a few are capable of bringing about destruction.

Thus, in the therapeutically suitable substance there must be present, in addition to the anchoring or haptophore group, which brings about the fixation, another group which brings about the destruction, and which, therefore, is characterized as the poisoning, or toxophore group. This concept exactly corresponds to the views which we have already held for years with respect to the toxins, in which we distinguish the presence of a haptophore group which causes the anchorage to the cell and also the formation of the antitoxins, and a toxophore group which brings about the injurious action on the cell. For the

---

62. Ehrlich, 'Infektionskrankheit' (n. 52), pp. 219–220; see also his notes of 6 February 1909, Ehrlich copybooks (n. 8), Ser. IV, No. IV, p. 324. Another metaphor that Ehrlich used was that one snares insects more easily with a bundle of lime twigs than with a single one. *Ibid.*, p. 479 (2 July 1909).
63. Ehrlich, 'Address' (n. 2), p. 57.

38

more complicated synthetic medicaments the assumption will have to be made that the haptophore group and the toxophore group are not directly connected with one another, but that they, as residues, are attached, like side-chains, to a chemical molecule. Thus, quite simply, the more complicated chemotherapeutic agents may be compared to a poison-arrow; the anchoring group of the medicament which anchors itself to the chemoreceptor of the parasite corresponds to the point of the arrow, the connecting link to the shaft, and the poison group to the arrow poison affixed to the shaft of the arrow. According to this scheme, in Salvarsan, dihydroxydiaminoarsenobenzene, the benzene nucleus would correspond to the shaft, the o-aminophenol group to the point, and the trivalent arsenic radicle to the poison. . . .

If, therefore, we poison a spirochaete with Salvarsan, at least two different chemical anchorages occur; first, the anchorage of the o-aminophenol group which primarily anchors the Salvarsan to the parasite. It is only in consequence of this anchorage that, second, the trivalent arsenic radicle is given the opportunity of entering into chemical combination with the arsenoceptor of the cell, and so of exerting its toxic action. The avidity of the arsenoceptor may, in itself, be so small that a reaction can take place only if favourable factors, which chemically must be regarded as steric facilitation, are operating. Examples of steric facilitations of this kind are frequently found in pure chemistry, e.g., in the chemistry of *ortho*-condensations. Thus the haptophore group of the arsenical primarily brings the arsenic into contact with the cell and secondarily provides an opportunity for its action.[64]

Even before Ehrlich had applied the receptor concept to drugs, as we have seen, he had argued that the search for specific medicaments should be based on searching for substances that possessed a particular affinity for a certain organ and then using such substances as vehicles to carry therapeutically active groups to the organ involved. Now, however, this concept was expressed in terms of chemoreceptors. Ehrlich felt that the chemotherapeutist must aim to discover for every type of parasite the characteristic haptophore group with the aid of which one could force a specific therapeutic radical (such as arsenic) upon the parasite. One must, in other words, learn what chemoreceptors are possessed by specific parasites. The ideal situation would be to find a chemoreceptor that is present only in the parasite and not in the cells of the host. Ehrlich expressed his views about such an ideal substance:

I have explained above that the parasites possess a whole series of chemoceptors which differ specifically from each other. Now, if we were to succeed in dis-

64. Ehrlich (n. 3), pp. 507–508.

Paul Ehrlich's Chemotherapy 39

covering among these a receptor which was not represented in the organs of the host, we would have the possibility of constructing an ideal medicament by selecting a haptophore group which fits exclusively this particular receptor of the parasites. A medicament provided with such a haptophore group would be entirely innocuous, because it is not anchored by the organs; it would, however, strike the parasites with full force, and, in this sense, correspond to the immune-substances, the antibodies discovered by Behring, which, in the manner of magic bullets, seek out the enemy. Let us hope that it will also be possible, chemotherapeutically, to score bull's-eyes in this way. I do not consider this at all improbable, since it can be shown that, with certain diseases, e.g., spirillosis of fowls, from a fiftieth to a hundredth part of the *dosis tolerata* of Salvarsan entirely frees the animals from the parasites and brings about a cure. Such a dose truly represents a zero dose, as the fowl cannot be harmed by it to the slightest extent. But such favourable circumstances have been encountered only very rarely up to the present; we shall have to be satisfied if we can obtain good therapeutic results with a tenth, or even a fifth or sixth, part of the *dosis tolerata*.[65]

As Ehrlich recognized, such ideal drugs would not be easy to find. We must often be satisfied to find substances that have a greater affinity for a particular chemoreceptor in a parasite than for the corresponding chemo-receptor in a human cell. A knowledge of the different chemoreceptors of a parasite, or what Ehrlich designated 'the therapeutic physiology of the parasite cell,' was for him 'a *sine qua non* for success in chemotherapy.' The larger the number of different chemoreceptors that could be demonstrated, the greater the possibility of successful chemotherapy.[66]

Ehrlich's theoretical view of chemotherapy came to be based on the chemoreceptor concept. And the chemoreceptor concept in turn was based on Ehrlich's concept of the cell as a giant protoplasmic molecule with chemical side chains involved in various biological functions (what he termed *partial functions* of the cell). Acknowledging that this view of the cell had long been accepted by Pflüger and others, he claimed for himself the credit for removing this idea from the realm of the theoretical and making it accessible to experimentation. He felt that his analysis of the cell into partial functions would be a lasting contribution to biology.[67] In his Nobel Prize Address of 1909 he stated:

Even now the time has come to find a way into the finest chemistry of cell life, and to dissect the inclusive concept of the cell into a large number of single

65. *Ibid.*, p. 510.
66. *Ibid.*, p. 507.
67. Letter from Paul Ehrlich to J. G. Adami, 17 March 1909, Ehrlich copybooks (n. 8), Ser. v, No. xxv, pp. 401–402.

40

and specific 'partial functions.' Since, however, everything that happens in the cell is essentially chemical in nature, and since the configuration of chemical structure lies beyond the limit of visibility, we shall have to make a search for other methods of investigation. This line of thought has not only a general importance for a true understanding of the phenomena of life; it is also fundamental to a truly rational application of medicinal remedies.[68]

In discussing the theoretical basis of his chemotherapy, mention should be made of two other concepts, or what Ehrlich called *therapeutic tactics*, which related to his understanding of drug action and guided his view of the practical application of chemotherapy. The first of these is his famous doctrine of *therapia sterilisans magna*, by which Ehrlich meant the elimination of all the parasites from the body by a single dose (or, at most, two doses). Ehrlich placed great emphasis on this goal, although he was not able actually to achieve it with Salvarsan in the treatment of syphilis. He seems to have been concerned to bring about the destruction of the parasites as quickly as possible and to avoid the possibility of having parasites that survived the first dose develop into a relapse strain that was resistant to the body's natural defense mechanisms and the drug.[69]

The other therapeutic tactic is combination therapy, that is, the use of two or more drugs in combination to treat a particular infection. The idea of combination therapy with chemotherapeutic agents was not original to Ehrlich. I have already mentioned Laveran's use of this procedure. But Ehrlich placed great emphasis on this tactic. Combination therapy should be carried out, in Ehrlich's view, with therapeutic agents that attack different chemoreceptors in the parasite. There would be no advantage, for example, to combining trypan red with trypan blue, since both drugs have the same point of attack. Combining Salvarsan with parafuchsin, however, can be effective because these substances attack entirely different chemoreceptors. Ehrlich noted that 'once we have come to know most of the chemoreceptors of a particular parasite—and this will be an arduous task requiring much hard work and thinking—we shall have tremendous possibilities [for] attacking with various agents simultaneously.' Such a combination therapy had two important advantages.

First, one might be able in this way to increase the therapeutic effect without increasing the toxicity towards the host. The reason for such a possibility was that the receptors for parafuchsin were likely to be in organs

68. Paul Ehrlich, 'On partial functions of the cell: Nobel lecture,' *Collected papers* (n. 2), III, 183–194, p. 183 (Nobelstiftelsen, Stockholm, *Les prix Nobel en 1908* [Stockholm, 1909]).
69. Ehrlich (n. 3), pp. 512–514; Ehrlich (n. 13), p. 292.

other than those for Salvarsan; hence the two drugs would be localized in different cells in the human body and their toxic effects on these cells would not be additive. On the other hand, both drugs would accumulate in the unicellular parasite, and their effects on the parasite would be additive. Combination therapy in this way made possible a cure with smaller doses of each drug, thus reducing the chances of toxic side effects.

Secondly, resistance was less likely to arise if two drugs were used. If parafuchsin and Salvarsan were used in combination, for example, those organisms that were resistant to one drug would most likely be destroyed by the other, and a relapse strain would be less likely to develop. Even if a relapse did occur, the organism seemed to be less resistant to the drug involved when combination therapy had been employed.[70]

The early successes in chemotherapy were concentrated in the area of diseases caused by protozoal-type microorganisms (for example, trypanosomes and spirochaetes), and significant progress was not made in the chemotherapeutic treatment of true bacterial infections until the development of the sulfa drugs in the 1930s. Sir Henry Dale suggested in his introduction to *The collected papers of Paul Ehrlich* that the publication by Ehrlich of the negative results of experiments with Bechhold on bacteria in 1906 seems to have discouraged him and others about the practicality of developing effective chemotherapeutic substances for bacterial infections.[71] I do not believe, however, that this was the case. As Dale himself pointed out, Ehrlich became so involved with Salvarsan from 1909 until his death that he did not have time for research in other areas.[72] But on several occasions Ehrlich expressed optimism concerning the successful application of chemotherapy to bacterial infections. He wrote to a colleague in 1909 that while he thought that the sterilization of bacteria within the body would be a very difficult task, he did not see it as impossible.[73] A few years later, he referred in a published lecture to some promising chemotherapeutic experiments that several investigators had carried out with bacteria and expressed the

---

70. Ehrlich (n. 3), pp. 514–515. The quotation is from p. 515. See also Ehrlich, 'Experimental' (n. 57), pp. 133–134.

71. Henry Dale, 'Introduction,' *Collected papers* (n. 2), III, 1–8, p. 5. Dale's claim has been repeated by M. P. Earles, 'Salvarsan and the concept of chemotherapy,' *Pharm. J.*, 1970, *204*, 400–402, p. 401. The publication that Dale referred to is H. Bechhold and Paul Ehrlich, 'Beziehungen zwischen chemischer Konstitution and Desinfektionswirkung: ein Beitrag zum Studium der "innern Antisepsis," ' *Collected papers* (n. 2), III, 64–80 (*Z. physiol. Chem.*, 1906, *47*, 173–199).

72. Dale (n. 71), p. 6. For a discussion of the problems surrounding Salvarsan that so absorbed Ehrlich's time and energy, see Marquardt, *Ehrlich* (n. 1), pp. 188–206.

73. Letter from Ehrlich to L. Krehl, 3 February 1909, Ehrlich copybooks (n. 8), Ser. v, No. xxv, pp. 274–275.

42

view 'that in the next five years we shall see very extensive advances in this field.'[74]

In the period from 1910 to 1930 a significant amount of research effort was devoted to attempts to find chemotherapeutic agents effective against bacteria, albeit without much success. The failure of such efforts certainly did lead in the 1920s to pessimism on the part of many scientists and physicians about the potential of bacterial chemotherapy.[75] This pessimism, however, owed more to the accumulation of negative findings over a period of years than it did to the publication of Ehrlich's disappointing results in 1906.

Ehrlich recognized that it was not necessary for a drug actually to kill the parasites in order for an infection to be eliminated from the body. There was evidence, he pointed out, that in some cases a drug prevented a microorganism from reproducing, and, by thus checking the infection, led to the eventual elimination of the parasite.[76] Sir Henry Dale has noted that since most of the antibacterial drugs discovered in recent decades act in this fashion (that is, they are bacteriostatic rather than bactericidal), it is unfortunate that Ehrlich did not find the time to follow up this concept. I do not think that Dale was justified in concluding that Ehrlich 'recognized this antireproductive effect as probably the most important factor in a practical chemotherapy.'[77] Neither Ehrlich's published writings nor the manuscript materials that I have examined devote a significant amount of attention to the antireproductive mechanism, and Ehrlich generally spoke in terms of a destruction of the parasites. The receptor theory could accommodate either mechanism, for the drug could be envisioned as either poisoning the microorganism or interfering with its ability to reproduce when it combined with the chemoreceptor. In either case the macroscopic result would be the same (assuming that the drug had been administered in time) —elimination of the parasite from the body of the host. While this question was thus not crucial to his general theory of drug action, it is certainly

74. Ehrlich (n. 3), pp. 516–517. The quotation is from p. 517.

75. For discussion of the growing pessimism, see Harry Dowling, *Fighting infection: conquests of the twentieth century* (Cambridge, Mass., 1977), pp. 105–107; and Iago Galdston, 'Some notes on the early history of chemotherapy,' *Bull. Hist. Med.*, 1940, *8*, 806–818, pp. 816–817. For a contemporary view of the research efforts in bacterial chemotherapy, see Henry Dale, 'Chemotherapy,' *Physiol. Rev.*, 1923, *3*, 359–393, pp. 363–367. Dale cited a significant number of studies, but concluded that the chemotherapy of bacterial infections 'cannot be said to have achieved, as yet, anything of practical importance' (p. 367).

76. Paul Ehrlich, 'Über die Neuesten Ergebnisse auf dem Gebiete der Trypanosomenforschung,' *Collected papers* (n. 2), III, 195–212, p. 209 (*Arch. Schiffs Tropenhyg.*, 1909, *13*, Suppl. 6, 91–116).

77. Dale (n. 71), pp. 4–6. The quotation is from p. 6.

the kind of fundamental scientific problem that would have interested Ehrlich, and Dale may have been correct in speculating that Ehrlich would have investigated the subject further had he not been diverted in the last years of his life from more basic research to the practical problems surrounding Salvarsan.[78]

Ehrlich's concept of chemotherapy and the practical success of Salvarsan stimulated a search for other effective chemotherapeutic agents as well as further research into the mechanism of drug action. The field of chemotherapy had been launched, and was to be guided by the general principles established by Ehrlich for many years to come. The theoretical basis of Ehrlich's chemotherapy, the side-chain theory, however, soon ran into difficulties. Even during his lifetime the view of the cell as a giant protoplasmic molecule with chemical side chains came under attack by such biochemists and physiologists as Frederick Gowland Hopkins and William Bayliss, and was eventually found untenable. Pharmacologists such as Walther Straub, Henry Dale, and Carl Voegtlin began to point out facts that were difficult to explain on the basis of the side-chain theory.[79] The basic concept of the drug receptor has, of course, survived to occupy a central place in theoretical pharmacology today, but in a form greatly modified from Ehrlich's conception of the chemoreceptor.

78. *Ibid.*, p. 6.
79. For a discussion of some of the criticisms of Ehrlich's theory, see Parascandola (n. 60).

VIII

The development of receptor theory

CONTENTS

In modern pharmacology the effects of drugs on biological systems are explained in many cases in terms of the interaction between the drug molecule and specific molecules or complex macromolecular structures in the cell which are termed 'receptors'. A.W. Cuthbert (1979) has called the last two decades in pharmacology 'the age of the receptor', and E.J. Ariëns (1979) has noted that for decades the receptor as an operational concept has been 'indispensable for discussing and understanding the mode of action of pharmaca.'

The concept of the drug receptor was first clearly developed at the beginning of the twentieth century by John Newport Langley (1852 – 1925) and Paul Ehrlich (1854 – 1915), working independently and from different approaches. It became firmly established in pharmacology largely through the work of A.J. Clark (1885 – 1941) in the 1920's and 1930's. The purpose of this chapter is to trace the development of receptor theory from its origins through its elaboration in a more quantitative form by Clark.

1. BACKGROUND

The fact that drugs may exert a selective action on specific organs has long been recognized empirically and expressed vaguely in the traditional designation of certain remedies as cordials, hepatics, etc. (Earles, 1961). Already in the seventeenth century Robert Boyle (1685) had tried to explain the specific effects of drugs in terms of the mechanical philosophy by suggesting that since the different parts of the body have different textures, it is not implausible that when the corpuscles of a medicine are carried by the body fluids throughout the organism they may, according to their size, shape and motion, be more fit to be detained by one organ than another.

Attempts were also made in the sixteenth and seventeenth centuries, under the influence of Paracelsus and his followers, to explain drug action in more chemical terms. The so-called iatrochemists, for example, tended to attribute most physiological and pathological phenomena (including pharmacological effects) to acid-base interactions. It was not until the nineteenth century, however, that the chemical approach to selective action achieved clearer and more specific expression. Around mid-century Jonathan Pereira (1854), not himself a convinced adherent of the chemical theory, explained this viewpoint as follows:

'The action of a medicine on one organ rather than on another is accounted for on the chemical hypothesis, by assuming the existence of unequal affinities of the medicinal agent for different tissues. Thus the action of alcohol on the brain is ascribed to the affinity of this liquid for the cerebral substance.'

Others suggested even more specifically that the physiological action of drugs was due in most cases to a chemical reaction between the drug and some constituent of the cell. For example, Thomas Fraser (1872) felt that pharmacological action was often, if not always, the result of a chemical reaction between the drug and certain constituents of the body, and Thomas Lauder Brunton (1871) postulated that certain chemicals enter into a reversible combination with the cell, altering its physical character and functional properties in the process. At the turn of the twentieth century, Sigmund Fränkel (1901) offered what was perhaps the clearest expression of the view that drugs combine with specific substances in the cell before the elaboration of the receptor theory by Ehrlich and Langley.

The above speculations arose largely out of a study of the relationship between chemical structure and pharmacological activity. Fraser, Brunton and Fränkel had all done significant work in this newly emerging field. Fraser, for example, had demonstrated in collaboration with Alexander Crum Brown that quaternary ammonium compounds were, in general, associated with a paralyzing action (Parascandola, 1971; Bynum, 1970). It is not surprising that the realization that the physiological action of a drug is dependent upon its chemical structure would lead to support for the concept that drugs act by combining chemically with cell constituents.

Further evidence for this view was provided by studies of the phenomenon of drug antagonism. The fact that one substance might counteract the physiological effects of another had been recognized for centuries in the concept of antidotes for poisons. In the nineteenth century, however significant attention began to be devoted to the physiological antagonism between specific drugs, e.g., opium and belladonna (Bennett, 1875; Bartholow, 1881). The English physiologist John Newport Langley was apparently the first to explain this antagonism in terms of a chemical competition for a specific cell constituent. In 1874, while still a student at Cambridge University, he began to investigate the action of pilocarpine on the heart at the suggestion of his mentor, Michael Foster. He also studied its effects on secretion, especially the secretion of saliva by the submaxillary gland. During the course of his work, he observed that atropine and pilocarpine were mutually exclusive in their actions on the gland. In a paper published in 1878, he explained this antagonism as follows (Langley, 1878):

'. . . we may, I think, without much rashness, assume that there is a substance or substances in the nerve endings or gland cells with which both atropine and pilocarpine are capable of forming compounds. On this assumption then the atropin or pilocarpin compounds are formed according to some law of which their relative mass and chemical affinity for the substance are factors.'

This statement certainly contains the germ of the receptor theory, but Langley did not follow it up for another quarter of a century.

2. EHRLICH AND THE RECEPTOR THEORY IN IMMUNOLOGY

In the same year that Langley published the above-mentioned paper (1878), Paul Ehrlich received his medical degree from the University of Leipzig. While still a medical student, Ehrlich became interested in the problem of selective action, an interest that was to culminate in the development of his receptor theory. Ehrlich (1906) himself recalled that this interest was aroused by reading a work on lead poisoning by Emil Heubel (1871). Heubel had demonstrated that the lead content of the various organs differed greatly in animals which had been subjected to lead poisoning. Immersing the organs of normal animals in dilute lead solutions, Heubel found, led to similar differences.

Ehrlich recognized that this technique might be used to ascertain the site of action of poisons. To identify the organs affected, however, was for Ehrlich only the starting point for an investigation. The brain, for example, is a complex structure made up of various tissues, and Ehrlich wanted to know in which cells of the organ the poison was concentrated. His attempts to determine this information with the aid of a microscope, however, resulted in failure.

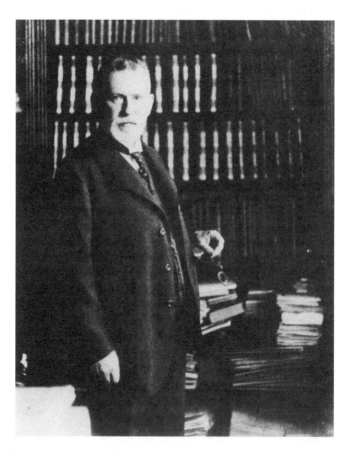

FIGURE 1. Paul Ehrlich (courtesy of the National Library of Medicine).

Intrigued by the question of the distribution of substances within the body, and convinced that distribution played a major role in governing pharmacological and toxicological action, Ehrlich soon tried another approach to investigating this problem. He decided to study the distribution of dyes in living tissues because here he could easily determine the distribution of a substance by its colour. His interest in dyes may well have been aroused by his cousin Carl Weigert, a pioneer in histological staining. The thesis that Ehrlich (1878) presented for his graduation in medicine at the University of Leipzig dealt with the theory and practice of histological staining. It is of interest to us here because it clearly demonstrates Ehrlich's early concern with selective affinity, in this case the affinity of particular dyes for certain types of tissues, and also his commitment to a chemical viewpoint. He argued that the process of staining was not merely the result of a physical adhesion of the dye to the tissue, but involved a chemical interaction between the two (probably similar to that involved in the formation of so-called 'double salts', i.e., the linking together of two apparently saturated compounds such as silver chloride and mercurous oxide).

Ehrlich's interest in dyes continued, and his 'Habilitationschrift' at the University of Berlin (Ehrlich, 1885a) was an investigation of the ability of different tissues to reduce certain dyestuffs. This work is important in the present context, however, largely because it concerns the first indication of his 'side-chain' theory of cellular action, a concept that played a very significant role in his later thinking about immunology and chemotherapy. Ehrlich adopted Edward Pfluger's view that protoplasm can be envisioned as a giant molecule consisting of a chemical nucleus of special structure which is responsible for the specific functions of a particular cell (e.g., a liver cell or a kidney cell), with attached chemical side chains. These side chains are more involved in the vital processes common to all cells, such as oxidation and nutrition. For example, he believed that some side chains probably consisted of 'combustible molecule-groups' that were consumed during the process of oxidation and then regenerated.

Ehrlich was later to apply the side chain theory to explain the process of immunization. In 1890, he was provided with laboratory space in Robert Koch's newly founded Institute for Infectious Diseases in Berlin and became actively involved in immunological research. His first account of the side chain theory of immunity was published in 1897.

Assume, Ehrlich (1897) postulated, that one of the 'receptive side chains' of the cell possesses an atom group with a specific combining property for a particular toxin, such as tetanus toxin. This side chain is normally involved in ordinary physiological processes, such as nutrition, and it is merely coincidental that it has the ability to combine with the toxin. Combination with the toxin, however, renders the side chain incapable of performing its normal physiological function. The cell then produces more of these side chains to make up for the deficiency, but it overcompensates so that excess side chains are produced, break away from the cell and are released into the bloodstream. These excess side chains in the blood are what we call antibodies or antitoxins. They neutralize the toxin by combining with it, thus preventing it from anchoring itself to the cell and exerting its poisonous effects. Ehrlich compared the interaction between toxin and side chain (or antitoxin) to that between a lock and a key, acknowledging his debt to Emil Fischer, who had earlier developed a 'lock and key' theory of enzyme action, for the analogy (see pp. 168 – 171).

Ehrlich (1897, 1898) went on to distinguish between what he called the 'toxophore' and the 'haptophore' groups of the toxin. The haptophore group is the group involved in binding the toxin to the side chain. Once the toxin is anchored to the cell, the latter comes under the influence of the toxophore group, which is responsible for the poisonous properties of the toxin. Ehrlich may very well have derived this concept from an analogy with dyes, where the chemical grouping responsible for colour is different from that responsible for fixing the dye to the fabric or tissue (see p. 160).

Ehrlich's theory became more elaborate as he struggled to explain various immunological phenomena, but we need not consider these modifications for our present purposes. Here we will just note that in 1900 Ehrlich introduced the term 'receptor' to refer to the 'receptive side chains' of the cell (Ehrlich, 1900a). We have considered his side chain theory of immunity only because this concept was later to be adapted to pharmacology. It must be stressed here, however, that Ehrlich did not apply the side chain theory to the question of drug action for some ten years. In fact, at first he specifically denied that drugs were bound to the cell in a manner similar to the binding of toxins. This fact has, with some exceptions (Blasko, 1969; Parascandola and Jasensky, 1974; Parascandola, 1980, 1981), generally been overlooked in accounts of Ehrlich's work.

3. EHRLICH CHANGES HIS MIND ABOUT DRUG RECEPTORS

Ehrlich's research in the 1890's was not limited to the field of immunology. The interest that he had developed in his medical school days concerning selective affinity had led him already in the 1880's to concern himself with the distribution of drugs as well as poisons and dyes. In the period 1885 – 1894, he published studies on the properties of various drugs, including iodine, thalline, methylene blue and cocaine (Ehrlich, 1885b, 1886; Ehrlich and Leppman, 1890; Gutmann and Ehrlich, 1891; Ehrlich and Einhorn, 1894).

These early studies reflect the interest in selective affinity and structure-activity relationships that was to continue to be exhibited in Ehrlich's later chemotherapeutic studies. For example, Ehrlich and Einhorn (1894) investigated the properties of cocaine and determined that the benzoyl radical was the portion of the molecule responsible for anaesthetic action (or, as Ehrlich phrased it, the 'anesthesiophore group' of the molecule). The chemical constitution of the drug molecule was also important, in Ehrlich's view, in determining the distribution of the substance in the body. At the time, he attributed the specific therapeutic action of a drug (such as anaesthetic properties) to the presence of a particular functional group, whereas he felt that the distribution of the drug depended upon the entire constitution or structure.

Although Ehrlich recognized the selective affinity of drugs for certain cells, and believed that this affinity was ultimately based on the structure of the molecule, he did not think it likely that a firm combination was formed between the drug and the cell, as in the case of toxins. He pointed out that many drugs can easily be extracted from tissues by solvents, thus they cannot be firmly bound. In addition, the action of many drugs is of a transitory character. Barring a few exceptions, chemically defined drugs and poisons, as opposed to foodstuffs and toxins, are not incorporated into the protoplasmic molecule by a chemical union. They do not possess haptophore groups and are not capable of evoking the production of antibodies (Ehrlich, 1902).

Ehrlich emphasized these points in his Croonian Lecture (Ehrlich, 1900b):

'If alkaloids, aromatic amines, antipyretics, or aniline dyes be introduced into the animal body it is a very easy matter, by means of water, alcohol, or acetone, according to the nature of the substance, to remove all these things quickly and easily from the tissues . . . We are therefore obliged to conclude that none of the foreign bodies just mentioned enter synthetically into the cell complex; but are merely contained in the cells in their free state. The combinations into which they enter with the cells, and notably with the not really living parts of them . . . are very unstable, and usually correspond only to the conditions in solid solutions, while in other cases only a feeble salt-like formation takes place . . .'

'Hence with regard to the pharmacologically active bodies in general, it was not allowable to assume that they possessed definite atom groups, which entered into combination with corresponding groups of the protoplasm.'

The specificity of drugs was thus not based on a specific affinity for a receptive side chain of the cell, as in the case of bacterial toxins. How then did Ehrlich explain the selective action of drugs? Here Ehrlich's work on dyes provided him with an analogy that he could apply to pharmacological agents.

The fixing of dyes, he noted, is not merely a mechanical or physical process involving surface attraction or absorption, but involves 'chemical' affinities in the broadest sense of the term. He discussed two current theories of the mechanism of dyeing, each of which might be correct in certain circumstances. The first of these involved the combination of the dye with a constituent of the fabric to form an insoluble, salt-like compound called a 'lake'. A similar process might occur, Ehrlich felt, in the tissues of the organism in the fixing of drugs. Cells which possessed constituents capable of forming a 'lake' with a particular drug could thus localize the substance.

Although the process involves chemical combination, it is quite different from Ehrlich's side chain or receptor concept. The drug is not thought to combine with the cellular protoplasm (note Ehrlich's reference in the above quotation to the 'not really living parts' of the cell). Instead, it is believed to react with a free substance in the cell, such as an acid, to form an insoluble complex which precipitates out of solution and is thus fixed in the cell.

The second theory of dyeing discussed by Ehrlich involved the formation of solid solutions, where the dye forms a homogeneous mixture with the substance of the fabric. He suggested that a similar process, involving the lipid portion of the cell, might be responsible for the fixing of certain drugs. We must assume, Ehrlich stated, 'that certain fat-like substances of the nervous system, as well as the fat of fat cells, possess a high solvent power, by means of which these soluble substances are anchored or accumulated in the tissue'. Again, this mechanism (based upon the physicochemical property of solubility) is quite different from the side chain theory, and does not involve chemical combination between an atom group of the drug and an atom group of the cell. Barring a few exceptions, Ehrlich argued, drugs do not enter into a 'chemical union' with the 'protoplasmic molecule' (Ehrlich, 1902).

In the case of drugs, Ehrlich believed at this time, there was no single definite 'haptophore' group that was responsible for fixing the drug in specific cells. Rather, the distribution of the drug depended upon the 'combined action of the separate components', and hence upon the 'entire constitution' of the molecule (Ehrlich, 1902). He further noted that whereas the haptophore groups of toxins exhibit a specific combining power towards certain atom groups of protoplasm, the ordinary functional groups of organic chemistry possess affinities for a large number of other groups. For example, aldehyde groups can unite with amino groups, methylene groups, etc. Their combining power is not specifically limited, hence the lock and key analogy (and the receptor concept) does not apply to drugs (Ehrlich, 1903).

Ehrlich's doubts about the probability of a 'true chemical combination' taking place between the drug and the cell were shared by many of his contemporaries. Chemical combination was generally thought of at the time essentially in terms of what we would call covalent and ionic bonds, which are not easily broken. Such concepts as hydrogen bonds and Van der Waals bonds had not yet been developed. It was thus hard to reconcile phenomena such as the ease with which many drugs could be washed out of tissues by solvents with the contemporary concepts of chemical bonding. Many pharmacologists leaned toward the view that drugs often induce their effects through their physical properties, by altering the surface tension, electrolytic balance, osmotic pressure, etc. of the cell, rather than through the formation of chemical bonds with protoplasmic constituents (Parascandola, 1974).

By 1907, however, Ehrlich had come to change his mind about the probable mechanism of the drug action. Already in 1906, he had accepted the view that a specific chemical group (the 'selective group'), rather than the entire structure of the molecule, is responsible for fixing drugs in particular cells (Ehrlich, 1906). And in his Harben Lectures of June, 1907, he fully embraced the receptor concept for drugs (Ehrlich, 1907b):

> 'I have now formed the opinion that some of the chemically defined substances are
> attached to the cell, by atom groupings that are analogous to toxin-receptors; these
> atom groupings I will distinguish from the toxin-receptors by the name of 'chemo-
> receptors'.'

What had happened to change Ehrlich's mind about the mechanism of drug action? Two important factors appear to have played a role in altering his thinking, the work of J.N. Langley and studies in Ehrlich's own laboratory on drug
resistance. Looking back at this period, Ehrlich (1914) later said:

> 'For many reasons I had hesitated to apply these ideas about receptors to chemical
> substances in general, and in this connection it was, in particular, the brilliant in-
> vestigations by Langley, on the effects of alkaloids, which caused my doubts to
> disappear and made the existence of chemoreceptors seem probable to me.'

We must thus turn back to Langley and consider these investigations to which
Ehrlich refers.

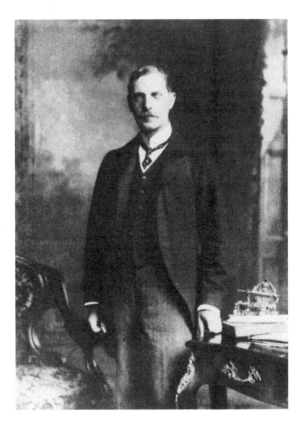

FIGURE 2. John Newport Langley (courtesy of the National Library of Medicine).

4. LANGLEY AND RECEPTIVE SUBSTANCES

After completing his medical degree at Cambridge University, John Newport Langley spent his entire career on the faculty of that institution. Beginning in the late 1880's, he became involved in a detailed study of the autonomic nervous system for which he eventually received widespread recognition. During the course of this research, he found that nicotine was a useful tool in the investigation of the structures and functions of the autonomic system. Some of his early experimental work in this area (Langley and Dickinson, 1889, 1890) suggested to him that the paralysis of sympathetic nerves caused by nicotine was due to a direct action of the drug on the nerve cells of the superior cervical ganglia, rather than on the peripheral endings of the sympathetic nerves. A decade later (Langley, 1901a), he was able to more convincingly demonstrate that the stimulation of sympathetic ganglia by nicotine, which preceded paralysis of the nerves, was due to a direct action on the nerve cells. Even after severing the preganglionic fibres and allowing the nerve endings to degenerate, nicotine still exerted its usual stimulating effect on the ganglia.

At about the same time, Langley (1901b) also reported on a study of the effects of supra-renal extract, which contained adrenaline as its active ingredient. His interest in this substance was probably motivated by the fact that it was known to produce certain effects similar to those resulting from stimulation of the sympathetic nerves. Supra-renal extract thus seemed like another potential tool for the investigation of the autonomic nerves. Although the fact that the extract produced effects similar to those produced by stimulating the sympathetic nerves might suggest that it acted on these nerves, Langley came to a different conclusion. He confirmed and extended the earlier observation of Lewandowsky that supra-renal extract continued to exert its effects after degeneration of the postganglionic sympathetic nerves had taken place. To Langley, this was strong evidence that the action must be directly on the tissues affected, such as unstriated muscle, rather than on the nerve endings.

Langley's controversial findings were challenged by Brodie and Dixon (1904), who argued that supra-renal extract acted either on the nerve endings or the 'connection link' between them. Elliot (1905) elaborated on this latter suggestion and developed a theory of the action of adrenaline on the 'myo-neural junction'. But Langley was convinced that there was more or less satisfactory evidence that a number of drugs and poisons act directly on tissues such as muscle and gland, rather than through the nerve endings or a hypothetical myoneural junction. It was in an attempt to provide further evidence for this point of view that he was led to develop the receptor theory, which was first described in a paper published in 1905 and in his Croonian Lecture of the following year (Langley, 1905, 1906).

In an effort to test his hypothesis on striated muscle tissue, Langley decided to investigate the muscular contraction that was known to be produced in fowl by injection of nicotine. Earlier this contraction had appeared to him to be largely due to a stimulation of the nerve endings (Langley, 1903). In 1905, however, he decided to examine this phenomenon in greater detail in connection with the developing controversy about the site of action of drugs such as nicotine and adrenaline. The injection of nicotine into the fowl caused certain muscles to contract, in fact to pass into a state of tonic rigidity. Nicotine, of course, also exerted a paralyzing action, when administered in sufficient quantities, by preventing stimulation of the motor nerve from having any effect upon the muscle. Yet Langley (1905, 1906) found that even after the nervous-muscular connection had been blocked by relatively large doses of nicotine, further administration of the drug still continued to cause muscular contraction. Could it be, he asked, that nicotine acted upon two different parts of the neuro-muscular mechanism, paralyzing the nerve endings (thus preventing nervous stimulation of muscle) while at the same time directly stimulating the muscle? Since the paralyzing effect of curare, like that of nicotine, was believed to be due to an action on the nerve endings, Langley reasoned that if the contraction caused by nicotine in fowls was really due to a direct action on the muscle cell it should not be antagonized by curare. He found to the contrary, however, that curare had a marked antagonizing effect; a sufficient dose of curare completely annulled the contraction produced by a small amount of nicotine and diminished that caused by a large amount. Further injection of nicotine once again resulted in contraction.

Langley investigated next the effects of these drugs when no nerve endings were present, i.e. after cutting the nerves to the muscle and allowing them to degenerate. He found that nicotine still produced contraction after section of the nerves, and, in fact, that curare continued to antagonize this contracting action. He could only conclude that both substances were capable of a direct action on the muscle cell.

To explain the observed antagonism between nicotine and curare, Langley (1905, 1906) returned to the suggestion he had made in 1878 when discussing the antagonism between atropine and pilocarpine. The two drugs must act on the same protoplasmic substance or substances in the muscle, and presumably this involved a combination of the alkaloid with protoplasm. In the presence of both nicotine and curare, which muscle-alkaloid compound is formed depends upon the amount of each alkaloid present and on their relative chemical affinities for the muscle substance.

Since the contracting effect of nicotine and the antagonistic effect of curare were apparently due to an action on the muscle, Langley (1905, 1906) questioned whether there was any justification for the accepted view that the paralyzing action of these compounds occurred at the nerve endings. He saw no need to postulate two different sites of action. Since the curare decreased the irritability of the muscle to the nicotine stimulus, he felt that it was not unreasonable to assume that it also decreased the irritability of the muscle to nervous stimuli, inducing paralysis in this fashion. Nicotine prevented stimulation of the nerves from causing contraction in the same manner, but it also had the ability of itself stimulating the contraction of muscle.

After a muscle had been paralyzed by curare or nicotine and it no longer reacted to nervous stimulation, the muscle could still be directly stimulated to contract, e.g., by an electrical current. The muscle substance with which these drugs combined, Langley reasoned, could thus not be the substance which actually contracts. Instead, nicotine and curare must combine with some other constituent of the muscle cell, and he called this unknown constituent 'receptive substance'. He postulated that the normal function of this receptive substance is to receive the stimulus from the nerve and transmit it to the contractile substance. By combining with the receptive substance, curare and nicotine might diminish its excitability or irritability, hence preventing nervous stimuli from having any effect (Langley, 1905, 1906). In 1906, he suggested alternatively that it was also possible that the transmission of an impulse from nerve to muscle does not take place via an electrical discharge, but involves the secretion of a special chemical substance at the end of the nerve. The receptive substance in the muscle cell combines with the chemical transmitter, forming a compound which stimulates the contractible substance. If curare or nicotine combine with the receptive substance, they prevent it from uniting with the transmitter substance and thus block the passage of nervous impulses (Langley, 1906). Since the contractile substance itself is not altered by these drugs, however, it can still be directly stimulated. The nicotine-receptive substance compound, although blocking nervous transmission, must have a certain ability to stimulate the contractive substance and cause contraction.

Langley felt that there was evidence to suggest that many other drugs and poisons, such as adrenaline, acted by combining with specific constituents of the cell. He generalized (Langley, 1905):

'I conclude then that in all cells two constituents at least must be distinguished, (1) substances concerned with carrying out the chief functions of the cells, such as contraction, secretion, the formation of special metabolic products and (2) receptive substances especially liable to change and capable of setting the chief substance in action. Further, that nicotine, curare, atropine, pilocarpine, strychnine, and most other alkaloids, as well as the effective material of internal secretions produce their effects by combining with the receptive substance, and not by an action on axon-endings if these are present, nor by a direct action on the chief substance.'

The fact that drugs produce different effects in different cells indicates that all cells do not possess the same receptive substance or substances. One would expect, however, that the receptive substances of the cells within a given class would be similar. Consequently, Langley argued, the fact that the effects of adrenaline on different tissues are always like those produced by stimulation of the sympathetic nerves does not mean that it acts by stimulating these nerves. The relationship of adrenaline to the sympathetic system could be explained by assuming that the presence of sympathetic nerves during the development of certain tissues created a certain chemical environment which led to the formation in these tissues of similar receptive substances, substances which had the ability to combine with adrenaline (Langley, 1905).

Langley (1905) also suggested that the receptive substances and the other substances responsible for carrying out the function of the cell need not actually be separate compounds. It is possible, he commented, that the receptive substance is a side chain on the contractile molecule. In his Croonian Lecture (Langley, 1906), he leaned towards the more general idea that all of these different substances (receptive substance, contractile substance, etc.) are 'radicles' or side chains of the protoplasmic molecule. Langley (1905) recognized and specifically mentioned the similarity of such views to Ehrlich's side chain theory of immunity. In his continued work on the receptive substance concept and its application to pharmacology, he moved more firmly towards the side chain model of Ehrlich. In one paper, Langley (1908) wrote:

'My theory of the action is in general on the lines of Ehrlich's theory of immunity. I take it that the contractile molecule has a number of 'receptive' or side-chain radicles, and that the nicotine by combining with one of these causes contraction and by combining with another, causes twitching . . .'

We must now return to Ehrlich and his development of the chemoreceptor concept for drugs.

5. EHRLICH'S CHEMORECEPTOR THEORY

Although Ehrlich himself admitted that Langley's work was instrumental in changing his mind about drug receptors, it is questionable whether he would have been prepared to accept Langley's views had not the studies being carried out in his own laboratory on drug resistance given him another reason for altering his ideas. It was in dealing with the phenomenon of drug resistance that he first applied the receptor concept to drugs.

About 1903, Ehrlich and his coworkers had begun in earnest their work in chemotherapy with a study of the effects of various chemicals in treating infections caused by trypanosomes, the microorganisms responsible for certain diseases such as sleeping sickness. Over the next few years, their work and that of other investigators established that there were three different classes of compounds which could attack trypanosomes (Ehrlich, 1907a):

1. arsenical compounds, such as atoxyl;
2. azo dyes, such as trypan red; and
3. basic triphenylmethane dyes, such as fuchsin.

In the period 1905 – 1907, experiments carried out by Franke, Röhl and

Browning in Ehrlich's laboratory demonstrated that a strain of trypanosomes which is susceptible to treatment with a particular drug, such as atoxyl, may, on continued exposure to that drug, develop a resistance to such treatment. In other words, a trypanosome strain is produced which no longer responds to treatment with the drug. Resistance was found not to be limited to the compound used to develop it, but to extend also to other compounds within the same chemical class. For example, the atoxyl-resistant strain exhibited a significant degree of resistance towards other arsenical compounds, such as acetylatoxyl, and the trypan-red resistant strain exhibited some resistance towards other azo dyes, such as trypan blue and trypan violet. The development of resistance towards one group of compounds (e.g., the arsenicals), however, did not increase resistance towards compounds of other classes (e.g., azo dyes).

In his first published report of these results, Ehrlich (1907a) offered a brief and somewhat vague explanation for this specificity, but one which would seem to suggest an acceptance of the receptor concept for drugs. He argued that one must imagine that the protoplasm of trypanosomes (and, in general, of all cells) must possess different 'places of attack' ('Angriffsstellen') for which specific types of drugs have particular affinities.

Ehrlich's first clear exposition of his concept of 'chemoreceptors' was in his previously mentioned Harben Lectures (Ehrlich, 1907b). As we have already noted, he pointed out in these lectures that he had come to believe that at least some drugs are bound to the protoplasm by certain atom groupings in a manner somewhat analogous to the binding of toxins. The chemoreceptors for drugs, however, were simpler in structure and less independent than the toxin receptors (e.g., they could not be separated from the cell to form antibodies).

A given drug or poison, Ehrlich continued, would only attack a cell (or a unicellular microorganism, such as the trypanosome) if the cell possessed chemoreceptors capable of combining with it. Like the 'nutrireceptors' that are attacked by microbial toxins, however, chemoreceptors are ordinarily engaged with the normal substances of nutrition or metabolism, and hence are present in all cells. Hence, Ehrlich explained, any chemical drug is likely to have an affinity for the cells of the host organism as well as for the parasite. In order for a drug to be an effective chemotherapeutic agent, it must have a greater affinity for the chemoreceptors of the parasite cells than for those of the host cells, or its 'parasitotropic' force must be greater than its 'organotropic' force. In other words, one must be able to produce a curative effect with a dose that is not injurious to the host.

The studies on drug resistance, Ehrlich (1907b) argued, supported the concept of chemoreceptors. The atoxyl-resistant strain, for example, was resistant to a number of arsenic compounds which otherwise possessed significant differences in their chemical characteristics. The arsenic acid radicle, however, represents a common point of attack in this series. It is bound to the cell by chemoreceptors. The trypanosome cell possesses other chemoreceptors which represent the points of attack for other poisons. The development of resistance could be readily explained by Ehrlich in terms of the receptor concept. The chemoreceptors of resistant trypanosome strains have somehow developed a reduced affinity for the drug, so that the distribution of the drug between the microorganisms and the host animal is shifted in the direction of the latter.

In his early discussions of the mode of action of arsenicals, Ehrlich emphasized the binding of the arsenic radicle to a chemoreceptor in the cell. He even speculated about the chemical nature of the 'arsenoreceptor', suggesting that it might be a hydroxyl or sulphydryl group, a remarkably accurate prediction, as Carl Voegtlin later showed that the chemical grouping involved in reacting with arsenic is indeed a sulphydryl group (Parascandola, 1977). But Ehrlich soon developed a more complex explanation of drug action involving more than one receptor for a given drug.

As Ehrlich (1909a) noted, if aromatic arsenic compounds were anchored to the cell exclusively through the trivalent arsenic atom bound on the phenyl residue and this anchorage was the determining factor in the action of this class of drugs, then one would expect that the simplest such compounds (such as phenylarsenic acid and arsenobenzene) would be the best substances for treatment. But this was not the case. In fact, the introduction of substituents in the *para*-position of the benzene ring in phenylarsenic acid greatly influenced toxicity and therapeutic action. For example, the introduction of an amino group in this position promotes the action of the drug.

In order to explain the fact that substitutions in the benzene ring, which do not affect the arsenic radicle itself, modify the action of the drug, Ehrlich (1909b) postulated that for complicated drugs other groupings in the molecule beside the arsenic residue are also involved in binding the drug to the cell. The addition, removal, or modification of such groups therefore affects the fixation of the compound to the cell and consequently its pharmacological action. The drug becomes successively fastened by its various groupings to the specific 'fangs' or 'snares' ('Fangen'), i.e., the chemoreceptors, of the protoplasm. Ehrlich, in his usual graphic way, compared the process to the mounting of a butterfly which is fixed first by the torso and then successively by the wings with pins.

He noted, however, that one can frequently determine experimentally a grouping which brings about the primary anchoring, and this grouping can be designated the 'primary haptophore'. In the drug arsenophenylglycine, for example, Ehrlich (1909b) felt that the acetic acid radicle was the group that primarily anchored the drug to the cell. Ehrlich was essentially applying the haptophore-toxophore concept that he utilized in immunology to the problem of drug action, with the stipulation that there could be more than one haptophore group involved in binding a drug.

This fact is perhaps most clearly seen in Ehrlich's discussion of the mode of action of Salvarsan, as expressed in his lecture before the International Congress of Medicine in 1913 (Ehrlich, 1914):

'Now, if we are to look for specific medicaments, the first condition is that they must possess a certain definite group which is chemically allied to one of the chemoreceptors of the parasites. This is only one of the prerequisites necessary for the medicament to be effective, but generally it is not sufficient in itself. Hundreds of substances may fix themselves to a parasite but only a few are capable of bringing about destruction.'

'Thus, in the therapeutically suitable substance there must be present, in addition to the anchoring or haptophore group, which brings about the fixation, another group which brings about the destruction, and which, therefore, is characterized as the poisoning, or toxophore group. This concept exactly corresponds to the views which we have already held for years with respect to the toxins, in which we distinguish the presence of a haptophore group which causes the anchorage to the cell and also the formation of the antitoxins, and a toxophore group which brings about the injurious action on the cell. For the more complicated synthetic medicaments the assumption will have to be made that the haptophore group and the toxophore group are not directly connected with one another, but that they, as residues, are attached like side-chains, to a chemical molecule. Thus, quite simply, the more complicated chemotherapeutic agents may be compared to a poison-arrow; the anchoring group of the medicament which anchors itself to the chemoreceptor of the parasite corresponds to the point of the arrow, the connecting link to the shaft, and the poison group to the arrow poison affixed to the shaft of the arrow. According to this scheme, in Salvarsan, dihydroxydiaminoarsenobenzene, the benzene nucleus would correspond to the shaft, the *o*-aminophenol group to the point, and the trivalent arsenic radical to the poison . . .'

'If, therefore, we poison a spirochaete with Salvarsan, at least two different chemical anchorages occur; first, the anchorage of the *o*-aminophenol group which primarily anchors the Salvarsan to the parasite. It is only in consequence of this anchorage that, second, the trivalent arsenic radical is given the opportunity of entering into chemical combination with the arsenoceptor of the cell, and so of exerting its toxic action. The avidity of the arsenoceptor may, in itself, be so small that a reaction can take place only if favourable factors, which chemically must be regarded as steric facilitation, are operating. Examples of steric facilitations of this kind are frequently found in pure chemistry, e.g., in the chemistry of *ortho*-condensations. Thus the haptophore group of the arsenical primarily brings the arsenic into contact with the cell and secondarily provides an opportunity for its action'.

Even before Ehrlich had applied the receptor concept to drugs, as we have seen, he had argued that the search for specific medicaments should be based on searching for substances that possessed a particular affinity for a certain organ and then using such substances as vehicles to carry therapeutically active groups to the organ involved. Now, however, this concept was expressed in terms of chemoreceptors. Ehrlich (1914) felt that the chemotherapeutist must aim to discover for every type of parasite the characteristic haptophore group with the aid of which one could force a specific therapeutic radicle (such as arsenic) upon the parasite. One must, in other words, learn what chemoreceptors are possessed by specific parasites. The ideal situation would be to find a chemoreceptor which is present only in the parasite and not in the cells of the host.

Of course, as Ehrlich (1914) recognized, such ideal drugs would not be easy to find. We must often be satisfied to find substances which have a greater affinity for a particular chemoreceptor in a parasite than for the corresponding chemoreceptor in a human cell. A knowledge of the different chemoreceptors of a parasite, or what Ehrlich designated as 'the therapeutic physiology of the parasite cell', was for him 'a *sine qua non* for success in chemotherapy'. The larger the number of different chemoreceptors that could be demonstrated, the greater the possibility of successful chemotherapy.

6. IMPACT OF EHRLICH-LANGLEY RECEPTOR THEORY

Langley and Ehrlich thus developed their versions of receptor theory from different backgrounds and for different purposes. Although they worked independently, each was influenced in some measure (as we have seen) by the work of the other. Langley's concept developed out of his investigations on the actions of nicotine and adrenaline, which were occasioned by his interest in the sympathetic nervous system. The receptor idea came to play an important part in his understanding of the interaction of nerves and other tissues, such as muscle. Ehrlich's theory developed out of his studies on drug resistance, which were a result of his interest in the chemotherapy of trypanosomes, and ultimately out of his side chain concept of cellular function. The receptor concept came to form the theoretical basis of his work in chemotherapy.

Langley's version of the theory focused on the action of drugs on animals, and dealt essentially with substances whose action was (in relative terms) readily reversible. In fact, the phenomenon of antagonism played a crucial role in the development of his ideas. On the other hand, Ehrlich's chemoreceptor concept was more concerned with the effects of chemicals on microorganisms (with the host animal playing a more indirect role). His studies came to focus on substances, such as the arsenicals, whose action was not readily reversible. It was the specificity of drug action that motivated his thinking, and the reversibility of drug action actually hindered for a time his adoption of the receptor theory.

Langley (1909) also tried to distinguish at one point between two different types of side chain radicles, 'receptive atom groups' and 'fundamental atom groups'. If a drug or poison combines with a 'receptive atom group', it may alter its function, but will not cause serious injury to the rest of the protoplasmic molecule (i.e., will not lead to the destruction of the cell). Since the combination of arsenic compounds with the chemoreceptors of trypanosomes results in the destruction of the microorganisms, these chemoreceptors must therefore represent 'fundamental atom groups'. Thus Langley's 'receptive class' actually excluded Ehrlich's chief example of a chemoreceptor. This distinction, however, would appear to be more semantic than substantive with respect to the overall concept.

The impact of the receptor theory of Ehrlich and Langley on pharmacology was very limited in their lifetimes. The science of pharmacology had not advanced far enough by the early decades of the twentieth century to permit a theory which dealt essentially with molecular mechanisms to be confirmed or denied by experimental means. More importantly, pharmacologists probably still had too much to learn about the action of drugs at the level of the organ (and even the organism) to be fruitfully guided in their research by a general and speculative theory of the interaction between the drug and the cell.

The receptor theory was by no means ignored, however, in the period between its introduction in the first decade of the century and Langley's death in 1925 (Ehrlich had died in 1915). Supporters and critics offered evidence for and against the theory, but pharmacologists could not come to a consensus concerning its validity and/or utility.

Those who supported the view that drugs act by combining chemically with protoplasmic constituents emphasized the specificity of drug action and the relationship between chemical structure and pharmacological action. Simon and Wood (1941a, b), for example, emphasized that the inhibiting effect of certain basic dyes on bacteria seemed to be intimately dependent upon the presence in the molecule of specific chemical groups (e.g., triphenylmethane, amino). They also stressed, as had Ehrlich, the specificity of drug resistance, and concluded that to 'explain these individual peculiarities upon a purely physical basis would certainly be difficult'. Schamberg, Kolmer and Raiziss (1917) also justified their support of Ehrlich's chemoreceptor hypothesis largely on the grounds of the importance of specific chemical moieties (e.g., the arsenic and amino groups) in determining the chemotherapeutic action of organic arsenicals (suggesting the presence of specific receptors).

A.V. Hill (1909), working in Langley's laboratory at Cambridge, offered some quantitative evidence in favour of the receptor theory. Hill studied the contraction of the rectus abdominus muscle of the frog caused by nicotine, and showed that the time curve of the reaction could readily be explained by assuming that the nicotine reacts reversibly with some constituent of the muscle,

$$N + A \rightleftarrows NA.$$

Although Hill was pursuing the general line of attack that was later to be taken up by A.J. Clark, his paper does not seem to have had a significant impact on the pharmacological field.

Critics of the receptor theory focused on several points. As noted earlier, many pharmacologists and other biomedical researchers doubted that drugs entered into a chemical combination with cellular constituents because of such facts as the ease with which most drugs could be washed out of tissues by solvents and the relatively transitory action of many drugs. Supporters of the 'physical' view, such as William Bayliss (1915), Walter Straub (1912) and Isidor Traube (1919), suggested that the action of most drugs could be attributed to their physical or physicochemical properties, such as solubility and conductivity. Under this approach, drugs were presumed to exert their effects by influencing the surface tension, electrolytic balance, etc. of the cell.

The physicochemical viewpoint downplayed chemical specificity. It was pointed out (Alsberg, 1921) that substances of very widely different chemical structure may have a similar physiological action, and that many chemically inert substances (e.g., hydrocarbons) exhibit significant pharmacological activity (Bayliss, 1915). The fact that changes in chemical structure may result in changes in pharmacological action was explained by noting that such structural changes also altered the physical properties of the molecule (Alsberg, 1921; Bayliss, 1915; Traube, 1919). Thus, chemical constitution affected physiological action only indirectly, through the modification of the molecule's physical properties. Specificity was reduced to physiochemical factors such as solubility. A drug might exert a specific effect on a given tissue, for example, because its solubility characteristics resulted in its accumulation in that tissue (Parascandola, 1974).

This controversy over the mechanism of drug action was part of a broader dispute at the time over the value of physical chemistry versus structural organic chemistry as explanatory models in the biological sciences. Immunology and biochemistry, for example, experienced similar debates to the one in pharmacology over related questions, such as the mode of action of enzymes or antibodies (Mazumdar, 1974; Kohler, 1975; Fruton, 1976). As the boundaries between 'physical' and 'chemical' forces came to be drawn less rigidly as a result of the work of Langmuir (1916) and others, the controversy eventually came to lose its meaning. Already during the period we are now considering, many investigators took an intermediate position in the controversy over drug action, noting that both physical and chemical factors were probably involved, with one or the other type perhaps dominating in certan cases (Barger and Dale, 1910; Greene, 1914; Sollmann, 1917), or pointing out (as Ehrlich himself had recognized) that processes such as adsorption could not be conceived of as purely 'physical' in nature (Dale, 1920; Storm van Leeuwen, 1924).

Another aspect of the Ehrlich-Langley theory which came under attack was the concept of chemical side chains. The view of the cell as a giant protoplasmic molecule was coming to be replaced in the early decades of the twentieth century by a more dynamic concept of the cell as a highly differentiated and coordinated system of enzymes and other molecules (Dixon, 1912; Hopkins, 1913; Bayliss,

1915; Teich, 1973). If a drug did combine chemically with some substance in the cell, it would have to be with a specific constituent (such as an enzyme) rather than with a side chain of the protoplasmic molecule as envisioned by Ehrlich. So, for example, when Carl Voegtlin identified the 'arsenic receptor' for organic arsenical drugs as a sulphydryl group in the 1920's, he envisioned this 'receptor' as a sulphydryl group on a glutathione molecule or a tissue protein (Parascandola, 1977).

Although the controversy surrounding the receptor concept stimulated some experimental research and sharpened the focus of discussions on the mechanism of drug action, the theory did not play a major role in the development of pharmacology before the 1930's. It remained too speculative and general for it to be universally accepted or exceptionally useful as a basis on which to build pharmacological theory and guide pharmacological research. In 1924, for example, Storm van Leeuwen (1924) discussed his researches on the interaction of alkaloids with blood serum, referring to the process as one of 'adsorption'. He was content, however, to leave the question of whether the combination of the drug and the serum was physical or chemical to the chemist, for he saw this question as immaterial to the pharmacological problem. What mattered to Storm van Leeuwen was that the combination was easily reversible and followed definite quantitative laws.

It was largely through the work of A.J. Clark in the 1920's and 1930's that the receptor theory became a generally accepted concept in pharmacology, and we must now turn our attention to Clark and his role in the receptor story.

7. A.J. CLARK AND RECEPTOR THEORY

Alfred Joseph Clark was trained in physiology at Cambridge University during the very period (1903 – 1907) when Langley was first elaborating his theory of receptive substances. He was later (1914) to also receive his M.D. from Cambridge. Walter Dixon, who taught pharmacology at Cambridge and at Kings College in London, first stimulated Clark's interest in pharmacology. At his suggestion, Clark studied the pressor action of tyramine in man, leading to his first pharmacological publication (Clark, 1910).

Clark's publications in the period 1912 – 1914, when he was working in the London laboratories of Dixon and Arthur Cushny, indicate that his interest in the mechanism of drug action at a cellular level developed early in his career. In these early papers, Clark (1912, 1913a, 1913b, 1914) focused on the action of inorganic ions and of various glycosides on the isolated heart. His experiments with the glycoside strophanthin confirmed the observations of Straub (1910) that very little of the drug entered the heart, indicating that the drug acted on this organ without actually penetrating the heart cells. Clark (1913b) concluded that it was probable 'that, as Straub suggested, strophanthin acts by altering the physical condition of the surface membrane of the cells, without entering into chemical combination with the cell constituents'. Thus early in his career Clark leaned towards the physicochemical view of drug action over the chemical receptor theory, at least in the case of strophanthin.

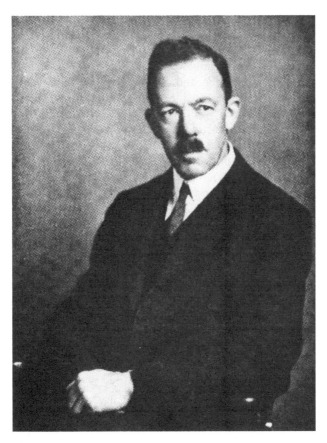

FIGURE 3. Alfred Joseph Clark (courtesy of Dr. David H. Clark).

Clark's work was interrupted at about this time by the outbreak of World War I. After four years of military service and a year of teaching at the University of Cape Town, South Africa, he was appointed to the chair of pharmacology at University College, London in 1919. Clark's efforts in the early 1920's essentially continued in the tradition of his earlier work, focusing at first on the effects of various ions on isolated organs and later on the action of organic drugs such as ergot and adrenaline (e.g., Clark 1921; Knaus and Clark,

1925). It was the study of one of these drugs, acetylcholine, that apparently led Clark to adopt the receptor theory.

It is not entirely clear what prompted Clark to investigate the action of acetylcholine. The drug's powerful pharmacological action had first been reported by Hunt and Taveau (1906), and was later studied more extensively by Dale (1914). At the time of Clark's work, however, it had not yet been demonstrated that it occurs naturally in the animal body, nor had it been positively identified as Otto Loewi's 'vagus substance' (Singer and Underwood, 1962). Clark (1926) himself stated in his first paper on the action of acetylcholine that it was especially well adapted for the study of the laws governing the reaction between drugs and cells for the following reasons: (1) it produces a graded response over a wide range of concentrations; (2) it affects a variety of tissues and produces different types of actions in different tissues; and (3) it acts rapidly and its action is quickly and completely reversible, so that large numbers of experiments can be performed on a single preparation.

He examined the action of the drug on two different muscles of the frog, the ventricle of the heart and the Rectus abdominus. Acetylcholine inhibits the contraction of the former and produces contraction of the latter. The experiments were done with isolated preparations of the muscles.

In both cases, Clark found that the relationship between the concentration and the action of the drug closely fitted the equation

$$K \cdot x = y/100 - y,$$

where x = concentration of the drug and y = action produced, expressed in terms of per cent of maximum action. It appeared improbable to him that the agreement between the measurements obtained and the formula was a chance one.

The simplest explanation for this equation, Clark suggested, would be 'to suppose that a reversible monomolecular reaction occurs between the drug and some receptor in the cells'. A similar type of curve, he pointed out, had been observed for the dissociation of oxyhaemoglobin in dilute solution (i.e., for the reaction between oxygen and haemoglobin, $O_2 + Hb \rightleftarrows HbO_2$). Clark (1933) later noted the similarity of this equation (and curve) to Langmuir's adsorption formula for freely reversible processes, such as the adsorption of gases by metal surfaces. All of these formulae can be derived from the law of mass action.

Clark (1926) also observed that there was no direct relationship between the amount of drug entering the cell and the amount of action produced. Recall that when he observed a similar phenomenon in the case of strophanthin a decade earlier, he used it as evidence against the idea that a chemical reaction takes place between the drug and some constituent of the cell. Now, however, he suggested that such a reaction might indeed take place if the receptor were on the surface of the cell and not inside it. In that case, the drug would not have to enter the cell in order to combine with the receptor.

With the aid of some clever calculations involving assumptions about such things as the space occupied by an acetylcholine molecule, Clark (1926, 1927) was able to convince himself that the drug did not act by simply covering the surface of the cell, but that it specifically reacted with only selected portions of the cell surface, i.e. the receptors.

But this evidence, however suggestive, was of a rather tenuous nature. Clark realized that the level of exactness in pharmacological data at the time was sufficiently low that one had to be careful in drawing conclusions simply on the basis of fitting data to mathematical formulae. This point was stressed by Clark (1932, 1933) several times in his writings. The fact that the assumption of a monomolecular reaction between a drug and a receptor on the cell would explain the curve obtained for the action of acetylcholine was not in itself proof that such a reaction takes place.

When Clark (1933) developed his version of the receptor theory more fully in his classic book, *The Mode of Action of Drugs,* he amassed other evidence to support his views. It was important to him that an explanation of drug action be based on a plausible physico-chemical model. There was no point, he stated, in fitting curves to a formula that did not express some possible physicochemical process (Clark, 1933).

Clark built his model of the mechanism of drug action on information from various fields. He felt, for example, that the process of catalysis provided an analogue for the receptor concept. The study of contact catalysis had recently shown, for example, that even in simple inorganic systems chemical reactions might be due to 'active patches' that covered only a small proportion of the surface of the catalyst. The proportion of the surface area occupied by these 'active patches' might range from 1/100 to 1/1000. These catalysts often selectively absorbed specific substances, and Clark (1933) pointed out the similarities between this process and that of specific drug action.

He also drew upon recent biochemical evidence to support his receptor concept (Clark, 1933). Contemporary research suggested that cellular oxidation occurred at specific centres on the cell surface and that the activity of certain large enzyme molecules, such as urease, depended upon the presence of a few active sites or receptors. In addition, he saw the receptor concept as fitting within the picture of the cell, then being developed by Rudolf Peters and others (Teich, 1973), as an organized network of protein molecules forming a three-dimensional mosaic extending throughout the cell. This conception of the cell structure made it possible to envision how a drug, by reacting with a relatively small number of receptor molecules on the cell surface, could alter the cell's activities by changing the surface pattern and thus affecting the orientation of the interior of the cell.

Clark (1933) also examined various alternatives to the receptor theory, such as Walter Straub's theory that the action of certain drugs depended upon the potential gradient between the concentrations of the drug inside and outside the cell. He found all of these alternative hypotheses less satisfying than the receptor concept, thereby strengthening his conviction that the receptor theory provided the best available explanation for the action of most drugs. Admitting the lack of direct evidence to support the receptor model, Clark (1933) therefore nevertheless adopted it as a basis for pharmacological theory.

'There is indeed very little direct evidence that the biological response is produced by a chemical reaction between the drug and the cell constituents. This assumption is chiefly justified by the facts that it is supported by much indirect evidence, and that there is no alternative hypothesis which has stronger evidence in its support'.

Four years later, in another monograph on *General Pharmacology,* Clark (1937) returned to his defense of the receptor theory. His treatment of the subject was basically similar to that in *The Mode of Action of Drugs on Cells,* except that he placed increased emphasis on the analogy between the reaction of drugs with receptors and the reaction of enzymes with substrates and poisons. No doubt Clark was influenced here by the extensive biochemical research on enzymes being carried out in the 1930's. An uncompleted and never published manuscript of a revised edition of *The Mode of Action,* which Clark (1941) was working on at the time of his death, devotes still greater attention to the study of enzymes and the significance of this subject for pharmacology. In the preface to this manuscript, Clark noted that since the first edition of the work, enzyme chemistry had developed very rapidly and the mode of action of drugs on enzymes had been extensively studied. Later in the text he stated that the poisoning of enzyme systems was one of the commonest means by which drugs act on living cells and he saw this subject as the 'most promising line of approach to the problem of the mode of action of drugs'.

In these later works, Clark (1937, 1941) also expanded his discussion of the organization of the cell based upon contemporary research. Admitting that our knowledge of this subject was imperfect, he emphasized that he felt it was necessary to postulate some sort of protoplasmic structure. It was difficult to conceive how the complex chain processes envisioned by contemporary biochemical theory could be carried out unless the different enzymes involved were oriented in some way. Clark assumed the cell to be a protein sol bounded by a surface membrane exhibiting marked selective permeability. He thought it likely that the cell surface consisted of a mosaic of proteins and lipids and that it contained many (though not necessarily all) of the enzymes essential for cell metabolism. In view of the highly specific nature of action of most drugs, he argued that it seemed probable that the receptors they combined with were parts of protein molecules (such as enzymes). Many of the receptors, he believed, were located on the cell surface.

It has often been pointed out in the pharmacological literature (e.g., Goodman and Gilman, 1965; Tallarida, 1981) that the classical receptor theory developed by Clark was an 'occupation theory', i.e., it assumed that the drug effect is proportional to the number of receptors occupied and that the maximal response occurs when all of the receptors are occupied. More recent work has challenged these assumptions. The concept of 'spare receptors', e.g., postulates that the maximal effect may be achieved when only a portion of the receptors is occupied, and 'rate theory' proposes that drug effect may be a function of the rate of drug-receptor combination rather than of the number of receptors occupied. It should be noted, however, that Clark himself, at least by 1937, admitted that it seemed improbable 'that the amount of biological effect produced is directly proportional to the number of specific receptors occupied by the drug'. The fact that a simple formula, such as that devised by Langmuir for the absorption of gases on metal filaments, could also express the concentration-action relations of many drugs in complex living systems was surprising, and Clark suggested that it probably represented an extreme simplification of the processes that actually occur. The simple end result was probably due in part to a mutual cancellation of independent variables and in part to the fact that the data are too inaccurate to demonstrate small deviations in the formula (Clark, 1937).

Recognizing the limitations of quantitative pharmacological data and the difficulty of attempting to prove a particular theory of the action of drugs on cells, Clark (1937) still felt that the effort was worth-while, 'even in our present incomplete state of knowledge'. The formulation of provisional hypotheses, he noted, provides an object for further research. 'The only danger is when such provisional hypotheses are mistaken for definitely established laws, and as a result inhibit rather than stimulate further investigation'. Therefore Clark emphasized the provisional nature of the theory that he had put forth.

Although contemporaries of Clark, such as J.H. Gaddum (1926, 1937), also contributed to the development of receptor theory in this period, it was largely through Clark's work that the theory became firmly established in pharmacological thought. It was not until after the Second World War, however, that receptor theory became a major focus of research interest in pharmacology. The work of Stephenson, Ariëns, Furchgott, Paton and others has led to further elaboration of the receptor concept, but these more recent developments are beyond the scope of this chapter.

8. ACKNOWLEDGEMENTS

Parts of this chapter were published earlier in modified form in Parascandola and Jasensky (1974), Parascandola (1980), Parascandola (1981) and Parascan-

154

dola (1982). The research was supported in part by grants from the National
Science Foundation (GS-41462) and the University of Wisconsin Graduate
School.

9. REFERENCES

Alsberg, C. (1921) J. Washington Acad. Sci. *11*, 321 – 341.

Ariëns, E.J. (1979) Trends Pharmacol. Sci. *1*, (inaug. issue), 11 – 15.

Barger, G. and Dale, H.H. (1910) J. Physiol. *41*, 19 – 59.

Bartholow, R. (1881) On the Antagonism between Medicine and between Remedies and Diseases. D. Appleton, New York.

Bayliss, W.M. (1915) Principles of General Physiology, pp. 17 – 20, 723 – 728, Longmans, Green and Company, London.

Bennett, J.H. (1875) Researches into the Antagonism of Medicines. J. and A. Churchill, London.

Blasko, H. (1969) In: Scientific Thought, 1900 – 1960: A Selective Survey, (Harré, R., Ed.), pp. 196 – 208, Clarendon Press, Oxford.

Boyle, R. (1685) On the Reconcileableness of Specific Medicines to the Corpuscular Philosophy. London.

Brodie, T.G. and Dixon, W.E. (1904) J. Phys. *30*, 476 – 502.

Brunton, T.L. (1871) Br. Med. J. *1*, 413 – 415.

Bynum, W.F. (1970) Bull. Hist. Med. *44*, 518 – 538.

Clark, A.J. (1910) Biochem. J. *5*, 236 – 242.

Clark, A.J. (1912) Proc. R. Soc. Med., Ther. Pharmacol. Sec. *5*, 181 – 197.

Clark, A.J. (1913a) J. Physiol. *47*, 67 – 107.

Clark, A.J. (1913b) J. Pharmacol. Exp. Ther. *4*, 399 – 424.

Clark, A.J. (1914) J. Pharmacol. Exp. Ther. *5*, 215 – 234.

Clark, A.J. (1921) J. Pharmacol. Exp. Ther. *18*, 423 – 447.

Clark, A.J. (1926) J. Physiol. *61*, 530 – 546.

Clark, A.J. (1927) J. Physiol. *64*, 123 – 143.

Clark, A.J. (1932) Pharm. J. *128*, 184 – 185.

Clark, A.J. (1933) The Mode of Action of Drugs on Cells. Edward Arnold, London.

Clark, A.J. (1937) In: Handbuch der experimentellen Pharmakologie, Vol. 4, (W. Heubner and Schüller, J., Eds.), Julius Springer, Berlin.

Clark, A.J. (1941) Unpublished manuscript for second edition of *The Mode of Action of Drugs on Cells,* in possession of D.H. Clark, Cambridge, England.

Cuthbert, A.W. (1979) Trends Pharmacol. Sci. *1* (inaug. issue), 1 – 3.

Dale, H.H. (1914) J. Pharmacol. Exp. Ther. *6*, 147 – 190.

Dale, H.H. (1920) Johns Hopkins Hosp. Bull. *31*, 373 – 380.

Dixon, W.E. (1912) Proc. R. Soc. Med., Sect. Ther. Pharmacol. *6*, 1 – 38.

Earles, M.P. (1961) Annal. Sci. *17*, 97 – 110.

Ehrlich, P. (1878) Contributions to the Theory and Practice of Histological Staining. M.D. Dissertation, University of Leipzig. In Himmelweit (1956), Vol. 1, pp. 65 – 98.

Ehrlich, P. (1885a) The Requirements of the Organism for Oxygen: An Analytical Study with the Aid of Dyes. In Himmelweit (1956), Vol. 1, pp. 433 – 496.

Ehrlich, P. (1885b) Ueber Wesen und Behandlung des Jodismus. In Himmelweit (1956), Vol. 1, pp. 530 – 534.

Ehrlich, P. (1886) Experimentelles und Klinisches über Thallin. In Himmelweit (1956), Vol. 1, pp. 542 – 551.

Ehrlich, P. (1897) The Assay of the Activity of Diptheria-Curative Serum and Its Theoretical Basis. In Himmelweit (1957), Vol. 2, pp. 107 – 125.

Ehrlich, P. (1898) Ueber die Constitution des Diphtheriegiftes. In Himmelweit (1957), Vol. 2, pp. 126 – 133.

Ehrlich, P. (1900a) On Haemolysins: Third Communication. In Himmelweit (1957), Vol. 2, pp. 205 – 212.

Ehrlich, P. (1900b) On Immunity with Special Reference to Cell Life. In Himmelweit (1957), Vol. 2, pp. 178 – 195.

Ehrlich, P. (1902) The Relations Existing between Chemical Constitution, Distribution and Pharmacological Action. In Himmelweit (1956), Vol. 1, pp. 596 – 618.

Ehrlich, P. (1903) Toxin und Antitoxin. Entgegnung auf Grubers Replik. In Himmelweit (1957), Vol. 2, pp. 391 – 394.

Ehrlich, P. (1906) Address Delivered at the Dedication of the Georg-Speyer Haus. In Himmelweit (1960), Vol. 3, pp. 53 – 63.

Ehrlich, P. (1907a) Chemotherapeutische Trypanosomen-Studien. In Himmelweit (1960), Vol. 3, pp. 81 – 105.

Ehrlich, P. (1907b) Experimental Researches on Specific Therapy. In Himmelweit (1960), Vol. 3, pp. 106 – 134.

Ehrlich, P. (1909a) Ueber der jetzigen Stand der Chemotherapie. In Himmelweit (1960), Vol. 3, pp. 150 – 170.

Ehrlich, P. (1909b) Chemotherapie von Infektionskrankheit. In Himmelweit (1960), Vol. 3, pp. 213 – 227.

Ehrlich, P. (1914) Chemotherapy. In Himmelweit (1960), Vol. 3, pp. 505 – 518.

Ehrlich, P. and Einhorn, A. (1894) Ueber die physiologische Wirkung der Verbindungen der Cocainreihe. In Himmelweit (1956), Vol. 1, pp. 567 – 569.

Ehrlich, P. and Guttmann, P. (1891) On the Action of Methylene Blue on Malaria. In Himmelweit (1960), Vol. 3, pp. 15 – 20.

Ehrlich, P. and Leppman, A. (1890) Ueber schmerzstillende Wirkung des Methylenblau. In Himmelweit (1956), Vol. 1, pp. 555 – 558.

Elliott, T.R. (1905) J. Physiol. 32,, 401 – 467.

Fränkel, S. (1901) Die Arzneimittel-Synthese auf Grundlage der Berziehungen zwischen chemischen Aufbau und Wirkung, pp. 13 – 41, Julius Springer, Berlin.

Fraser, T. (1872) Br. Med. J. 2, 401 – 403.

Fruton, J. (1976) Science 192, 327 – 334.

Gaddum, J.H. (1926) J. Physiol. 61, 141 – 150.

Gaddum, J.H. (1937) J. Physiol. 89, 7P – 9P.

Goodman, L.S. and Gilman, A.G. (1965) The Pharmacological Basis of Therapeutics, 2nd Edn., p. 18, MacMillan, New York.

Greene, C.W. (1914) Handbook of Pharmacology, pp. 3 – 7, William Wood, New York.

Heubel, E. (1871) Pathogenese und Symptome der chronischen Bleivergiftung: experimentelle Untersuchungen. Hirschwald, Berlin.

Hill, A.V. (1909) J. Physiol. 39, 361 – 373.

Himmelweit, F. (Ed.) (1956 – 1960) The Collected Papers of Paul Ehrlich, 3 Vols., Pergamon Press, London.

Hopkins, F.G. (1913) Nature 92, 213 – 223.

Hunt, R. and Taveau, R de M. (1906) Br. Med. J. 2, 1788 – 1791.

Knaus, H.H. and Clark, A.J. (1925) J. Pharmacol. Exp. Ther. 26, 347 – 358.

Kohler, R. (1975) J. Hist. Biol. 8, 275 – 318.

Langley, J.N. (1878) J. Physiol. 1, 339 – 369.

Langley, J.N. (1901a) J. Physiol. 27, 224 – 236.

Langley, J.N. (1901b) J. Physiol. *27*, 237 – 256.
Langley, J.N. (1903) J. Physiol. *30*, 221 – 252.
Langley, J.N. (1905) J. Physiol. *33*, 374 – 413.
Langley, J.N. (1906) Proc. R. Soc. *78B*, 170 – 194.
Langley, J.N. (1908) J. Physiol. *37*, 285 – 300.
Langley, J.N. (1909) J. Physiol. *39*, 235 – 295.
Langley, J.N. and Dickinson, W.L. (1889) Proc. R. Soc. *46*, 423 – 431.
Langley, J.N. and Dickinson, W.L. (1890) Proc. R. Soc. *47*, 379 – 390.
Langmuir, I. (1916) J. Am. Chem. Soc. *38*, 2221 – 2295.
Mazumdar, P. (1974) Bull. Hist. Med. *48*, 1 – 21.
Parascandola, J. (1971) Pharm. Hist. *13*, 3 – 10.
Parascandola, J. (1974) Pharm. Hist. *16*, 54 – 63.
Parascandola, J. (1977) J. Hist. Med. *32*, 151 – 171.
Parascandola, J. (1980) Trends Pharmacol. Sci. *1*, 189 – 192.
Parascandola, J. (1981) J. Hist. Med. *36*, 19 – 43.
Parascandola, J. and Jasensky, R. (1974) Bull. Hist. Med. *48*, 199 – 220.
Pereira, J. (1854) The Elements of Materia Medica, 4th Edn., Vol. 1, p. 91, Longman, Brown, Green and Longmans, London.
Schamberg, J.F., Kolmer, J.A. and Raiziss, G.W. (1917) Am. J. Syphilis *1*, 1 – 41.
Simon, C.E. and Wood, M. (1914a) Am. J. Med. Sci. *147*, 247 – 260.
Simon, C.E. and Wood, M. (1914b) Am. J. Med. Sci. *147*, 524 – 540.
Singer, C. and Underwood, E.A. (1962) A Short History of Medicine, 2nd Edn., pp. 564 – 577, Clarendon Press, Oxford.
Sollmann, T. (1917) A Manual of Pharmacology. pp. 75 – 78, W.B. Saunders, Philadelphia.
Storm van Leeuwen, W. (1924) J. Pharmacol. Exp. Ther. *24*, 25 – 32.
Straub, W. (1910) Biochem. Z. *28*, 392 – 407.
Straub, W. (1912) Verh. Ges. dtsch. Naturforsch. Aerzte *84*, 192 – 214.
Tallarida, R.J. (1981) Trends Pharmacol. Sci. *2*, 231 – 234.
Teich, M. (1973) In: Changing Perspectives in the History of Science: Essays in Honour of Joseph Needham (Teich, M. and Young, R., Eds.), pp. 439 – 471, Heinemann, London.
Traube, J. (1919) Biochem. Z. *98*, 177 – 196.

IX

JOHN J. ABEL AND THE EARLY DEVELOPMENT OF PHARMACOLOGY AT THE JOHNS HOPKINS UNIVERSITY*

When the funds became available to open The Johns Hopkins University Medical School in 1893, the so-called "Big Four" (Welch, Osler, Halsted and Kelly) already had positions at The Johns Hopkins Hospital. It was necessary, however, to secure faculty for the pre-clinical sciences of anatomy, physiology, and pharmacology to round out the staff of the Medical School. Franklin Mall was appointed in anatomy and William Howell in physiology. For pharmacology, the science involving the study of the physiological action of drugs and poisons, the University turned to John Jacob Abel (1857–1938), then Professor of Materia Medica and Therapeutics at the University of Michigan.

The modern science of pharmacology was still a relatively young discipline in 1893, and hardly existed at all in the United States at that time. Although the word "pharmacology" dates back at least to the seventeenth century, experimental pharmacology did not emerge as a distinct discipline until the nineteenth century. Originally the term pharmacology was used in a much broader sense to refer to the study of essentially all aspects of knowledge about drugs: their origin, composition, physical and chemical properties, physiological effects, therapeutic uses, and modes of preparation and administration. Sometimes the term "materia medica" was used synonymously with pharmacology, but often materia medica was more narrowly defined as the subfield of pharmacology that dealt with the natural history of medicines. The other two subdivisions of pharmacology in this classification scheme were pharmacy (the preparation and storage of medicines) and therapeutics (the use of medicines in treating illness).

In the nineteenth century, that portion of the science of drugs which concerned itself with the investigation of their physiological effects was sometimes labeled "pharmacodynamics." During the course of the century, however, the term pharmacology came to be used increasingly to refer to

* Revised version of a paper presented at the 53rd annual meeting of the American Association for the History, of Medicine, Boston, Massachusetts, 2 May 1980. The research for this paper was supported by NIH Grant LM03300 and by a grant from the University of Wisconsin Graduate School. Part of the work was carried out while the author was Visiting Associate Professor at the Johns Hopkins Institute of the History of Medicine. The author wishes to thank the staff of the institute and of the Alan Mason Chesney Archives of The Johns Hopkins Medical Institutions for the facilities and assistance that they provided, and for permission to use the John J. Abel Papers, now housed in the Chesney Archives.

this narrower subdivision of pharmacodynamics.[1] The older, broader meaning of pharmacology has largely become obsolete, and today the discipline is frequently defined as the study of the interaction of chemicals with living matter (or in similar terms).[2]

Experiments on the physiological effects of drugs and poisons upon animals and humans were carried out even in antiquity, but the birth of experimental pharmacology as a science is usually associated with the work of the French physiologist François Magendie in the early nineteenth century. Magendie's investigations of the mode of action of strychnine-containing arrow poisons were elegant models of pharmacological experimentation. The research of Magendie and other physiologists, such as Claude Bernard (whose studies on curare and carbon monoxide established the mechanism of action of these poisons), provided pharmacology with some of the techniques and concepts that it needed in order to develop.[3]

Yet it was not in France but in the Germanic universities, that pharmacology was to establish itself first as an independent discipline, which was related to, but distinct from, physiology. The German Rudolf Buchheim established what appears to have been the first institute of pharmacology in 1847 at the University of Dorpat. Although Dorpat was in Russian-governed Estonia, the university was essentially German in language, faculty and curriculum.

Chairs of materia medica had, of course, existed in medical schools long before the mid-nineteenth century. Materia medica largely concerned itself, however, with the origin, constituents and preparation of drugs rather than with their physiological effects. It was more closely allied to botany, chemistry and pharmacy than it was to physiology.

Buchheim called for an independent, experimental discipline of pharmacology, arguing that the investigation of the action of drugs was a task for the pharmacologist rather than for the chemist or pharmacist. At first, his pharmacological laboratory and institute had to be located in his home, but eventually he was provided with the necessary facilities at the university. Of

---

[1] On the history of the term "pharmacology," see Melvin P. Earles, "Studies in the Development of Experimental Pharmacology in the Eighteenth and Early Nineteenth Centuries" (Ph.D. diss., University College, London, 1961), p. 11; Gert Preiser, "Zum Geschichte und Bildung der Fermini Pharmakologie und Toxikologie," *Medizinhist. J.*, 1967, *2*: 124–34; *A New English Dictionary on Historical Principles* (Oxford: At the Clarendon Press, 1909), 7: 768; *Encyclopedia Britannica*, 11th ed. (Cambridge: Cambridge University Press, 1911), 21: 347.

[2] See, for example, Andres Goth, *Medical Pharmacology: Principles and Concepts*, 8th ed. (St. Louis: C. V. Mosby, 1976), p. 1.

[3] On the beginnings of experimental pharmacology, see Earles, "Experimental Pharmacology," and J. E. Lesch, "The Origins of Experimental Physiology and Pharmacology in France, 1790–1820" (Ph.D. diss., Princeton University, 1977). For recent discussions of two eighteenth-century predecessors of Magendie whose pharmacological studies were far more careful and systematic than those of most of their contemporaries, see Karl-Werner Schweppe and Christian Probst, "Die Versuche zur medikamentösen Karzinomtherapie des Anton Störck (1731–1803): Ein Beitrag zur Geschichte der experimentellen Arzneimittelforschung in der älteren Wiener medizinischen Schule," in *Festschrift für Erna Lesky zum 70. Geburtstag*, ed. by Kurt Ganzinger, Manfred Skopec and Helmut Wyklicky (Vienna: Brüder Hollinek, 1981), pp. 105–22, and P. K. Knoefel, "Felice Fontana and poisons," *Clio Medica*, 1980, *15*: 35–65.

the students who received research training in Buchheim's laboratory, the most important was undoubtedly Oswald Schmiedeberg.

Schmiedeberg, who succeeded Buchheim at Dorpat in 1866, became the most influential pharmacologist of his generation and helped to establish firmly the subject as an autonomous discipline. Schmiedeberg's pharmacological institute at Strasbourg, where he moved in 1872, became a mecca for students of pharmacology from all over the world. It has been estimated that about 120 students from some twenty different countries worked in his laboratory, and that his students later occupied approximately forty academic chairs. He was also the cofounder and coeditor of the first journal of experimental pathology and pharmacology. It was one of Schmiedeberg's students, John J. Abel, who was eventually to play the key role in the transmission of the new science to the United States.[4]

In 1876, the year in which Abel embarked upon his undergraduate studies at the University of Michigan and four years after Schmiedeberg's move to Strasbourg, The Johns Hopkins University opened its doors. From the beginning, the plans for the University called for the establishment of a medical school. Although the medical school was not scheduled to open until The Johns Hopkins Hospital was completed, the University Trustees created a Medical Faculty in 1883 to develop the plans for medical education. The original Medical Faculty consisted of University President Daniel Coit Gilman, Professor of Chemistry Ira Remsen, Professor of Biology H. Newell Martin and Dr. John Shaw Billings of the office of the Surgeon General in Washington.[5]

In the few years since its opening, The Johns Hopkins University had already acquired a reputation for excellence in graduate study and research. Not surprisingly, the organizers of the medical school felt that it was "very desirable to afford special opportunities for study, and to encourage research in the scientific branches of medicine." Among the scientific branches singled out for study by the Medical Faculty at their first meeting in January 1884 was "the Physiological action of drugs."[6]

It seems clear that at the very outset the Medical Faculty favored the new science of pharmacology, the teaching of which had not yet been established at any American university, over the traditional materia medica. As taught in American medical schools in the late nineteenth century, "materia medica remained an empirical and traditional study, didactic in presentation, relying largely on botanical or alphabetical arrangements that depended upon memorization as the chief educational method." The teaching of materia

---

[4] On Buchheim and Schmiedeberg, see Gustav Kuchinsky, "The influence of Dorpat on the emergence of pharmacology as a distinct discipline," *J. Hist. Med.,* 1968, *23:* 258–71; Marianne Bruppacher-Cellier, *Rudolf Buchheim (1820–1879) und die Entwicklung einer experimentellen Pharmakologie* (Zurich: Julius Druck, 1971); Jan Koch-Weser and Paul Schechter, "Schmiedeberg in Strassburg, 1872–1918: the making of modern pharmacology," *Life Sci.,* 1978, *22:* 1361–71.

[5] Alan Chesney, *The Johns Hopkins Hospital and The Johns Hopkins University School of Medicine: A Chronicle,* 2 vols. (Baltimore: The Johns Hopkins Press, 1943–1958), 1: 76–79.

[6] *Ibid.,* p. 79.

medica was frequently combined with responsibilities for a variety of other subjects, such as botany, chemistry, hygiene, medical jurisprudence, and therapeutics, suggesting that the subject did not occupy a place of prestige in the medical curriculum.[7]

Physiologist H. Newell Martin probably played an instrumental role in the Medical Faculty's decision to incorporate research and teaching in pharmacology into the program of the new Medical School. In an address delivered before the Medical and Chirurgical Faculty of Maryland in 1885, entitled "The Study of the Physiological Action of Drugs," Martin clearly presented the case for the importance of the new discipline.

> I have selected as my topic *Pharmacology*—that branch of science which is concerned with the investigation of the action of drugs on the healthy body— because I believe that it is destined in the near future to acquire an importance in regard to therapeutics which is not yet properly appreciated.
>
> Pharmacology can hardly be said to have existed in ancient medicine, nor indeed until the present century. . . .
>
> There are, at present, a small number of laboratories devoted entirely to such work on the continent of Europe; not one, I think, in the United States. Such investigations are, of course, often made here in physiological laboratories, but usually as a secondary matter and for purposes with no direct therapeutic end in view. I believe that as regards the advancement of medical art, there is nothing at present more desirable than an increase of well-equipped workshops, in which men already trained in chemistry, in physiology, in pathology, shall investigate the action of substances, with a view to discover whether they may be useful as medicines, and in what pathological conditions they may be rationally expected to prove of benefit.[8]

Apparently the decision was made to try to secure an established scholar, either Thomas Lauder Brunton of London or Horatio C. Wood of Philadelphia.[9] Although Brunton and Wood can perhaps be considered to be transitional figures between materia medica and pharmacology, rather than modern pharmacologists in the Schmiedeberg mold, they were clearly two of the most prominent pharmacological investigators in the Anglo-American scientific community. Both were medical practitioners as well as scientists, and both had broad interests that transcended several medical disciplines. But both men recognized the significance of experimental pharmacology and contributed to research in the discipline. Brunton was a physician and Lecturer in Materia Medica at St. Bartholomew's Hospital and Wood was

---

[7] David Cowen, "Materia Medica and Pharmacology," in *The Education of American Physicians: Historical Essays*, ed. by Ronald Numbers (Berkeley: University of California Press, 1980), pp. 95—105. The quotation is from p. 105.

[8] H. N. Martin, "The study of the physiological action of drugs," *Trans. Med. Chir. Fac. Maryland*, 1885, *88*: 81, 90. I wish to thank A. McGehee Harvey for calling my attention to this paper.

[9] J. S. Billings to D. E. Gilman, 15 May, 29 September 1884, Founding Documents, Alan Mason Chesney Medical Archives, The Johns Hopkins Medical Institutions, Baltimore. All of the manuscript materials cited in the discussion of the efforts to appoint a professor of pharmacology in the 1880s are from two folders labeled "Appointment of Matthew Hay as Professor of Pharmacology" and "Executive Committee Proposals to Dr. Hay."

Professor of Nervous Diseases, Materia Medica, Pharmacy and General Therapeutics at the University of Pennsylvania Medical School.[10]

Hopkins was unable, however, to obtain either man for the position. While in Britain in the summer of 1884, Billings discussed the question of the professorship in "experimental pharmacology" with several colleagues in London and Edinburgh, including Brunton and Thomas Fraser, Professor of Materia Medica and Therapeutics at the University of Edinburgh. They recommended Matthew Hay, who was then Professor of Medical Jurisprudence and Toxicology at the University of Aberdeen, very highly. Hay had received his medical degree at Edinburgh in 1878, and had served as an assistant to Fraser. Billings had an opportunity to interview Hay, and "was much pleased with him." He informed President Gilman that, apart from Wood and Brunton (whom he was satisfied could not be secured), he felt there was "no better man available for the place than Dr. Hay," and recommended his appointment.[11]

In October 1884, Billings wrote to Hay that he had been authorized to offer him the "chair of Pharmacology and Experimental Therapeutics (the precise title to be determined hereafter)."[12] Hay was offered an annual salary of $4,000, with an understanding that he would not engage in private medical practice.[13] He was ready to accept the offer, but raised the question as to whether he might not be allowed to devote an hour a day, or every other day, to private consulting practice, which he felt sure would not interfere with his university duties.[14] The Executive Committee of the Board of Trustees, however, denied Hay's request. The Committee believed that medical education in the United States suffered from the fact that the chairs were almost always filled by practitioners, resulting in the scientific work of the schools of medicine being "less efficient than it should be." They thought it best to initiate their own medical school by appointing several teachers who would not be engaged in medical practice.[15] Thus from the very beginning, the policy of full-time professorships in the pre-clinical sciences, then a novelty in the United States, was established at The Johns Hopkins University School of Medicine.[16]

[10] On Brunton see the article by W. F. Bynum in *Dictionary of Scientific Biography,* 16 vols. (New York: Charles Scribner's Sons, 1970–1980), 2: 547–48. On Wood, see the article by Glenn Sonnedecker in *ibid.,* 14: 495–97 and G. B. Roth, "An early American pharmacologist, Horatio C. Wood (1841–1920)," *Isis,* 1939, *30:* 38–45.

[11] See note 9. See also Matthew Hay to J. S. Billings, 11 May 1884, Founding Documents; Simon Flexner and J. T. Flexner, *William Henry Welch and the Heroic Age of American Medicine* (New York: Viking Press, 1941), pp. 490–91.

[12] J. S. Billings to Matthew Hay, 11 October 1884, Founding Documents.

[13] D. C. Gilman to Matthew Hay, 4 December 1884, Founding Documents; "Memorandum of proposals made to Dr. Hay by the Executive Committee," 1 December 1884, Founding Documents.

[14] Matthew Hay to D. C. Gilman, 9 February 1885, Founding Documents.

[15] "Minute of the Executive Committee," 2 March 1885, Founding Documents. A copy of this document is attached to the memorandum cited in note 13. A second untitled, undated copy is also contained in this collection.

[16] Because the Hay case is of interest from the point of view of the full-time issue, it receives significant attention in Chesney, *Johns Hopkins,* 1: 86–89.

As The Johns Hopkins Hospital was not scheduled to open until the autumn of 1887, and instruction in the medical school would not commence until that time, it was decided not to begin Hay's appointment until 1 January 1887. In fact, Hay never took up the Hopkins position. In August 1886 he wrote to Gilman resigning the chair because of "private and personal matters."[17] No immediate effort was made to replace Hay for it soon became apparent that the medical school would not be able to open on schedule. The University's income was severely reduced as a result of the financial difficulties of the Baltimore and Ohio Railroad, in which much of its endowment was invested, and the opening of the medical school was delayed until 1893 when funds were obtained from other sources.[18] It was at that time that John Abel was invited to join the Hopkins faculty.

When Billings wrote to Hay to offer him the professorship of pharmacology in the fall of 1884, Abel had just recently left The Johns Hopkins University, after a year of post-graduate study, to continue his education in Germany. Abel was born on a farm near Cleveland, Ohio, in 1857, the descendant of German immigrants.[19] He received his undergraduate education at the University of Michigan, where he began his studies in 1876, but interrupted them for three years (1879–1882) for financial reasons.

It was during this hiatus in his academic education, while he was serving as a teacher and principal and later as superintendent of schools in La Porte, Indiana, that he made the decision to study medicine. Abel began to devote some of his spare time to the reading of medical books. From the beginning, he was apparently more inclined towards medical research than practice, and recognized the need for a solid education if he were ever to achieve his goal of contributing significantly to this field.[20] In the summer of 1881, he wrote to Mary Hinman, his fiancée, a teacher in the La Porte school system:

> It will be necessary to extend our apprenticeship over as many years as possible after leaving La Porte in order that part of the work that I have laid out this summer may be accomplished. I should be almost certain of finally seeing my great desire accomplished—that I might work out something—a masterpiece of some kind, in the medical line that will help people along a little—if I could have a few years of such unobstructed, uninterrupted quiet digging as I now enjoy. Of course, I would have to precede this period of digging with a training in laboratories such as I have not enjoyed.[21]

When Abel returned to Ann Arbor to complete his last year in 1882–1883, he spent part of his time studying physiology, anatomy and physiological chemistry with Victor Vaughan and Henry Sewall in the medi-

---

[17] Matthew Hay to D. C. Gilman, 14 August 1886, Founding Documents.

[18] On the financial difficulties of the University at this time, see Chesney, *Johns Hopkins*, 1: 95–97.

[19] For general biographical and bibliographical information about Abel, see the article by Charles Rosenberg in the *Dictionary of Scientific Biography*, 1: 9–12.

[20] Correspondence between John Abel and Mary Hinman, 1881–1882, John J. Abel Papers, Chesney Archives. For example, see John Abel to Mary Hinman, 22 June 1881.

[21] John Abel to Mary Hinman, 24 July 1881, Abel Papers.

cal school. Upon graduating from Michigan in 1883, he married Mary Hinman and they went to Baltimore, where Abel pursued his interest in physiology in Newell Martin's laboratory at Johns Hopkins. Even while still in Michigan, Abel had been intrigued by the prospect of studying in Germany, and in August of 1884 he and his wife sailed for Europe.[22] Before leaving the United States, he spent part of that summer in the laboratory of Horatio C. Wood in Philadelphia, where he received his first exposure to pharmacological research.[23]

In going to Germany to continue his education, Abel was of course choosing a path followed by numerous other American students of medicine in this period. His original plan was to spend two years studying medicine and biomedical science in Germany, then to return to the United States to obtain a Ph.D.[24] But Abel soon fell in love with Europe and the opportunities offered to him for study and research, and his stay abroad extended to six and a half years. During that time he studied at about half a dozen universities in Germany, Austria and Switzerland.[25]

Abel began his European apprenticeship by undertaking physiological research in the laboratory of Carl Ludwig at Leipzig. He soon came to feel that his preparation for such work was inadequate, and so decided to embark upon more basic medical studies.[26] After further study at Leipzig, and brief stints in Heidelberg and Wurzburg, the Abels moved in 1887 to Strasbourg, where John Abel received his M.D. the following year.

One of the motivating forces behind Abel's move to Strasbourg was a desire to study in the laboratory of the noted physiological chemist, Felix Hoppe-Seyler. Abel was beginning to recognize the important role that chemistry seemed destined to play in medicine. Fellow students warned him, however, that Hoppe-Seyler was too busy to devote much time to his pupils, and they advised him instead to work with the pharmacologist Oswald Schmiedeberg, who was also well versed in physiological chemistry.[27] Abel spent about a year working in the laboratory of the eminent pharmacologist.

After a period of clinical work in Vienna, Abel went to Bern, Switzerland, in 1890 to obtain biochemical training with Marcel von Nencki. In the meantime, Mary Abel returned to the United States, where she helped Ellen Richards to establish the New England Kitchen, designed to educate the poor about nourishing, yet low-priced foods, in Boston.[28] Abel had begun in

---

[22] Abel was thinking about the possibility of going to Germany for advanced study as early as 1882, see John Abel to Mary Hinman, 26 August 1882, Abel Papers.

[23] See letters from John Abel to Mary Abel, June 1884, Abel Papers.

[24] Mary Abel to unknown person, 12 May 1884, and John Abel to G. S. Hall, June 1888, Abel Papers.

[25] Abel's desire to prolong his period of study abroad as long as possible, and his respect for the scientific work being carried out in the Germanic countries, is adequately documented in his letters from this period in the Abel Papers.

[26] John Abel to H. C. Wood, 24 June 1888, and John Abel to G. S. Hall, June 1888, Abel Papers.

[27] Ibid.

[28] Mary Abel's letters to her husband in 1889–1890, Abel Papers, describe her work at the New England Kitchen. On Ellen Richards, see Caroline Hunt, *The Life of Ellen H. Richards* (Boston: Whitcomb and Barrows, 1912).

1888 to contact some of his former teachers (such as Wood and Sewall) about possible positions in the States, and his wife, after her return home, also began to make inquiries on his behalf. By this time, Abel was convinced that his future lay in the application of chemistry to physiology and/or the related fields of pathology and pharmacology.[29]

Abel had tentatively accepted a position (arranged through Mrs. Abel) as an assistant to Francis Williams, Professor of Therapeutics at the Harvard Medical School, when he received in the summer of 1890 a letter from Victor Vaughan of the University of Michigan asking: "How would the chair of materia medica and therapeutics suit you, say with physiological chemistry attached?"[30] The man who had been teaching materia medica (along with ophthamology and aural surgery) at Michigan had recently been fired over a disagreement with the Board of Regents.[31] Both Abel and his wife had contacted his former teacher, Vaughan, earlier that summer about a possible position at Michigan, and their inquiries had obviously arrived at an opportune moment.[32]

After conferring with von Nencki, Abel decided to accept the Michigan position. He wrote to his wife: "Chemistry is as necessary in Pharmacology or what we call Therapeutics as it is in Physiological Chemistry. And I know that I can make vastly more out of Pharmacology in the States."[33] Abel received permission to delay the start of his appointment for six months so that he could continue his studies abroad, and he finally arrived in Ann Arbor to take up his teaching duties in January 1891. It was decided that Vaughan would continue to teach physiological chemistry, and Abel's responsibilities would be limited to pharmacology.[34]

John Abel brought with him to Michigan the German tradition of experimental pharmacology, as developed by Buchheim and Schmiedeberg. He immediately converted the traditional, didactic materia medica course into a pharmacology course which included experimental demonstrations. He soon developed advanced laboratory courses on the methods of modern pharmacology and on the influence of drugs on tissue metabolism. Abel also promptly established a research laboratory in which to carry out his own scientific investigations. Although Abel's official title was Professor of Materia Medica and Therapeutics, his appointment at Michigan represents the establishment of the first chair of modern pharmacology in the United States.[35]

---

[29] See, for example, John Abel to Henry Sewall, June 1888, Abel Papers. See also note 26.

[30] Victor Vaughan to John Abel, 1 July 1890, Abel Papers.

[31] For a discussion of the circumstances leading to Abel's call to Michigan see Henry Swain, E. M. K. Geiling and Alexander Heingartner, "John Jacob Abel at Michigan: the introduction of pharmacology into the medical curriculum," *Univ. Mich. Med. Bull.,* 1963, *29:* 1–14. Vaughan's recollection of how he came to decide to hire Abel, quoted on p. 6, would appear, on the basis of manuscript evidence, to be inaccurate.

[32] John Abel to Victor Vaughan, 1 June 1890 and Mary Abel to Victor Vaughan [June 1890], Abel Papers.

[33] John Abel to Mary Abel, 24 July 1890, Abel Papers.

[34] Victor Vaughan to John Abel, 1 August 1890, Abel Papers. On the appointment with Williams, which Abel eventually declined in favor of the Michigan offer, see the correspondence of Mary Abel with Francis Williams and John Abel, June–August 1890, Abel Papers.

[35] For a fuller discussion of Abel's work at Michigan, see Swain, Geiling and Heingartner, "Abel at Michigan."

In a lecture delivered to the Michigan State Pharmaceutical Association in 1891, Abel discussed his view of the new discipline of pharmacology.

Briefly, this science tries to discover all the physical and chemical changes that go on in a living thing that has absorbed a substance capable of producing such changes, and it also attempts to discover the fate of the substance incorporated. It is not therefore an applied science, like therapeutics, but it is one of the biological sciences, using that word in its widest sense. . . . Its growth is intimately connected with that of physiology.[36]

He went on to note that Buchheim and others had developed pharmacological laboratories where experimenters could build up their science "undisturbed by the intrusive demands of practical utility" (i.e., the demands of therapeutics). He was quick to point out, though, that once pharmacology was placed on a firm basis, it would automatically yield results of value to the practical man.[37]

At the same time, The Johns Hopkins University finally was making preparations to open its medical school. Efforts were being made to complete the assembling of a faculty of high quality. At a meeting of the existing medical faculty on 12 January 1893, it was agreed that it would be desirable to appoint an instructor in pharmacology (among other subjects) before the opening of the medical school.[38] Abel's name must already have been in the minds of some of those present, for the very next day, Osler wrote to him and asked: "On what terms could you be dislocated?" Osler added that he felt that no one in the country had a better training in pharmacology than Abel.[39]

Several members of the medical faculty were familiar with Abel's work. Newell Martin knew him well, of course, since Abel had spent the 1883–1884 academic year working in his laboratory. At that time, Abel had also come into contact with Gilman and Remsen, though probably only casually.[40] He had also written to Martin, Gilman and Welch in 1888, when he was seeking his first position, and outlined in detail his European studies and his career plans.[41]

Both Osler and Welch were acquainted with Abel and respected his work. Welch had first met Abel in Ludwig's laboratory in Leipzig in 1885.[42] In response to some reprints that Abel sent him in 1893, Welch replied: "Your work is of a high order and so far as I know the only work in just the same direction which is done in this country."[43] Osler and Abel first met on a steamer bound for Europe in June 1892.[44] Even before their first meeting,

---

[36] John Abel, "The methods of pharmacology, with experimental illustration," *Pharm. Era,* 1892, 7: 105.
[37] *Ibid.*
[38] "Medical Faculty Advisory Board Minutes," 12 Jan. 1893, vol. 1, p. 26, Chesney Archives.
[39] William Osler to John Abel, 13 Jan. 1893, Abel Papers.
[40] D. C. Gilman to John Abel, 5 July 1882; Ira Remsen to John Abel, 28 May 1884; John Abel to D. C. Gilman, 18 June 1888, Abel Papers.
[41] John Abel to William Welch, 18 June 1888; John Abel to D. C. Gilman, 18 June 1888; John Abel to H. N. Martin, June 1888, Abel Papers.
[42] John Abel to William Welch, 18 June 1888, Abel Papers.
[43] William Welch to John Abel, 14 May 1892, Abel Papers.
[44] John Abel to Mary Abel, June 1892, Abel Papers.

however, they had been in touch through correspondence, and Osler had expressed admiration for Abel's work.[45]

Abel was thus a logical choice for the pharmacology chair. Because of delays in reaching agreement with Mary Garrett about the terms of her bequest, which was to provide the funding enabling the medical school to open, an official offer could not be made to Abel until March. After clarifying a few questions concerning salary and funding for laboratory help and supplies, Abel happily accepted the position. In his letter, Osler had erroneously referred to a professorship of materia medica, and Abel requested in his reply that the title be changed to materia medica *and pharmacology*.[46]

When Abel arrived in Baltimore to take up his duties in September of 1893, his actual title was Professor of Pharmacology. Abel was later to state that, so far as he could determine, this was the first chair in the country to carry the title "pharmacology."[47] The term "pharmacology" had been used earlier as part of a combined title (e.g., chemistry, pharmacology and materia medica),[48] but Abel's chair at Hopkins was most probably the first to carry the sole designation "pharmacology" in which the word was intended explicitly in its modern sense.

Abel was called upon to teach physiological chemistry in his first year, as no one had yet been hired for that task, and as the pharmacology course was to be taught in the second year of the medical curriculum. Physiological chemistry at Hopkins remained nominally under his jurisdiction until 1908, when a separate department was created with Walter Jones as head. Jones had been hired as an assistant to Abel, and by 1899 had apparently taken over the major responsibility for the course.[49]

The pharmacology course taught by Abel at Hopkins for the first time in 1894 included not only experimental demonstrations, as at Michigan, but also laboratory work carried out by the students themselves. Students were divided into groups of four and investigated the effects of various drugs on anesthetized laboratory animals. Laboratory work also played a significant part in the instruction in toxicology offered under Abel's direction.[50]

Abel continued to pursue the experimental investigations that he had begun at Michigan, and soon became engaged upon studies in a new field, hormone research, that was to occupy a major part of his attention during the rest of his career. Among the more significant contributions from his laboratory over the next several decades were the isolation of epinephrine

[45] William Osler to John Abel, 26 March 1892, Abel Papers.
[46] William Osler to John Abel, 2 March 1893 and John Abel to William Osler, 7 March, 16 March 1893, Abel Papers. It is clear that the title was intended to be pharmacology rather than materia medica. See "Medical Faculty Advisory Board Minutes," 2 March 1893, vol. 1, p. 40. See also note 38.
[47] John Abel to W. L. Bierring, 18 February 1924, Abel papers.
[48] For example, Silas H. Douglass was Professor of Chemistry, Pharmacology and Materia Medica at the University of Michigan in 1850. See Cowen, "Materia Medica," p. 99.
[49] Chesney, *Johns Hopkins,* 1: 227–28; 2: 95–100.
[50] *The Johns Hopkins Medical School, Announcement for 1894–95,* pp. 14–15, Chesney Archives; John Abel, "On the teaching of pharmacology, materia medica and therapeutics in our medical schools," *Phila. Med. J.,* 1900, 6: 384–90.

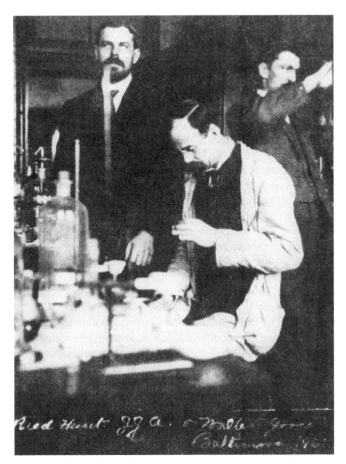

Fig. 1. (L. to R.) Reid Hunt, John J. Abel and Walter Jones in Abel's laboratory at The Johns Hopkins University, 1901. (Courtesy of the Alan Mason Chesney Archives.)

in the form of its benzoyl derivative (1897) and the crystallization of insulin (1926).[51]

Abel's laboratory also played a key role in the training of pharmacologists to fill the positions that eventually began to open in academic, industrial and government institutions. Numerous letters from deans and other administrators asking Abel to recommend a candidate for an opening in pharmacology may be found in the Abel Papers.[52] In the last decade of the

[51] For a good overview of Abel's research accomplishments, see Carl Voegtlin, "John Jacob Abel, 1857−1938," *J. Pharmacol. Exp. Ther.*, 1939, *67*: 373−406. On the insulin work, see Jane Murnaghan and Paul Talalay, "John Jacob Abel and the crystallization of insulin," *Perspect. Biol. Med.*, 1967, *10*: 334−80.

[52] For example, David Jordan to John Abel, 8 April 1910; M. Bye to John Abel, 8 Sept. 1919; C. H. Whipple to John Abel, 26 November 1915, Abel Papers.

nineteenth century and the early years of the twentieth century, Abel's laboratory was one of the few centers, and certainly the most prominent one, where an advanced student might study pharmacology in the United States. (Perhaps the only alternatives at first were the laboratories of Torald Sollmann at Western Reserve University and of Arthur Cushny, Abel's successor at the University of Michigan.) Among the pharmacologists who worked with Abel in the pre-World War I period were: Reid Hunt, who later became Professor of Pharmacology at Harvard; Arthur Loevenhart, who became the first Professor of Pharmacology at the University of Wisconsin; Carl Voegtlin, who succeeded Reid Hunt as Chief of the Division of Pharmacology of the Public Health Service's Hygienic Laboratory and later became first Head of the National Cancer Institute; A. C. Crawford, who became Professor of Pharmacology at Stanford; and H. G. Barbour, who became Professor of Pharmacology at Yale.[53]

These individuals did not receive their pharmacological training through formal graduate study. In fact, Abel was opposed to the establishment of a Ph.D. program in pharmacology, and such a program was not instituted at Hopkins during his tenure there. He felt that the ideal education for a pharmacologist was a solid grounding in chemistry and physics followed by training in medicine (preferably to the level of the M.D. degree).[54] Those who went to work in Abel's laboratory usually already had an advanced degree when they joined his staff. Crawford, Loevenhart, Hunt and Barbour, for example, all had earned their M.D. degrees before entering Abel's laboratory (and Hunt had a Ph.D. as well). Voegtlin came to Abel with a Ph.D. in chemistry and some medical training.

Abel's protégés were thus essentially postdoctoral workers who assisted in the teaching of medical students and carried out researches in his laboratory. Their training in pharmacology was achieved through their opportunity to work in an active research laboratory in the field and to participate in the teaching of the subject. As Abel's career progressed, much of the teaching of pharmacology at Hopkins came to be carried out by his co-workers.[55]

Almost all of his former associates also stress the importance of the famous lunch table discussions on their scientific development. Typically everyone brought their own fare to these daily luncheons in the laboratory, except for some items provided by general collection (such as tea and cookies) and occasional delicacies contributed by Mrs. Abel. The luncheons were not only attended by Abel and his co-workers, but often by other members of the Hopkins faculty as well. In addition, visiting scientists sometimes joined the luncheon group. Much of the discussion centered around

[53] A number of former students of Abel discussed their experiences working in his laboratory in "Centenary of the birth of John Jacob Abel," *Bull. Johns Hopkins Hosp.*, 1957, *101*: 297–328.

[54] For Abel's views on the training of pharmacologists, see John Abel to Abraham Flexner, 12 March 1920, and 5 June 1922; John Abel to Charles Erlanger, 20 January 1921; John Abel to M. M. Zinninger, 14 October 1929; and John Abel to George Roth, 28 November 1930, Abel Papers.

[55] E. M. K. Geiling, "John Jacob Abel, decade, 1923–1932," *Bull. Johns Hopkins Hosp.*, 1957, *101*: 318.

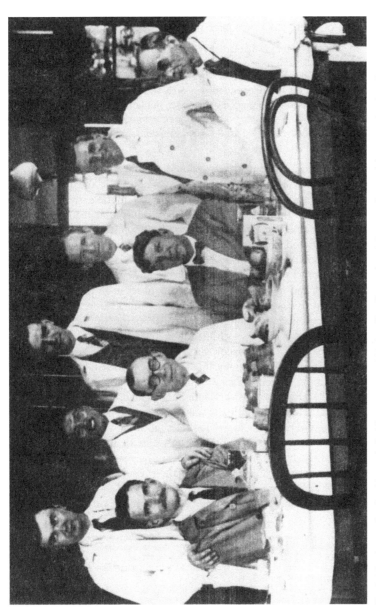

Fig. 2. The famous lunch table in Abel's laboratory, ca. 1925. Standing (L. to R.): J. V. Supniewski, Y. Ishikawa, Frederick Bell, Vincent Vermooten, David Campbell. Seated (L. to R.): C. A. Rouiller, E. M. K. Geiling, W. W. Ford, John J. Abel. (Courtesy of the Alan Mason Chesney Archives.)

IX

the latest developments in pharmacology, biochemistry and related sciences, but the conversations could also range from the arts to sailing. The current researches of the participants naturally received significant attention.[56] One of Abel's associates later wrote:

> In passing I might say that Dr. Abel's lunch table was an institution in itself. At lunch he inculcated into us, his assistants, the highest ideals of medicine, acquainted us with the great leaders of medicine, inspired us to think for ourselves and started us off on independent research which he supervised unselfishly, without exploitation, and guided our steps to publication. If in my eight years at Hopkins, had I done nothing but attend the professor's luncheons, I would have acquired a liberal education and learned, in addition, the secrets of successful graduate teaching.[57]

Another significant contribution of Abel to the professionalization of pharmacology was his role as the principal founder of the first national pharmacological society and journal in this country. In the early years of the twentieth century, a number of American medical schools made the transition from materia medica to modern pharmacology.[58] Pharmacologists were also beginning to find a place in government and industrial laboratories.[59] As the first decade of the new century drew to a close, American pharmacology had progressed in its search for a separate identity to the point where its practitioners felt the need for a separate organization of pharmacologists. Not surprisingly, it was John Abel who took the initiative in this direction.

Abel had been instrumental in the formation of the American Society of Biological Chemists in 1906, and already at that time he had in mind a similar organization for pharmacologists.[60] He began to communicate with his colleagues about this idea. In early 1908 he wrote to Torald Sollmann: "It is high time that we started a society. Our subject is suddenly getting popular. Twenty years ago there was very little interest taken in it." He went on to say that medical schools were finally waking up to the need for the subject, and that during the past year there had been about ten openings for pharmacologists in universities and not enough "good men" to fill them. A specialized society, he felt, would give young pharmacologists an opportunity to present research papers and discuss their results and views with their colleagues. He also believed that there was a need for a journal in the field and indicated to Sollmann that he was working on this problem as well.[61]

---

[56] On the famous Abel lunch table, see, for example, *ibid.*, p. 317; Samuel Amberg, "John Jacob Abel, decade, 1893–1903," *Bull. Johns Hopkins Hosp.*, 1957, *101*: 301–2; Paul Lamson, "John Jacob Abel—A portrait," *ibid.*, 1941; *68*: 140–41.

[57] Leonard Rowntree, "John Jacob Abel, decade, 1903–1913," *Bull. Johns Hopkins Hosp.*, 1957, *101*: 307.

[58] Cowen, "Materia Medica," pp. 109–10.

[59] For example, the Division of Pharmacology of the Hygienic Laboratory, United States Public Health Service was established in 1904. See R. C. Williams, *The United States Public Health Service, 1798–1950* (Washington, D.C.: Commissioned Officers Association of the United States Public Health Service, 1951), p. 244.

[60] William Gies to John Abel, 23 December 1906, Abel Papers.

[61] John Abel to Torald Sollmann, 16 January 1908, Abel Papers.

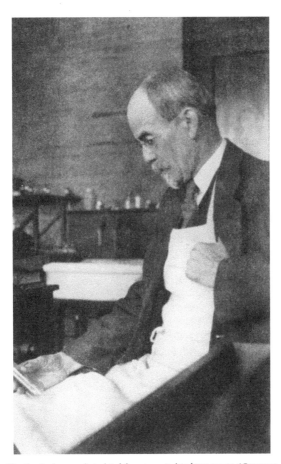

Fig. 3. Abel at work in his laboratory in his later years. (Courtesy of the Smithsonian Institution.)

On 28 December 1908, when the American Physiological Society and the American Society of Biological Chemists were meeting in Baltimore, eighteen men interested in pharmacology met at Abel's invitation in his laboratory to found the new society. It was a most appropriate place to establish the organization, to which the name "American Society for Pharmacology and Experimental Therapeutics" was given. As one would expect, Abel was made the first president of the society, while his former students Reid Hunt and Arthur Loevenhart became secretary and treasurer respectively.[62]

[62] On the founding of the Society, see K. K. Chen, ed., *The American Society for Pharmacology and Experimental Therapeutics, Incorporated: The First Sixty Years, 1908–1969* (Bethesda, Maryland: American Society for Pharmacology and Experimental Therapeutics, 1969), pp. 5–7. There are numerous documents related to the founding of the Society in the Abel Papers and in the "Minutes and Records" of the Society at its headquarters in Bethesda.

At the organizational meeting, Abel announced that he was establishing the *Journal of Pharmacology and Experimental Therapeutics* and invited the members of the society to become collaborators in this project. Although the *Journal* did not become the official organ of the society until 1933, when the society took over its ownership from Abel, the relationship between the two was a close one from the beginning. Abel served as editor of the publication from its founding in 1909 until his retirement from the chair of pharmacology at Hopkins in 1932. His successor as editor was the man who succeeded him in the chair at Hopkins, his former student E. K. Marshall, Jr.[63]

By 1909, American pharmacologists thus had their own national professional society and their own specialized journal, signs that pharmacology was achieving status as an independent scientific discipline in the United States. John J. Abel, and his laboratory at The Johns Hopkins University, played a crucial role in that process. Recognizing his contributions to the discipline, his colleagues came to regard him as the "Father of American Pharmacology."[64]

---

[63] On the history of the *Journal*, see Maurice Seevers, "Publications," in Chen, ed., *American Society*, pp. 123–31. The Abel Papers and the "Minutes and Records" of the American Society for Pharmacology and Experimental Therapeutics also contain numerous materials on the development of the *Journal*.

[64] On the one-hundredth anniversary of Abel's birth, a memorial volume was published under the title of *John Jacob Abel, M.D., Investigator, Teacher, Prophet, 1857–1938: A Collection of Papers by and about the Father of American Pharmacology* (Baltimore: Williams and Wilkins, 1957). Abel was widely recognized as the "founder" of American pharmacology by his contemporaries, and has continued to be so regarded by pharmacologists today.

X

Development of Pharmacology in American Schools of Pharmacy *

by John Parascandola and John Swann

THE SCIENCE of pharmacology occupies an important place in today's pharmacy curriculum. It has been referred to by pharmaceutical educators as being the "focus of the curriculum thrust" towards biological science and "the key to the development of the pharmacist's clinical role."[1] One pharmacy school dean has commented that:

> For practicing pharmacists, it is pharmacology which is the most important and indeed the keystone course in the curriculum. In any school of pharmacy where it is taught at a lower level than to medical students, it is a disservice to the profession and a betrayal of the student's trust. The practicing pharmacist must be an expert on drugs, and pharmacology is the bulwark of this expertise.[2]

Pharmacology did not always occupy such an honored place in pharmaceutical education. When the relatively new science of pharmacology was struggling to establish itself in the United States around the turn of the twentieth century, it found its first academic home in schools of medicine. American schools and colleges of pharmacy were slower to make the transition from courses in traditional materia medica to those in modern pharmacology than were their counterparts in the field of medicine. At the time an extensive understanding of the physiological action of drugs did not seem essential for the practicing pharmacist. As the perceived role and the education of the pharmacist evolved during the course of the twentieth century, a knowledge of pharmacology came to be viewed as a necessary part of the pharmacist's training. The purpose of this paper is to trace the development of pharmacology in American pharmaceutical education.

Pharmacology Emerges as a Discipline

Although the word "pharmacology" dates back to at least the seventeenth century (as a general term referring to the study of drugs), modern pharmacology did not emerge as a distinct discipline until the nineteenth century. Experiments on the physiological effects of drugs and poisons upon animals and humans have been sporadically performed since antiquity, but the birth of the science of experimental pharmacology is generally associated with the work of the French physiologist Francois Magendie in the early nineteenth century.

It was in the Germanic universities, however, rather than in France, that pharmacology first clearly established itself as an independent discipline,

* Presented before the Section on Contributed Papers, American Institute of the History of Pharmacy, Las Vegas, April 27, 1982. This publication was supported in part by NIH Grant LM03300 from the National Library of Medicine.

related to but distinct from physiology. The German Rudolf Buchheim appears to have founded the first institute of pharmacology at the University of Dorpat in 1847. Although Dorpat was in Russian-governed Estonia, the university was essentially German.

Chairs of materia medica had existed in medical schools long before the mid-nineteenth century, but materia medica had concerned itself largely with the origin, constituents, preparation and traditional therapeutic uses of drugs rather than with their physiological action. It was more closely allied to botany, chemistry and pharmacy (as well as practical therapeutics) than it was to physiology. Buchheim called for an independent, experimental discipline of pharmacology.

Buchheim's student and successor at Dorpat, Oswald Schmiedeberg, probably did more than any other single individual to establish pharmacology as an autonomous discipline, especially after his move to Strassburg in 1872. Schmiedeberg's pharmacological institute at Strassburg became a mecca for students of pharmacology from all over the world. It has been estimated that about 120 students from some twenty different countries worked in his laboratory, and that his students later occupied approximately forty academic chairs. Schmiedeberg was also the cofounder and coeditor of the first journal of experimental pathology and pharmacology *(Archivs für experimentelle Pathologie und Pharmakologie)*.[3]

It was one of Schmiedeberg's students, John J. Abel, who played the key role in the transmission of the new science of experimental pharmacology from Germany to the United States. Appointed Professor of Materia Medica and Therapeutics at the University of Michigan in 1891, Abel immediately transformed the traditional, didactic materia medica course for medical students into a modern pharmacology course which included experimental demonstrations. Two years later he moved to the newly-established medical school of The Johns Hopkins University where his laboratory became the center of American pharmacology.[4]

A number of other American medical schools began to make the transition from materia medica to pharmacology around the turn of the twentieth century.[5] The famous Flexner Report of 1910 on medical education stressed

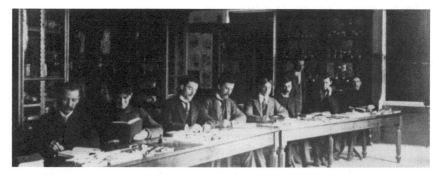

Pharmacy students at the University of Wisconsin studying crude drug samples for their materia medica course, 1894-95. (Courtesy of F. B. Power Pharmaceutical Library, University of Wisconsin.)

the importance of pharmacology for rational therapeutics and referred to materia medica as a subject "now much shrunken."[6] Pharmacologists were also beginning to find a place in government and industrial laboratories at about this time. By the close of the first decade of the twentieth century, pharmacology had become sufficiently well established as a discipline in the United States to have its own national society (American Society for Pharmacology and Experimental Therapeutics) and specialized journal *(Journal of Pharmacology and Experimental Therapeutics).*

Materia Medica and the Traditional Pharmacy Curriculum

Until the late nineteenth century, the standard curriculum in American schools of pharmacy consisted of three subjects: materia medica, pharmacy and chemistry. Courses in materia medica generally embraced a wide variety of topics related to the study of drugs, including aspects of botany, pharmacognosy, toxicology, pharmacology and therapeutics. No doubt the course varied considerably from school to school depending upon the instructor. Whatever its exact nature, however, it would appear that the typical pharmacy school course in materia medica in the late nineteenth century devoted more attention to the origin, cultivation, commerce, identification, preservation, physical properties and chemical constituents of drugs than to their physiological action and therapeutic uses.[7]

Surveying the development of materia medica in American schools of pharmacy in the nineteenth century, historian of pharmacy J. Hampton Hoch concluded that as pharmacists increasingly replaced physicians as teachers of the subject as the century progressed, "it permitted the development of a kind of materia medica which placed more emphasis on pharmacognosy and less on therapeutics."[8] In 1892, Edward Kremers of the University of Wisconsin drew a distinction between "pharmaceutical materia medica" for pharmacy students and "medical materia medica" for medical students.[9] A decade earlier, in a discussion of pharmaceutical education in the United States, Oscar Oldberg of the Chicago College of Pharmacy had already emphasized the different needs of medical and pharmacy students with respect to the teaching of materia medica.

For the information of prospective students of pharmacy, who frequently study materia medica in the dispensatories and in works on materia medica and therapeutics prepared for the use of students of medicine, and in the hope of being able to relieve them of much useless labor by pointing out particularly the kind of information they should acquire as well as the kind of study they may safely omit, we will state, that the physical properties, microscopical structure, and chemical constituents of drugs are always much more thoroughly taught in a college of pharmacy than in a medical college; while the medical properties and uses, which are all-important in the course of materia medica in a medical college, are necessarily and properly passed over very briefly in a college of pharmacy. Thus, while a whole lecture may be devoted to the physiological effects and the therapeutic properties and uses of opium when the lecture is given the students of medicine, the lecturer on pharmacognosy may very properly limit his remarks on the action and uses of that drug, important as it is, to less than a hundred, or even less than fifty words. Therapeutics, in other words, is not taught in the colleges of pharmacy, because practicing pharmacists as such have no use for it.[10]

To Oldberg and many of his contemporaries, an intimate knowledge of the physiological and therapeutic action did not seem essential in light of the traditional role of the pharmacist as a compounder and dispenser of medicines. Rather, said Oldberg, materia medica should convey to the student of pharmacy "such an intimate knowledge of the drugs as will enable their certain identification, and the unfailing recognition and selection of good and pure drugs."[11] The noted pharmacist John Maisch also stressed the greater value of pharmacognosy over pharmacology for the pharmacist: "Whatever views may be held, regarding the necessity for the apothecary, of a thorough knowledge of the physiological action of medicines upon man and animals, it must certainly be granted that a knowledge of the botanical, physical, histological, chemical and commercial relations and of the proper doses of drugs, is of by far greater importance to the apothecary and druggists."[12]

Toward the end of the century, led by state universities such as Michigan and Wisconsin, many American pharmacy schools began to develop a curriculum that gave greater emphasis to basic science and laboratory experience. Instruction in schools of pharmacy was placed on essentially a full-time basis, in place of the traditional pattern of evening lectures. With the development of a full-time, laboratory science-based curriculum, more specialized subjects, branching off the old trio of omnibus courses, were introduced. Courses such as analytical chemistry, organic chemistry, physics, toxicology, botany, pharmacognosy and physiology found their way into the pharmacy programs of at least the stronger institutions.[13]

By the 1890's at least a few educators, as will be discussed in the next section, were arguing the desirability of incorporating pharmacology into the pharmacy curriculum. Even Oldberg, who a decade earlier had deemphasized the pharmacist's need for knowledge of the physiological and therapeutic effects of drugs, had a change of heart. He expressed concern that in reacting against the medically-oriented materia medica courses taught by physicians, many pharmacy schools had gone too far in almost entirely eliminating instruction in "pharmacodynamics" (a term commonly used to designate the study of the physiological action of drugs, i.e., pharmacology in the modern sense of the word). While extended reference to the application of medicines to the treatment of disease was not appropriate for pharmacy students, Oldberg now felt that an elementary course in pharmacodynamics, adapted to the need of pharmacists, merited a place in the pharmacy curriculum.[14]

But courses in pharmacology did not find a home in most schools of pharmacy for many years to come. Descriptive pharmacognosy continued to dominate instruction in the field of materia medica. A number of reasons were offered in opposition to devoting significant attention to pharmacology in the pharmacy curriculum. As suggested before, there was a feeling on the part of some pharmacists and educators that pharmacology, like therapeutics, belonged to the realm of the physician rather than that of the pharmacist. Professor William Simon of the Maryland College of Pharmacy, for example, stated in 1892:

> The division of labor between the physician and the pharmacist, points out clearly the field each one has to cultivate. The manufacture and the dispensing of medicines is the proper field of the pharmacist, and for this he neither requires a study of the physiological actions, changes, and processes in the animal body, nor does he necessarily require a detailed knowledge of the therapeutic action of the medicines he dispenses.[15]

Echoing this view in commenting on Simon's paper, A. H. Elliott of the New York College of Pharmacy noted that the province of the pharmacist is "the manufacture of medicines and a knowledge of their properties and constituents" and that he should not "encroach upon the domain of the physician" by putting too much emphasis on physiology and therapeutics.[16] In a similar vein, a critic of the 1910 *Pharmaceutical Syllabus* (discussed in the next section) argued that the 80 hours devoted to physiology, toxicology, posology, pharmacodynamics and therapeutics in the proposed curriculum was "an unnecessary waste of time from the standpoint of the utility." He added that unless the object was to qualify druggists to prescribe medicines, as English apothecaries did, then the total time spent on these subjects could be reduced to no more than 20 to 30 hours.[17]

The concern about the proper domain of the pharmacist versus the physician is also reflected in the discussion of therapeutic incompatibilities in pharmacy textbooks of the period. Caspari, for example, stated that since therapeutic incompatibility depended upon antagonism between the physiological or medical actions of drugs, it did "not properly belong to the domain of the pharmacy" but was "solely in the hands of the physician." Similarly, Remington commented that this form of incompatibility did not often require the aid of the pharmacist, for "the correction of the fault lies solely within the province of the physician." Scoville also saw therapeutic incompatibility as being "beyond the ken of pharmacists." Typically these textbooks urged the pharmacist to use caution in questioning the knowledge of the physician in such matters.[18]

It was also argued that if the pharmacist acquired too much knowledge of the physiological action and therapeutic uses of drugs, he would be tempted to indulge in counter prescribing.[19] Another justification for opposing the introduction of a pharmacology course into the pharmacy curriculum was the problem of finding time for it. Even as dedicated an educational reformer as Edward Kremers felt that time could not be spared from the other subjects in the curriculum to enable a satisfactory course in pharmacology to be offered.[20] Finally, there were those who felt that the pharmacy curriculum overemphasized theoretical as opposed to practical training, an attitude which scarcely encouraged the addition of coursework in a subject whose direct relevance to pharmacy practice was, at the time, questionable.[21]

Pioneer Teaching of Pharmacology in Pharmacy Schools

Recommendations that pharmacology should become a part of the pharmacy curriculum emerged as early as the 1890's. For example, in 1892 a physician named R. H. Brown claimed that pharmacists who were ignorant of pharmacology were not worthy of the profession. Brown reasoned that since toxicology was generally considered to be an appropriate subject for pharmacy students then pharmacology should likewise be accepted. A knowledge of the toxic actions of substances was incomplete, he argued, without some understanding of their physiological actions in controlling diseases. Moreover, pharmacology contributed to the preparation of thoroughly educated graduates, thus assuring them of rewarding positions.[22]

At the 1897 meeting of the American Pharmaceutical Association, Alfred R. L. Dohme, of the pharmaceutical firm Sharp & Dohme and President of the Maryland Pharmaceutical Association, offered several reasons why pharmacology should be adopted by colleges of pharmacy. Pharmacology not only broadened the pharmacist's knowledge of drugs and created a new field of work for him, but more significantly it allowed him to prevent therapeutically incompatible prescriptions (a function which, as has been previously noted, some of Dohme's colleagues did not see as falling within the sphere of pharmacy). Against those who argued that the curriculum was already too crowded to allow for the introduction of a new subject, Dohme countered that the pharmacy student typically had only five subjects to study, as opposed to up to fifteen subjects for the medical student and about ten subjects for the law student.[23]

It is not surprising, however, that most pharmacy schools did not offer significant instruction in pharmacology in this early period, when the discipline was only first becoming established in American medical schools by John J. Abel and his colleagues. Unlike medical schools, schools of pharmacy did not have a tradition of teaching physiology and other biological sciences. Pharmaceutical educators had several reasons, as already discussed, for rejecting pharmacology. Yet the subject did find a home at the time in some far-sighted schools of pharmacy, most notably at the University of Michigan and the University of Nebraska.

The University of Michigan School of Pharmacy pioneered in the development of a basic science-oriented curriculum from its founding in 1868. The man chiefly responsible for this innovation was the physican-chemist Albert Prescott, Dean of the Michigan pharmacy faculty. According to Prescott, the thoroughly-trained pharmacist had to be prepared to dispense and prepare galenical, natural and synthetic drugs; to assay drugs for quality, purity and strength; and to give advice as needed to the medical profession and the public (as the chemist of the community). To fulfill these demands, Prescott felt that it was the duty of the pharmacy college to offer, in addition to the traditional pharmacy courses, extensive laboratory work and instruction in the basic sciences.[24]

Throughout the 1880's, the materia medica course in the pharmacy curriculum at Michigan was taught by faculty in the medical school, and included "lectures on the physiological action of drugs." In 1891, the school of pharmacy catalog listed, for the first time, a course that bore the title "Pharmacology and Therapeutics" (in addition to the materia medica course).[25] It was no accident that the introduction of this subject coincided with Abel's arrival at Michigan. During his first year, Abel taught a course in pharmacology for third-year medical students, dental students and pharmacy students. The course involved experimental demonstrations by the instructor, but not laboratory work on the part of the students. Apparently Abel soon came to feel, however, that the pharmacy and dental students did not possess sufficient knowledge of physiology and medicine for the course.[26] In any case, the 1892-1893 pharmacy school catalog now clearly labeled the course in "Pharmacology and Therapeutics" as an elective (which had not been the case the previous year).[27] Presumably the course referred to was still Abel's course in the medical school, in which selected pharmacy students apparently were allowed to enroll, but it is difficult to be sure since the catalog does not identify the instructor.

The catalog for 1895-1896, by which time Abel had left Michigan, listed for the first time a laboratory course in pharmacology taught by Abel's successor in the medical school, Arthur Cushny. The course was an elective "obtained only by permission," and appears to have been aimed at students taking the optional four-year Bachelor of Science in Pharmacy Degree rather than at students in the standard two-year program. The lecture course in "Pharmacology and Therapeutics" was no longer shown in the catalog. Beginning in 1901, the University also offered a three-year course in pharmacy, with the last year devoted to studies in pharmacology, bacteriology, physiology, physiological chemistry and related subjects.[28]

Michigan was not the only American school of pharmacy to offer substantial instruction in pharmacology in the last decade of the nineteenth century. When Clement Lowe (Ph.G., M.D.) became Professor of Materia Medica at the Philadelphia College of Pharmacy in 1897, for example, he appears to have given significant emphasis to the physiological action of drugs in his materia medica course. By 1905, the Univerity of North Carolina was requiring of its pharmacy students a course on "Materia Medica and Pharmacology," taught by a physician, which gave particular attention to the physiological action of remedies and "the indications for their rational use."[29]

Pharmacology thus began to find a niche in the pharmaceutical curriculum of at least a few schools. With the appointment of Rufus A. Lyman as Dean of the University of Nebraska School of Pharmacy, pharmacology found a great defender and popularizer. In 1908, Lyman, a physician and Professor of Physiology and Pharmacology at the University of Nebraska School of Medicine, accepted an offer to organize a school of pharmacy at Nebraska. According to Lyman, the average pharmaceutical curriculum of the day was "the most devitalizing nonstimulating setup" that he had ever seen. His plans to "vitalize pharmacy" involved the introduction of much more biological science into the curriculum. Among the courses included in the curriculum of the new school were zoology, bacteriology, physiology and pharmacology. Lyman considered the latter subject "absolutely necessary in order to make it possible for pharmacists to practice their profession intelligently."[31]

The Nebraska pharmacology course, which was required for the two-, three-, and four-year programs, consisted of four hours each of lectures and laboratory for one semester. Nebraska was apparently the first American school of pharmacy to require a course in pharmacology that included both lectures and laboratory work as a part of the two-year program. The course was not taught in the medical school (as it was at Michigan), but in the school of pharmacy by Lyman himself.[32]

When Lyman attempted to share his belief in the importance of pharmacology with other pharmaceutical educators, his views were apparently not greeted with general enthusiasm. For example, his paper on the value of experimental pharmacology in the pharmacy curriculum at the 1910 meeting of the American Pharmaceutical Association was not received very favorably. Lyman later recalled (although perhaps with exaggeration) that one vocal critic "thought I was insane and made a motion not to receive the paper or have it printed in the Proceedings of the Association." Just as the motion was about to be passed, according to Lyman, Henry Kraemer, Professor of Pharmacognosy at the Philadelphia College of Pharmacy and editor of the College's *American Journal of Pharmacy,* intervened and invited Lyman to publish his paper in the *Journal.*[33]

Lyman's paper appeared in the *American Journal of Pharmacy* in November of 1910.[34] Here he argued that both physicians and pharmacists should be knowledgeable about the physiological action of drugs. Lyman also suggested that pharmacology would provide the pharmacist with at least the general principles of the physiological standardization procedures in the pharmacopeia and would enhance his standing in the eyes of the physician and the public. Pharmacology was not just a desireable addition to the curriculum, according to Lyman, but a fundamental ingredient of pharmaceutical education.

> I can see no reason why, at least, the fundamentals of experimental pharmacology could not be taught to students of pharmacy. They should, at least, be shown that drugs do induce physiological changes, that these changes are inducted by action upon certain part or parts of the organism, and that such action may be used as a means of classification and standardization. If such a movement could be made general, it would give a wonderful impetus to a science which is full of promise for improving both medical and pharmaceutical practice.[35]

Years later Lyman reflected on what he believed were the two main forces working against the inclusion of pharmacology in the pharmaceutical curriculum ever since he presented his paper in 1910. The first force was ignorance: "For a quarter of a century I have listened to arguments in the American Association of Colleges of Pharmacy against the education of the pharmacist. The attitude has always been that it is dangerous to teach the pharmacist anything." Arguments against introducing courses such as bacteriology or pharmacology because these would offend the medical community were forwarded, not by physicians, Lyman said, but by "the ignorant pharmacist or his ally."[36] The second force was the idea that the introduction of a pharmacology course would be far too expensive for pharmacy schools. For example, the Chairman of the Syllabus Committee in the early 1930's cast the deciding vote against making pharmacology a required subject, because he felt too many schools could not afford to adopt it. But Lyman had pointed out in 1910 that most of the equipment for a pharmacology laboratory could be found in a physiology laboratory. Thus, even if schools did not already have programs in physiology, pharmacy schools could develop programs in both physiology and pharmacology (the former was a prerequisite of the latter anyway) at a fairly reasonable cost.[37]

Rufus Lyman pioneered the introduction of biological sciences into the pharmaceutical curriculum. Although Nebraska was not the first school to offer instruction in pharmacology, it was the first to grant experimental pharmacology a major place in the required two-year pharmacy curriculum. Lyman's course was based upon physiology as a prerequisite, and involved extensive laboratory work as well as four hours of lectures weekly. Lyman himself became a valuable crusader for the field. Although his recommendations concerning pharmacology were not immediately adopted by most schools, in time pharmacy educators came to agree with his view that the subject was indeed vital to pharmacy.

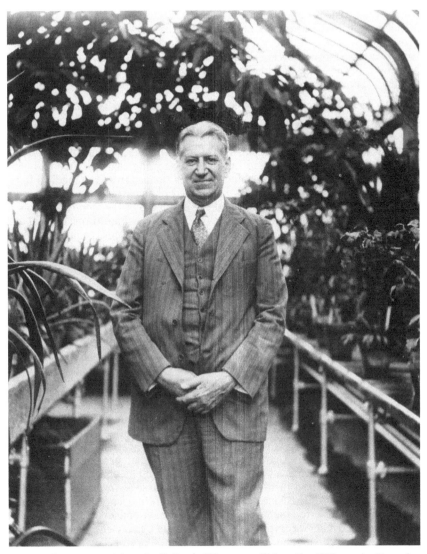

Rufus A. Lyman on a visit to the College of Pharmacy, University of Minnesota, November, 1933. (Courtesy of F. B. Power Pharmaceutical Library, University of Wisconsin.)

During the same year that Lyman's paper appeared in the *American Journal of Pharmacy*, the National Syllabus Committee issued the first edition of *The Pharmaceutical Syllabus* (1910). This guide to the pharmacy curriculum recommended that pharmacology be offered during the second year of study for a total of 35 clock hours (out of 500 total hours), far below what Nebraska required of its students, and no mention was made of laboratory work. When the second edition of the *Syllabus* appeared in 1913, the recommended time to be spent on pharmacology had been doubled, reflecting a growing awareness of the value of the subject even in this brief period of time.[38] Lyman's advocacy may well have helped create this awareness. By the beginning of the First World War, pharmacology was thus slowly beginning to find a home in American schools and colleges of pharmacy.

Growth of Pharmacology Between Two World Wars

The efforts and recommendations to include pharmacology in the pharmaceutical curriculum continued to grow after the First World War. In 1919, Henry J. Goeckel presented a paper to the American Pharmaceutical Association's Section on Education and Legislation, arguing that the time had come for biological, chemical, and technical studies to pass from the medical to the pharmacy schools. He specifically mentioned pharmacology in this connection. In the first place, he believed that the emphasis of the medical schools on these sciences came at the expense of the more important clinical and diagnostic studies. Also, sciences such as pharmacology required a more thorough background in pharmacy and chemistry than the medical schools were offering; of course, this was not a problem in pharmacy schools. According to Goeckel, pharmacy schools would be the training grounds for a new member of the field of health care in the near future, the "hospital pharmacologist":

> With the rapid advance in biological and physiological research, the time is not far off when a trained pharmacologist will be one of the regular staff of every first-class hospital. His duties will be to advise the staff as to what remedies, and what particular form of the same and what method of application are advisable. Such a hospital or community pharmacologist will also need to see that the various preparations are correctly prepared by the supply house, hospital apothecary or nurse, as the occasion requires.[39]

William H. Zeigler, Professor of Pharmacology and Materia Medica at the School of Pharmacy and Medical College of the University of South Carolina, was also a strong supporter of pharmacology in the pharmaceutical curriculum. Like Rufus Lyman, Zeigler believed that pharmacology was as necessary to the pharmacist as to the physician, and he urged that laboratory instruction be required in the pharmacology course.[40] In his address as the retiring President of the American Conference of Pharmaceutical Faculties in 1925, Zeigler presented his views on the position of pharmacology in the new three-year pharmacy program. He said it should occupy eight percent of the total time the student spent in the classroom or laboratory, or 180 hours, over the second and third years.[41] Physiology was an essential prerequisite to an intelligent study of the physiological action of drugs, according to Zeigler, and the School of Pharmacy at South Carolina (much like Nebraska) indeed required didactic and experimental work in physiology before the pharmacology course.[42]

The third edition of *The Pharmaceutical Syllabus* (1922) increased the suggested time devoted to pharmacology dramatically, compared to earlier editions. For the three-year program in pharmacy, the Pharmaceutical Syllabus Committee recommended that the course in materia medica – which included pharmacology – be offered for 15 clock hours in the first year, 75 hours in the second year, and 75 hours also for the final year.[43]

The American Conference of Pharmaceutical Faculties (ACPF), in 1917, established six sections within the Committee on Questions and Examinations "to consider the larger question of teaching, as well as of [uniform] examination." One of the sections was called "Physiology and Pharmacology, including Biological Assaying and Experimental Pharmacology," certainly an indication of the growing interest in pharmacology.[44] Two years later the section on Physiology and Pharmacology, after examining the requirements for pharmacology at several schools, published its own suggestions for the time to be devoted to this science in schools of pharmacy. The section concluded that 12 to 15 hours should be sufficient in the two-year course "to enable the student to intelligently understand what is meant when matters of drug action and drug uses are discussed." However, the section expected the three- and four-year courses to provide enough instruction in pharmacology (e.g., 45-60 hours of laboratory work alone in the three-year program, and as much above 60 hours in the four-year program as possible) "to enable the student to accept positions in pharmacodynamic laboratories."[45]

In 1920 A. Richard Bliss, Jr., Professor of Pharmacology at the School of Medicine of Emory University and later the Dean of the School of Pharmacy of the University of Tennessee, published the first detailed survey of the status of pharmacology in schools of pharmacy. Based on data gathered from questionnaires and catalogs from 51 pharmacy schools, Bliss showed that about half of these schools taught pharmacology. Of the 26 schools offering pharmacology, 17 gave the subject as a separate course and nine presented it as part of another course (e. g., materia medica). Although 25 schools did not offer pharmacology, 13 of these expressed a desire to add it to their curricula. A few of the pharmacy schools offered pharmacology through medical schools, and Bliss saw no problem with this approach. However, the pharmacy school-medical school affiliation was not always a friendly and beneficial one for the pharmacy students. For example, Melvin R. Gibson, editor of the *American Journal of Pharmaceutical Education*, related his experience as a pharmacy student at the University of Illinois: "During the lectures in pharmacology [at the medical school] the pharmacologists cast snide remarks at the pharmacy students . . . . The pharmacy students instead of becoming proud of their profession, were made painfully aware it did not enjoy the respect of the medical profession."[46]

Of the schools offering pharmacology, the average number of hours devoted to lecture and laboratory were 40 and 19, respectively, a total of almost 60 clock hours. Although Bliss felt that the total number of hours was sufficient, he was dissatisfied with the small amount of time that students were spending in the laboratory. The experimental work should have accounted for one-half to two-thirds of the time devoted to pharmacology, according to Bliss. He pointed out that a majority of the 26 schools (about 62%) were offering only didactic work, and that at least some were probably simply giving the uses of drugs and calling such instruction "pharmacodynamics."[47] However, 76% of the schools Bliss surveyed in 1920 either taught at least some pharmacology or wished to add the course to their program; clearly educators believed pharmacology should become a part of the pharmaceutical curriculum.[48]

Shortly after the appearance of Bliss' papers a group of educators from the University of Pittsburgh and the University of Buffalo, in collaboration with the American Association of Colleges of Pharmacy, the National Association of Boards of Pharmacy, and the National Association of Retail Druggists, began a study of the functional role of the pharmacist and the curriculum necessary to fulfill that role. The study culminated in 1927 with the publication of *Basic Material For a Pharmaceutical Curriculum*. This so-called Charters Survey recognized "that it is absolutely essential for [the pharmacist] to have a rather wide and intimate acquaintance with the fundamental sciences upon which the art depends," and included pharmacology among these fundamental sciences.[49] The Charters Survey had a revitalizing effect on the profession of pharmacy, and its specific influence on the teaching of pharmacology in schools of pharmacy was also dramatic. As Rufus Lyman related several years later: "I have been criticized by other schools as overloading the curriculum with physiology and pharmacology. This continued until the Charters Study was made and the attitude of the pharmacists of the country was changed entirely."[50] By the end of the 1920's, with support from the influential Charters Survey and the *Pharmaceutical Syllabus,* pharmacology was becoming more firmly established in schools of pharmacy.

Pharmacology made further inroads into the pharmaceutical curriculum during the 1930's. In 1932 A. R. Bliss, by this time the Dean of the School of Pharmacy of the University of Tennessee, published another article in support of pharmacology, with suggestions for operating the course. Bliss believed that pharmacology would not only safeguard the pharmacist from his own errors in compounding prescriptions, but it would also help him to recognize the errors of physicians when they wrote therapeutically incompatible prescriptions. Thus, pharmacology would be in the best interest of the public in the end. Bliss echoed the Charters Survey in his desire to have instruction in pharmacology solid in the essentials rather than exhaustive in its coverage of most of the drug armamentarium. In this way it would be more profitable to the pharmacist and more economical to the pharmacy school to emphasize a "synthetic conception" of the actions of drugs. That is, Bliss preferred the pharmacological treatment of groups of drugs rather than individual medicaments. This group approach would make a much greater and more enduring impression on the pharmacist.[51] In the same year, the National Pharmaceutical Syllabus Committee published the fourth edition of *The Pharmaceutical Syllabus,* with its recommended curriculum for a new four-year program. Pharmacology (including therapeutics, toxicology, and posology) occupied 96 clock hours of lectures in the *Syllabus,* but the Committee also suggested laboratory work in pharmacology – a total of 32 hours.[52]

Others also commented on the necessity of pharmacology in the early and mid-1930's. For example, pharmacologist Marvin R. Thompson of the Maryland School of Pharmacy believed that the rise of the prepackaged drug industry made it necessary for pharmacy schools to offer experimental pharmacology to their students in order to supply the manufacturers with qualified

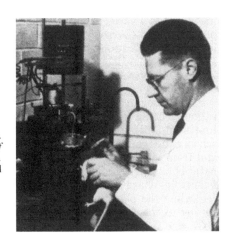

James Dille in the pharmacology laboratory. From *University of Washington College of Pharmacy, Announcements, 1945-1946.* (Courtesy of F. B. Power Pharmaceutical Library, University of Wisconsin.)

personnel for the necessary pharmacological standardizations of their products.[53] It was sometimes argued, however, that the ability to do bioassay work was of little value to the retail pharmacist, who did not have the facilities to perform biological standardizations in the pharmacy.[54]

In 1936 the Dean of the School of Pharmacy at the North Pacific College of Oregon, A. O. Mickelsen, offered some reasons why pharmacology was indeed vital to the professional pharmacist. For one thing, Mickelsen argued: "To be in a position to give definite information regarding the desired drug, its action, use and contraindications is bound to bring professional business to the pharmacist." Mickelsen thus envisioned the pharmacist, trained in pharmacology, as a drug expert and drug counselor. Like Bliss, he also felt that pharmacology would help the pharmacist recognize and prevent therapeutically incompatible prescriptions and those directing an overdose. Pharmacology would even be beneficial to the detail man, since "the selling point [of a drug] is pharmacology."[55]

Another indication of the growing status of pharmacology in the 1930's was the establishment of what was apparently the first name chair devoted to the subject in an American school of pharmacy. The Emerson chair in the University of Maryland School of Pharmacy, funded by a gift from Captain Isaac E. Emerson of the Emerson Drug Company, was actually announced in the school catalog for 1929. It was not until 1931, however, that Marvin R. Thompson was appointed Emerson Professor of Pharmacology. Thompson had received the Ebert Prize of the American Pharmaceutical Association in the previous year for his work on the pharmacology of ergot, and was only 26 at the time that he assumed the Emerson chair. He taught several courses in pharmacology and bioassay, as well as physiology, at Maryland.[56]

James Dille, a pharmacologist at the University of Washington, published an extremely important survey of pharmacology in pharmacy schools in 1938.[57] Dille's survey was far superior to Bliss's paper of 1920. He went beyond the questions Bliss had asked—how many schools taught pharmacology, in which years was it offered, and for how many clock hours—and investigated a variety of other topics such as the different titles used for the pharmacology courses, the textbooks used, the status of laboratory instruction, the qualifications of pharmacology teachers and the teaching responsibilities of pharmacology instructors. Using the extensive data that he collected, Dille was able to examine key problems and to assess the development of pharmacology as a discipline in schools of pharmacy.

Dille began planning for his 1938 survey as early as March of 1936, his rationale being that "if pharmacology is to grow in the field of pharmacy the first step is to take stock, hence the survey."[58] He collected his data from school catalogs, letters, questionnaires sent to the deans of pharmacy schools, and from visits to the schools.[59] Basically, Dille wanted to evaluate: 1) the nature of undergraduate work, 2) the laboratory facilities of the schools, 3) the faculty in pharmacology, 4) research, and 5) the philosophy of the deans regarding the place of pharmacology in the curriculum. Dille presented his survey to the American Association of Colleges of Pharmacy in August of 1937, and in the following year it was published in the *American Journal of Pharmaceutical Education*.[60]

Of the 55 members of the AACP, Dille found that almost all (approximately 50 schools) taught at least some pharmacology. Thirty-five of the Association schools offered basic pharmacology for at least one semester, including 21 that taught it for a year or more. To gain some impression of the nature of the undergraduate work in pharmacology, Dille examined the number of schools giving pharmacology as part of another course, the texts used, and the relationship of the courses to the recommendation in *The Pharmaceutical Syllabus*. Thirteen of the schools surveyed taught the subject with another course, which Dille believed was an inadequate way to treat the principles of pharmacology, considering the attention they required. Based on the texts used for pharmacology courses, Dille found a wide variation in the subject matter of the courses, since some schools employed "elementary" texts while others used "ponderous" ones. The pharmacology programs that adopted *The Pharmaceutical Syllabus* as a guide were wholly unsatisfactory, according to Dille, because the *Syllabus* itself left a great deal to be desired:

> At the present time the section on pharmacology is a heterogenous mass of unrelated material jumbled together without order or attention to logical classification. The group names are for the most part obsolete and undue importance is given to insignificant groups. It provokes contempt from a pharmacologist and the most encouraging thing about it is that many pharmacology teachers do not follow the syllabus.[61]

Dille also determined the number of schools giving laboratory work in the basic pharmacology course as another measure of the type of undergraduate work in pharmacology. Twenty-three schools offered a pharmacology laboratory, and of these several sent their students to a medical school pharmacology department. Like Bliss, Dille saw some advantages in pharmacy students taking pharmacology in medical schools. For example, the economic burden on the pharmacy schools would be significantly reduced, and the students would have the opportunity to come into contact with pharmacology specialists. However, there were also some problems, such as the possibility of emphasizing the pharmacological needs of the medical students over the needs of the pharmacy students, and the chance that pharmacy would begin to regard pharmacology as a medical discipline. Only sixteen pharmacy schools offered laboratory instruction within the school itself.[62]

Dille discovered some serious problems regarding the teachers of pharmacology. Few of them had any experience in pharmacology or even in physiology. Moreover, they were often required to teach a variety of courses in addition to pharmacology, many of which were unrelated to or only remotely related to pharmacology (e.g., bacteriology, botany, and public health). Pharmacology teachers in 13 schools taught from five to seven subjects in addition to pharmacology; only in three schools did teachers devote themselves solely to pharmacology. Such a situation could only exist, according to Dille, at the expense of pharmacology or the other subjects: "If a man must teach, in addition to pharmacology, five or six other subjects the only conclusion tenable is that every subject must have very low standards or that one has been developed to the exclusion of the others. Such a situation is incompatible with real education."[63] Pharmacy school deans and others who shaped the educational policies on pharmacology generally supported the admission of the subject to the curriculum but, according to Dille, most believed a lecture course in general pharmacology with a few demonstrations would be sufficient.[64]

It is safe to say that by the end of the 1930's pharmacology truly became a part of the pharmaceutical curriculum. About the time of World War I the main debate was whether or not schools should adopt this subject. By the beginning of World War II the problem was not so much *whether* pharmacology should be taught but *how* it should be taught. In the early 1920's about half of the pharmacy schools offered pharmacology, as Bliss pointed out, but by the late 1930's Dille demonstrated that almost every pharmacy school gave at least some pharmacology. Still, less than half of them offered laboratory work in pharmacology, and the course was often taught by someone who was not a pharmacologist and who was responsible for instruction in several different subjects.

Pharmacology After World War II

In the post-World War II period, the science of pharmacology has firmly established itself as one of the cornerstones of pharmaceutical education. When the revised tentative fifth edition of *The Pharmaceutical Syllabus* was issued in 1945, it contained a recommendation that a minimum of 112 didactic hours and 80 laboratory hours of instruction be devoted to pharmacology in the required curriculum.[65] A survey of American pharmacy schools conducted in 1945-1946 indicated that many schools were not meeting this suggested minimum, especially with respect to the laboratory hours. On the other hand, a large majority of schools were offering significant instruction in the subject. All but nine schools offered at least 64 hours of didactic instruction and all but ten schools offered at least 32 hours of laboratory work. In addition, some pharmacological instruction was also no doubt included in the separate courses in toxicology, posology, etc. that were taught at some institutions.[66]

The immediate postwar period also saw the initiation in 1946 of the most ambitious survey of American pharmacy undertaken to date.[67] One outgrowth

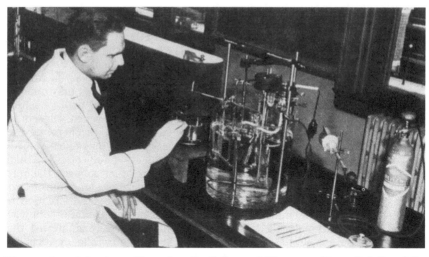

Pharmacology laboratory, Massachusetts College of Pharmacy. From *Bulletin of the Massachusetts College of Pharmacy*, Vol. 31, No. 1, March, 1942, p. 42. (Courtesy of F. B. Power Pharmaceutical Library, University of Wisconsin.)

of the Pharmaceutical Survey was the report, published in 1952, on *The Pharmaceutical Curriculum*, which an historian of American pharmaceutical education has called "the single most influential force on curriculum construction for at least two decades after its appearance."[68] What did this landmark work have to say concerning pharmacology?

Pharmacology was termed "one of the fundamental supporting sciences of pharmacy." The pharmacist required a knowledge of pharmacology in order that he might consult with and advise physicians, critically evaluate drug literature and labeling, make decisions involving legal regulation of drugs, and supply information to the public concerning the action of drugs. The report emphasized that changes in pharmaceutical practice and the field of service envisioned for the pharmacist in the future made substantial training in pharmacology a necessity.

The Pharmaceutical Curriculum reported that every approved college of pharmacy included some instruction in pharmacology in its curriculum, and that the median number of semester hours devoted to the subject was seven. Occasionally, however, it was found that the term "pharmacology" was used for a course whose description clearly indicated that it actually consisted of "outmoded descriptive content of materia medica instead of dynamic modern materials from the field of experimental pharmacology." The report recommended that materia medica should be dropped from the curriculum, and that the course in pharmacology should carry six semester hours of credit, consisting of 64 hours of didactic instruction and 96 hours of laboratory work.[69]

Since most schools by the early 1950's appeared to be devoting significant time in the curriculum to pharmacology, concern about the teaching of the subject came to center more around the quality of the instruction and the instructor. *The Pharmaceutical Curriculum,* for example, complained that the lack of adequately trained personnel had limited and retarded the development of instruction in pharmacology in colleges of pharmacy.[70] In 1951, Richard Deno of the Rutgers University College of Pharmacy evaluated the credentials of teachers of pharmacology in American colleges of pharmacy. Defining "professional pharmacologists" as those who had graduate training in the subject, held memberships in relevent scientific societies, and published in pharmacological journals, he found that 34 of the 72 accredited colleges were served by professionals. Included in this total of 34, however, were 14 colleges in which the pharmacology course for pharmacy students was taught in the medical school. At the other colleges of pharmacy, the subject was taught by personnel whom Deno categorized as "semi-professionals" (those who had some training and interest in the subject, but were not very active in research or publication) or by "pinch hitters" (those who had little or no advanced training in the subject and contributed little or nothing of an original nature).[71]

A few years earlier, Ewart Swinyard and L. David Hiner of the University of Utah had lamented the fact that schools of pharmacy often employed only one person to teach both pharmacognosy and pharmacology. Under such conditions, they felt, one or the other subject had to suffer. They called for a revision of the by-laws of the American Association of Colleges of Pharmacy to require member colleges to have at least one full-time teacher of professional rank for each of these subjects. Swinyard and Hiner particularly stressed the fact that changes in pharmaceutical practice required more emphasis on the biological sciences, and that to be a real ally to the physician "the pharmacist must be as well grounded as the physician in all the basic sciences and be able to discuss therapy with him without any sense of inferiority."[72]

Suggestions that the role of the pharmacist was undergoing change and that he should serve as more of an advisor on drugs to the physician and the patient, like those noted by Swinyard and Hiner and by the authors of *The Pharmaceutical Curriculum,* were given new meaning as the concept of clinical pharmacy began to emerge more clearly in the 1960's. The patient-oriented, clinical approach to pharmacy, with its emphasis on the role of the pharmacist in insuring safe and effective use of drugs, called for a greater knowledge of biomedical science and therapeutics. Pharmacology's place within the pharmacy curriculum has obviously been strengthened by these developments.[73]

A survey of pharmacy schools conducted in 1976 revealed that the average number of clock lecture hours of pharmacology was 118. In addition, pharmacology laboratory was a core requirement in 71% of the schools responding.[74] All but about ten American colleges of pharmacy offer their own instruction in pharmacology, rather than arranging for such coursework through the medical school.[75] Many pharmacy schools offer graduate degrees in pharmacology, with a national total of about 270 students enrolled in such programs in 1978.[76] Pharmacological research is being actively pursued today by numerous well-qualified pharmacologists based in schools of pharmacy.[77] Over the course of the twentieth century, pharmacology has thus progressed

X

from a subject whose relevance to the pharmacist was in question to one which now occupies a central place in the pharmacy curriculum.

Notes and References

1. Robert Talbot and Charles Walton, "An Integrated Approach to Instruction in Pharmacology and Therapeutics," *Am. J. Pharm. Educ.*, 40 (1976): 369; Lawrence Weaver, "The Importance of Pharmacology and Toxicology to the Pharmacist in the Delivery of Improved Patient Care," *ibid.*, 35 (1971): 734.

2. Linwood Tice, "Pharmacy Education for Today and the Future,' paper presented at the Medical College of South Carolina, October 28, 1966, pp. 6-7. Copy in Kremers Reference Files, at C31(a)I, F. B. Power Pharmaceutical Library, University of Wisconsin-Madison.

3. On the early development of pharmacology see Melvin Earles, "Studies in the Development of Experimental Pharmacology in the Eighteenth and Early Nineteenth Centuries" (Ph.D. diss., University College, London, 1961); J. E. Lesch, "The Origins of Experimental Physiology and Pharmacology in France, 1790-1820" (Ph.D. diss., Princeton University, 1977); Gustav Kuchinsky, "The Influence of Dorpat on the Emergence of Pharmacology as a Distinct Discipline," *J. Hist. Med.*, 23 (1968): 258-71; and Jan Koch-Weser and Paul Shechter, "Schmiedeberg in Strassburg, 1872-1918: The Making of Modern Pharmacology," *Life Sci.*, 22(1978): 1361-71.

4. On Abel's role in the development of American pharmacology, see John Parascandola, "John J. Abel and the Early Development of Pharmacology at the Johns Hopkins University," *Bull. Hist. Med.*, 56(1982): 512-527.

5. For an overview of the history of teaching of pharmacology in American medical schools, see David L. Cowen, "Materia Medica and Pharmacology," in Ronald Numbers, ed., *The Education of American Physicians: Historical Essays* (University of California, Berkeley, 1980), pp. 95-121.

6. Abraham Flexner, *Medical Education in the United States and Canada.* (Carnegie Foundation for the Advancement of Teaching, New York, 1910), pp. 63-5.

7. On the teaching of materia medica in American schools of pharmacy, see J. Hampton Hoch, "A Survey of the Development of Materia Medica in American Schools and Colleges of Pharmacy from 1821 to 1900," *Am. J. Pharm. Educ.*, 12 (1948): 148-61; and Glenn Sonnedecker, "American Pharmaceutical Education before 1900" (Ph.D. diss., University of Wisconsin, 1952), pp. 423-33. An examination of the collection of pharmacy school catalogs in the F. B. Power Pharmaceutical Library, University of Wisconsin-Madison also provides valuable information on materia medica courses.

8. Hoch, "Development of Materia Medica," 152.

9. Edward Kremers, "Notes on Pharmaceutical Education: The Study of Materia Medica," *Proc. Am. Pharm. Assoc.*, 40 (1892): 309-17.

10. Oscar Oldberg, *Pharmaceutical Education in the United States* (Cowdrey, Clark and Co., Chicago, 1884), pp. 6-7.

11. *Ibid.*, p. 7.

12. [John Maisch], review of *Eleventh Annual Report of the Alumni Association of the Philadelphia College of Pharmacy* (1875), *Am. J. Pharm.*, 47 (1875): 236.

13. Sonnedecker, "American Pharmaceutical Education," pp. 423-33, 454-7; Hoch, "Development of Materia Medica," 154-61.

14. [Oscar Oldberg], "Anatomy, Physiology and Therapeutics in Pharmaceutical Schools" (editorial), *Apothecary* (Chicago), 2 (1892): 23-6.

15. W. Simon, "The Three Years' Course in Colleges of Pharmacy," *Proc. Am. Pharm. Assoc.*, 40 (1892): 301.

16. A. H. Elliott, discussion, *ibid.*, 302-3.

17. Quoted in H. L. Taylor, "Schools and Colleges of Pharmacy," *Pharm. Era*, 45 (1912): 707.

18. Charles Caspari, Jr., *A Treatise on Pharmacy for Students and Pharmacists*, 4th ed. (Lea and Febiger, Philadelphia, 1910), p. 369; Joseph P. Remington, *The Practice of Pharmacy*, 5th ed. (J. B. Lippincott, Philadelphia, 1907), p. 1183; Wilbur Scoville, *The Art of Compounding*, 4th ed. (P. Blakiston's Sons, Philadelphia, 1914), pp. 321-2. For another example of this view, see A. B. Stevens, *A Manual of Pharmacy and Dispensing* (Lea and Febiger, Philadelphia, 1909), pp. 404-5.

19. Comment by Charles Caspari, Jr., on L. E. Sayre, "To What Extent Should Pharmacy be Taught Medical Students? To What Extent Should the Action of Medicines be Taught Pharmacy Students?" *Proc. Am. Pharm. Assoc.*, 40 (1892): 309; anonymous comment quoted in H. H. Rusby, "What Shall We Teach," *J. Am. Pharm. Assoc.*, 7(1918): 1072.

20. Quoted in Bernard Fantus, "Report of the Section on Physiology and Pharmacology (including Bio-Assay) of Committee on Questions and Examinations of the American Conference of Pharmaceutical Faculties,"

J. Am. Pharm. Assoc., 8 (1919): 501. See also [Edward Kremers], "The Dilemma of the Pharmacy Professor," 12-page typescript, Kremers Reference Files, at C31(a)I, p. 11.

21. For examples of such criticisms of the curriculum, see Otto Wall, "Pharmaceutical Education and Legislation," *Proc. Am. Pharm. Assoc.*, 54 (1906): 166-8, and Henry Henkin, "What Ails the Druggist?" *Drugg. Circ.*, 55 (1909): 250-1.

22. R. H. Brown, "Physiology and Pharmaco-Dynamics in Schools of Pharmacy," *Apothecary* (Chicago), 2 (1892): 9-10. See also J. O. Schlotterbeck, "Pharmacognosy – Its Scope and the Methods of Teaching It," *Pharm. Era*, 11 (1894): 249.

23. Alfred R. L. Dohme, "The Desirability of Incorporating Pharmacology in Courses at Pharmaceutical Colleges," *Proc. Am. Pharm. Assoc.*, 46 (1898): 482-6. Two years earlier Dohme proposed a two-year course, which included pharmacology, leading to the Ph.G. degree; see *idem*, "Outline of a Course in Pharmacy Leading to the Degree of Graduate in Pharmacy," *Proc. Am. Pharm. Assoc.*, 43 (1895): 436-7.

24. *University of Michigan Catalogue of the Officers and Students for 1868-9, with a General Description of the University* (Ann Arbor: University of Michigan, 1869), p. 56; Glenn Sonnedecker, revisor, *Kremers and Urdang's History of Pharmacy*, 4th ed. (Philadelphia: J. B. Lippincott, 1976), pp. 232-3; and A. B. Prescott, "School of Pharmacy of the University of Michigan," *Merck's Market Report*, (no. 7) 1 (1892): 10.

25. See, e.g., *Annual Announcement of the School of Pharmacy of the University of Michigan*, 1881-82, p. 6; *ibid.*, 1882-83, pp. 8-9; *School of Pharmacy of the University of Michigan. Register of Alumni and Annual Announcement*, 1891-92, p. 15.

26. Henry Swain, E. M. K. Geiling and Alexander Heingartner, "John Jacob Abel at Michigan: The Introduction of Pharmacology into the Medical Curriculum," *Univ. Michigan Med. Bull.*, 19 (1963): 10.

27. *Michigan, Annual Announcement*, 1892-93, p. 14.

28. *Ibid.*, 1895-96, pp. 17-20; *ibid.*, 1901-02, p. 11.

29. *The University of North Carolina Record Describing the Departments of Medicine and Pharmacy*, April, 1905, p. 21.

30. On Lyman and the organization of the pharmacy school at Nebraska, see Jennie Tom, "Rufus Ashley Lyman, Pioneer in Pharmacy," *Pharm. Hist.*, 14 (1972): 90-4, 111.

31. "An Informal Talk by Doctor R. A. Lyman to the Third Year Pharmacy Students at the College of Pharmacy, University of Washington," May 11, 1953 (unpublished 12-page typescript, Rufus A. Lyman Papers, AIHP Collection, State Historical Society of Wisconsin, Madison, Box 44), p. 7.

32. *Bulletin of the University of Nebraska: Annual Catalog of the School of Pharmacy*, 1910-11, pp. 13-4, 18.

33. Rufus Lyman to James Dille, March 27, 1936 (Lyman Papers, Box 23).

34. Rufus A. Lyman, "Experimental Pharmacology: An Essential in the Pharmaceutical Curriculum," *Am. J. Pharm.*, 82 (1910): 510-6.

35. *Ibid.*, p. 515. Lyman came to believe that the ability to carry out the physiological standardizations of the pharmacopeia would be the most significant factor in the decision of schools of pharmacy to adopt pharmacology. See Rufus Lyman to James Dille, Feb. 1, 1937 (Lyman Papers, Box 23).

36. Rufus Lyman to James Dille, July 2, 1936 (Lyman Papers, Box 23).

37. *Ibid.*; Lyman to Dille, March 27, 1936; and Lyman, "Experimental Pharmacology," 515.

38. *The Pharmaceutical Syllabus*, 1st ed. (n.p.: New York State Board of Pharmacy, 1910), p. 14, and *The Pharmaceutical Syllabus*, 2nd ed. (n.p.: Pharmaceutical Syllabus National Committee, 1913), p. 25.

39. Henry J. Goeckel, "Pharmaceutical Education and Opportunities," *J. Am. Pharm. Assoc.*, 8 (1919): 931-2 (quotation is from p. 932).

40. See W. H. Zeigler, "The Teaching of Pharmaco-Dynamics in Schools of Pharmacy," *American Conference of Pharmaceutical Faculties: Proceedings*, 1919: 66.

41. William H. Zeigler, "Pharmaceutical Education of the Future," *Pharm. Era*, 61 (1925): 260.

42. Zeigler, "Teaching of Pharmaco-Dynamics," 66, and *idem*, "The Teaching of Physiology and Pharmacology in Schools of Pharmacy," *J. Am. Pharm. Assoc.*, 16 (1927): 246-8. Rufus Lyman claimed (in Lyman to Dille, March 27, 1936) that South Carolina did not offer physiology prior to the pharmacology course. However, based on an examination of the school's course announcements, and in light of Zeigler's papers above, Lyman must have been mistaken.

43. *The Pharmaceutical Syllabus*, 3rd ed. (n.p.: Pharmaceutical Syllabus Committee, 1922), insert between pp. 14 and 15. The *Syllabus* included pharmacology, therapy-dynamics, posology, and toxicology in the materia medica course, but did not specify what proportion of the total time each of these should receive.

44. *American Conference of Pharmaceutical Faculties: Proceedings*, 1916: 112 (quotation), and *ibid.*, 1917: 200-1.

45. *Ibid.*, 1919: 84-5.

46. A. Richard Bliss, "Pharmacodynamics in the Schools and Colleges of Pharmacy," *J. Am. Pharm. Assoc.*, 9 (1920): 378-83, 386-7, and Melvin R. Gibson to Rufus A. Lyman, quoted in "Dr. Lyman Comments," ca.

X

1947 (unpublished 10-page typescript, Lyman Papers, Box 44), pp. 4-5.

47. Bliss, "Pharmacodynamics," 381-2, and *idem*, "Experimental Pharmacodynamics for Students of Pharmacy," *J. Am. Pharm. Assoc.*, 9 (1920): 1067-70.

48. Bliss, "Experimental Pharmacodynamics," 1067, 1070-5.

49. Sonnedecker, *History of Pharmacy*, pp. 252-3; Robert G. Mrtek, "Pharmaceutical Education in These United States – An Interpretive Historical Essay of the Twentieth Century," *Am. J. Pharm. Educ.*, 40 (1976): 342, 344; and W. W. Charters, A. B. Lemon, and Leon M. Monell, *Basic Material for a Pharmaceutical Curriculum* (New York: McGraw-Hill, 1927), pp. 13 (quotation), 156.

50. Lyman to Dille, March 27, 1936.

51. A. Richard Bliss, Jr., "The Term 'Pharmacology,' Its Meaning, and the Scope and Content of a Course in Pharmacology for Pharmacy Students," 21 (1932): 389-90, and Charters, Lemon, and Monell, *Pharmaceutical Curriculum*, p. 156.

52. *The Pharmaceutical Syllabus*, 4th ed. (n.p.: National Pharmaceutical Syllabus Committee, 1932), p. 136.

53. Marvin R. Thompson, "The Importance of Experimental Pharmacology and Its Possibilities in the Pharmaceutical Curriculum," *J. Am. Pharm. Assoc.*, 22 (1933): 237.

54. See, e.g., [James Dille], Summary of Interviews and Evaluations of Pharmacology Programs at Various Pharmacy Schools, ca. 1936 (untitled 8-page typescript, Lyman Papers, Box 24), and Otto Augustus Wall, "Pharmaceutical Education and Legislation, *Proc. Am. Pharm. Assoc.*, 54 (1906): 166-7.

55. A. O. Mickelsen, "A Greater Knowledge of Pharmacology Is Essential to the Professional Pharmacist," *J. Am. Pharm. Assoc.*, 25 (1936): 999-1001.

56. "Chosen Emerson Chair Incumbent," *Pharm. Era*, 68 (1931): 16; *Catalogue of the School of Pharmacy, University of Maryland*, 1929-30, p. 4; and *ibid.*, 1931-32, pp. 4, 19. Although the 1931-32 catalog gives Thompson's title as Emerson Professor of Physiology, Pharmacology and Therapeutics, subsequent catalogs list him as Emerson Professor of Pharmacology, and this is the title that he gave in his scientific publications. The original announcement in the 1929-30 catalog, before Thompson was appointed, gave the title as Emerson Professor of Pharmacology and Therapeutics.

57. James Dille, "A Study of the Teaching of Pharmacology in Colleges of Pharmacy," *Am. J. Pharm. Educ.*, 2 (1938): 8-31.

58. James Dille to Rufus Lyman, March 23, 1936 (Lyman Papers, Box 23).

59. *Ibid.;* [Dille], Summary of Interviews and Evaluations; James Dille to Rufus Lyman, June 22, 1936 (Lyman Papers, Box 23); Dille, "Teaching of Pharmacology," 9; and James Dille to Rufus Lyman, Nov. 18, 1936 (Lyman Papers, Box 23). Attached to the last letter are copies of the cover letter and tentative questionnaire which Dille planned to send to the deans of pharmacy schools.

60. Dille to Lyman, March 23 and Nov. 18, 1936; Dille, "Teaching of Pharmacology," 9; and *idem*, "A Detailed Study of the Teaching of Pharmacology in Colleges of Pharmacy: A Report to the American Association of Colleges of Pharmacy, August 16, 1937" (copy in Kremers Reference Files, at A(2): Dille, James M.).

61. Dille, "Teaching of Pharmacology," 9-14 (quotation is from p. 14).

62. *Ibid.*, pp. 15-9. In 1939 Dille published a paper on the basic objectives of an undergraduate pharmacology laboratory and a general outline of groups of drug actions that the students should have covered in the laboratory. See *idem*, "The Nature of Laboratory Work in Pharmacology for Pharmacy Students," *Am. J. Pharm. Educ.*, 3 (1939): 72-8.

63. Dille, "Teaching of Pharmacology," 23-7 (quotation is from pp. 26-7). Not surprisingly, Dille's statement drew some fire. For example, Frederick Marsh, Professor of Pharmacognosy and Biology at Creighton, responded to the statement in Dille's original report to the AACP ("If a man must teach, in addition to pharmacology, five or six other subjects, the only conclusion tenable is that every subject must have very low standards."): "I resent this accusation deeply, and if I thought it were necessary I might submit plenty of evidence attesting its falsehood." See Frederick Marsh to James Dille, Sept. 14, 1937 (copy in Lyman Papers, Box 23), and Dille, "Detailed Study of Pharmacology," p. 15-16; cf. James Dille to Frederick Marsh, Sept. 18, 1937 (copy in Lyman Papers, Box 23).

64. Dille, "Teaching of Pharmacology," 28-30, and James Dille to Rufus Lyman, June 22, 1936 (Lyman Papers, Box 23).

65. *The Pharmaceutical Syllabus*, tentative fifth edition, revised (n.p.: National Pharmaceutical Syllabus Committee, 1945), p. 126.

66. Hugh Vincent, "A Quantitative Survey of the 1945-46 Pharmacy Curricula. I. Comparison with the Requirements of the Pharmaceutical Syllabus," *Am. J. Pharm. Educ.*, 10 (1946): 20-1.

67. See Edward C. Elliot, dir., *The General Report of the Pharmaceutical Survey, 1946-49*, (Washington, D.C.: American Council on Education, 1950).

68. Lloyd E. Blauch and George L. Webster, *The Pharmaceutical Curriculum: A Report Prepared for the Committee on Curriculum, American Association of Colleges of Pharmacy* (Washington, D.C.: American

Council on Education, 1952). The quotation is from Mrtek, "Pharmaceutical Education," 357.

69. Blauch and Webster, *Pharmaceutical Curriculum*, pp. 123-4, 126-33.

70. *Ibid.*, p. 133.

71. Richard A. Deno, "Needs of Our Colleges of Pharmacy," *Am. J. Pharm. Educ.*, 15 (1951): 534-6.

72. Ewart A. Swinyard and L. David Hiner, "A Plea for the Complete Separation of Pharmacognosy from Pharmacology in the Instructional Program," *Am. J. Pharm. Educ.*, 11 (1947): 719-24 (quotation is from p. 723).

73. On the development of clinical pharmacy, see, e.g., Don C. McLeod, "Clinical Pharmacy: The Past, Present and Future," *Am. J. Hosp. Pharm.*, 33 (1976): 29-38, and Donald C. Brodie and Roger A. Benson, "The Evolution of the Clinical Pharmacy Concept," *Drug Intelligence and Clinical Pharmacy*, 10 (1976): 506-10.

74. Norman Katz, Hemendra Bhargava, Donald Walter and Robert Warwick, "Status of Undergraduate Pharmacology Laboratories in Colleges of Pharmacy in the United States," *Am. J. Pharm. Educ.*, 42 (1978): 17-21.

75. *Ibid.*, p. 18; and Tom S. Miya and R. Craig Schnell, eds., *Survey of Pharmacology and Toxicology Departments. II. Schools of Pharmacy in North America* (n.p.: n. pub., 1975), p. ii.

76. John Schlegel, "Enrollment Report on Graduate Degree Programs, Fall, 1978," *Am. J. Pharm. Educ.*, 43 (1979): 280-94.

77. For detailed information on instructional and research programs in pharmacology in American and Canadian schools of pharmacy, see Miya and Schnell, *Survey of Pharmacology*.

The Beginnings of Pharmacology in the Federal Government

ALTHOUGH experiments on the action of drugs and poisons on humans and animals have been carried out since antiquity, the modern science of experimental pharmacology did not emerge as a distinct discipline until the nineteenth century. Its beginnings are associated with the work of the French physiologists François Magendie and Claude Bernard, who perfected many of the techniques and developed many of the concepts that shaped the new science. But it was in the Germanic universities that pharmacology, the study of the physiological effects of drugs and poisons, first became established as an independent discipline in the second half of the nineteenth century. In the medical school curricula of these universities pharmacology replaced the traditional didactic courses in materia medica, which involved a descriptive approach to the origins, composition, physical and chemical properties, therapeutic uses, and modes of preparation and administration of drugs.[1]

The science of pharmacology was brought to the United States by John Jacob Abel, who had studied medicine and biomedical science in European universities for some six and one-half years during the 1880s. His return to this country to accept the chair of materia medica and therapeutics at the University of Michigan in 1891 marks the beginning of the teaching of modern experimental pharmacology in America, in spite of the traditional title of his position. Two years later Abel joined the faculty of the new medical school at The Johns Hopkins University as professor of pharmacology.[2]

During the last decade of the nineteenth century and the first decade of this century, other American medical schools made the transition from materia medica to pharmacology. (This transition generally took place somewhat later at American schools of pharmacy, as John Swann and I have discussed.[3]) In his classic 1910 report on medical education, Abraham Flexner stressed the value of pharmacology as a basis for rational therapeutics. A solid grounding in the science would enable physicians to prescribe more wisely, basing their decisions on scientific knowledge rather than on empirical traditions or the claims of drug manufacturers.[4]

The new science also began to make its way into non-academic laboratories as well in this period. For example, Parke Davis and Company apparently hired the first pharmacologist to be employed by an American pharmaceutical firm in 1894. When the newly founded Rockefeller Institute for Medical Research was opened in 1904, one of its divisions was devoted jointly to physiology and pharmacology. By 1908 American pharmacology had progressed in its search for a separate identity to the point where its practitioners felt the need for an organization of their own, and the American Society for Pharmacology and Experimental Therapeutics was founded in that year. The following year the first American journal devoted to the new field began, the *Journal of Pharmacology and Experimental Therapeutics;* another sign that pharmacology was well on its way to becoming an established discipline in this country.[5]

Experimental pharmacology also entered the scientific laboratories of the Federal government during this same period. Of the eighteen founding members of the American Society for Pharmacology and Experimental Therapeutics, for example, five worked for the Federal government.[6] The focus of this paper is the early development of pharmacology within the Federal government, with special emphasis on the two agencies where the science especially flourished, the Hygienic Laboratory of the Public Health Service, and the Bureau of Chemistry of the Department of Agriculture. Pharmacology still plays a major role today in the agencies that grew out of these institutions: the National Institutes of Health, successor to the Hygienic Laboratory, and the Food and Drug Administration, which was created to assume the regulatory functions of the Bureau of Chemistry.

The Hygienic Laboratory

The first appointment of a pharmacologist in a Federal agency appears to have been in the Hygienic Laboratory in 1904. The Hygienic Laboratory had been established in Staten Island, New York, by the Marine Hospital Service (later the Public Health Service) in 1887, largely to undertake bacteriological work in connection with public health. In 1891 the Laboratory was moved to Washington, D.C. Almost no original research was carried out in the first decade or so of the Laboratory's existence, but laws passed in 1901 and 1902 reorganized the Laboratory and greatly strengthened its research function. The 1902 act authorized the creation of three new divisions. The existing program was designated the Division of Pathology and Bacteriology, and new Divisions of Chemistry, Pharmacology, and Zoology were created. The establishment of pharmacology as one of the divisions demonstrates the growing recognition of this relatively new discipline in America.[7]

The individual appointed to head the Division of Pharmacology was Reid Hunt, who began work at the Hygienic Laboratory on March 1, 1904.[8] Hunt had studied physiology under Henry Newell Martin and William H. Howell at Johns Hopkins University, where he received his Ph.D. in 1896. He also held an M.D. from the College of Physicians and Surgeons in Baltimore. In 1898, Hunt joined Abel's staff in the Department of Pharmacology at Johns Hopkins,

becoming associate professor in 1901. He spent much of his time in 1902 and 1903 working in the Frankfurt laboratory of Paul Ehrlich, the founder of modern chemotherapy.[9]

The new Division of Pharmacology divided its work between research and practical applications of pharmacological knowledge and techniques. The examination of drugs for strength and purity, for example, occupied a significant portion of the staff time in the Division. The medical purveyor of the Public Health Service sent samples of drugs to the pharmacological laboratory for testing against the standards set in the *United States Pharmacopoeia*. The Pharmacology Division then made recommendations as to whether the drugs should be accepted or rejected. In fiscal year 1905, for example, the Division tested 289 drug samples, and found that about a third of them did not meet acceptable standards.[10]

The Division also soon became involved in a major way in public service work with two private professional medical bodies concerned with the quality of the country's drug supply. The problem of the control and standardization of drugs had become an important issue in the United States in the early years of this century.

PUBLIC HEALTH SERVICE
Hygienic Laboratory
Milton Rosenau, Director
Division of Pathology and Bacteriology
Division of Chemistry
Division of Pharmacology
1904, Reid Hunt, Head
1913, Carl Voegtlin, Head
Division of Zoology

Concern over drug adulteration and patent medicine quackery contributed to the movement for a national pure food and drug law, culminating in the passage of the Pure Food and Drugs Act of 1906. Clearly the new science of pharmacology, involving experimental investigations of the action of drugs and poisons, was relevant to food and drug issues.

Since its founding in 1820, the *United States Pharmacopoeia* had attempted to establish standards for drugs, although these standards were not legally enforceable by the Federal government until the passage of the 1906 Act. The *Pharmacopoeia* was not published by a government agency, but by a private body (called "the United States Pharmacopoeial Convention" since 1900) consisting of physicians and pharmacists, which was responsible for periodically revising the work. Almost from its beginning the Division of Pharmacology cooperated with the Pharmacopoeial Convention, and with committees of the American Medical Association and the American Pharmaceutical Association that were concerned with the *Pharmacopoeia*, in efforts to improve drug standards.[11] For example, Hunt and his colleagues undertook experimental work on the standardization of thyroid preparations, and the Division published a bulletin in 1905 on changes in the eighth decennial revision of the *Pharmacopoeia*.[12]

Milton Rosenau, Director of the Hygienic Laboratory, strongly supported this cooperation with the *Pharmacopoeia*. He believed that the Division of Pharmacology was "peculiarly fitted" for work on physiological standards for drugs and chemicals and that both the Division and the *Pharmacopoeia* stood to benefit from close relations between them.[13] In his annual report for 1909, Surgeon General Walter Wyman of the Public Health Service also argued the case for the involvement of the Hygienic Laboratory in pharmacopoeial work, largely on the grounds that the 1906 Act had made the standards of the *Pharmacopoeia* legally enforceable under Federal law.[14]

The Division of Pharmacology also became involved in the work of another body concerned with the quality and safety of drugs, the American Medical Association's Council on Pharmacy and Chemistry. The Council had been created in 1905 to investigate the composition and standing of proprietary medicines. The Council made recommendations, for example, as to whether or not certain proprietary medicines deserved the patronage of physicians and pharmacists, and whether or not the AMA's journal should accept advertising for these products. Beginning in 1907, the Council issued *New and Nonofficial Remedies*, an annual publication that provided physicians and pharmacists with information on drug products not included in the

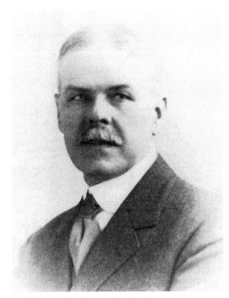

Reid Hunt, the first professional pharmacologist in Federal government service, headed the Hygienic Laboratory's Division of Pharmacology from 1904 to 1913.

United States Pharmacopoeia or the *National Formulary*.[15]

From its establishment in early 1905, the Council included Martin Wilbert, a pharmacist in the Hygienic Laboratory's Division of Pharmacology, as a member. A year later, the Division's head, Reid Hunt, joined Wilbert as a member of the Council, and remained one for thirty years. The Division of Pharmacology undertook various investigations for the Council, examining the composition, activity or toxicity of specific drug products.[16]

The Division of Pharmacology was also sometimes called upon to assist other government agencies. For example, Division staff cooperated on a number of occasions with the Bureau of Chemistry of the Department of Agriculture in connection with the evaluation of drugs or chemicals, since the Bureau was responsible for the enforcement of the 1906 Food and Drugs Act (see below). Other agencies as-

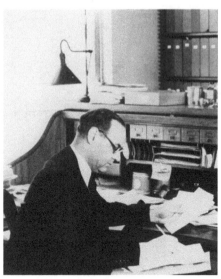

Carl Voegtlin, Hunt's successor at the Hygienic Laboratory, at work at his desk at the National Institute of Health in the 1930s.

sisted by the Division included the Army (testing the physiological activity of certain suprarenal preparations), the Interior Department (examining the radioactivity of the waters of Hot Springs, Arkansas), and the Post Office Department (in connection with the exclusion from the mails of certain fraudulent medicines).[17]

Basic Research

In addition to these activities, which were more or less directly related to public health and the enforcement of drug standards, the Division also engaged in a significant amount of basic research in pharmacology. At first the practical work of the Division occupied almost all of Hunt's attention. The Division's report for 1905, for example, noted that there had been little time during the year for systematic research work.[18] In March of that year, Director Rosenau complained to the Surgeon General:

Dr. Hunt has a special genius for original research in physiological chemistry and has many problems in mind which offer results of the greatest value if he could be relieved of most of the routine work of examining drugs and chemicals.[19]

Later reports of the Division indicate that research soon became one of its important functions. Hunt and his colleagues explored such subjects as the physiology and pharmacology of thyroid preparations and the pharmacology of alcohol.[20] The most significant research to come out of the Division in its early years was Hunt's study with Taveau on the physiological action of choline derivatives in the period 1906–1911. In the course of this work, they observed the remarkable activity of acetylcholine, reporting that this substance was 100,000 times more potent itself than choline in lowering the blood pressure.[21] It was not until the 1920s, however, that the role of acetylcholine in the chemical transmission of nervous impulses was established through the work of Otto Loewi in Austria and Henry Dale in England.

On the basis of these many activities, especially those concerned with public health, Hunt argued successfully for expansion of the staff of the Division. For example, W. Worth Hale, who had received an M.D. degree from the University of Michigan in 1904, joined the staff as assistant pharmacologist in 1908.[22] Arrangements were also made for academic scientists to spend time working in the Division on a temporary basis. For example, Cornell University pharmacologist Robert Hatcher spent the summer of 1909 working in the Hygienic Laboratory on the determination of some of the physical constants of pharmacopoeial substances, and pharmacologist C. W. Edmunds of the University of Michigan spent the summer of 1910 there working on methods for the standardization of ergot. Such arrangements helped to forge closer ties between the Division and university centers of pharmacological research.[23]

In 1913, Reid Hunt left the Hygienic Laboratory to become professor of pharmacology at Harvard University. His successor was another protegé of John Abel, Carl Voegtlin, who later became the first head of the National Cancer Institute. While at the Hygienic Laboratory, Voegtlin carried out important research on the chemotherapy of organic arsenic compounds.[24]

It was also during Voegtlin's tenure that the Division of Pharmacology became more directly involved with the Biologics Control Act of 1902. Under this law, the Hygienic Laboratory issued licenses for the production of vaccines, antitoxins, and analogous pharmaceutical products of biological origin and periodically tested commercial preparations of these substances to ensure that they met established standards for potency and purity. This work was done in the Division of Pathology and Bacteriology. In 1919, however, arsphenamine (Salvarsan) and related organic arsenic compounds used in the treatment of syphilis and other diseases were brought under the provisions of the 1902 Act (even though they were chemical rather than biological products) because of the difficulty of obtaining uniform preparations of these drugs. Voegtlin's laboratory was responsible for developing the chemical and pharmacological tests used for this purpose.[25]

The Bureau of Chemistry

The other Federal agency where the science of pharmacology began to make its impact felt at an early date was the Bureau of Chemistry of the Department of Agriculture. Physician and chemist Harvey Wiley, who had served as Chief of the Bureau from 1883, was the major figure responsible for the passage of the 1906 Food and Drugs Act. The enforcement of the provisions of the Act had been placed in the hands of Wiley's Bureau of Chemistry, and he recognized early the need for a pharmacologist to help in carrying out these regulatory responsibilities.

In March of 1908, pharmaceutical chemist Lyman Kebler, Chief of the Bureau of Chemistry's Division of Drugs, wrote to John Abel seeking his advice on the employment of a pharmacologist:

We are desirous of securing some one qualified in pharmacology and would ask if you are acquainted with any one whom you would care to recommend for our work. It is chiefly in connection with the enforcement of the Food and Drugs Act.[26]

Abel recommended a former associate of his, A. C. Crawford, who was then employed by the Department of Agriculture's Bureau of Plant Industry.[27] Either Kebler did not accept this advice or Crawford did not accept the job, for in June of that year William Salant was appointed to head the newly-created pharmacological laboratory in the Bureau's Division of Drugs.[28] Salant received an M.D. from the College of Physicians and Surgeons at Columbia University and then spent the next several years as an assistant in physiology or physiological chemistry at the

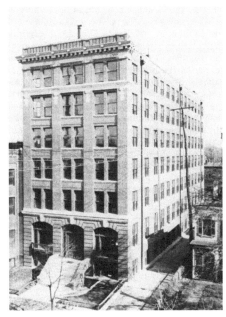

This building housed a number of laboratories that were part of the Bureau of Chemistry, including the Pharmacological Laboratory.

Cornell and Columbia medical schools, while also carrying out research under grants from the Rockefeller Institute for Medical Research. He was serving as an adjunct professor at the University of Alabama when he was hired by the Bureau of Chemistry.[29]

The first research carried out in the Bureau's pharmacological laboratory seems to have grown largely out of regulatory concerns. For example, among the subjects extensively studied in the early years of the laboratory were the physiological effects of extracts of bleached and unbleached flour and the pharmacology and toxicology of caffeine.[30] Both of these studies were directly related to court cases in which the Bureau was involved. Wiley opposed the common practice of bleaching flour with nitrogen peroxide on the grounds that it involved the use of an objectionable substance for the unethical purpose of concealing an inferior product. The studies of the pharmacological laboratory on flour were obviously designed to determine

183

whether the bleached flour might have undesirable physiological effects. Wiley also objected to the addition of caffeine to Coca Cola, arguing that it was an added poisonous ingredient. Again, the pharmacological laboratory carried out research on the pharmacology and toxicology of caffeine in support of Wiley's regulatory efforts.[31] In discussing the work of the laboratory, the 1911 report of the Bureau clearly stated that: "Much of the information acquired on the physiological effect of various drugs and chemicals was used in connection with the enforcement of the food and drugs act and the preparation of expert testimony along these lines."[32]

Although practical concerns motivated much of the research of the pharmacological

istry, it should be noted that a biochemist-pharmacologist, Carl Alsberg, succeeded Wiley as Chief of the Bureau in 1912. Alsberg gave the Bureau more of a research orientation during his tenure, which lasted until 1921.[34]

Some pharmacological work was also carried out in two other divisions of the Department of Agriculture in the first decade of the century. The pharmacological research in the Bureau of Plant Industry involved the study of poisonous plants, an interest of the Bureau since 1894. Even before the Bureau hired a pharmacologist, a botanist on its staff collaborated with Reid Hunt, while he was still at Johns Hopkins, and with another pharmacologist, Torald Sollmann of Western Reserve, on studies of poisonous

DEPARTMENT OF AGRICULTURE		
Bureau of Chemistry	**Bureau of Plant Industry**	**Bureau of Animal Industry**
1883–1912, Harvey Wiley, Chief		
1912–1921, Carl Alsberg, Chief		
DIVISION OF DRUGS		
Lyman Kebler, Chief	*1904–1908 Albert C. Crawford, pharmacologist*	
Pharmacological Laboratory		
1908, William Salant, Head	*1908, Carl Alsberg*	*1908, Albert C. Crawford moves from Bureau of Plant Industry*

laboratory, the results were sometimes of broader scientific interest, and Salant and his colleagues (like Hunt and his co-workers) reported some of their work at professional meetings and in the scientific literature.[33] On the whole, however, the Bureau of Chemistry's pharmacological laboratory was less oriented towards basic research than the Hygienic Laboratory's Division of Pharmacology, and neither Salant nor his immediate successors ever achieved the status in the field enjoyed by Hunt and Voegtlin, both of whom eventually served as presidents of the American Society for Pharmacology and Experimental Therapeutics. Before leaving the subject of the Bureau of Chem-

plants about 1902. Albert C. Crawford, mentioned above, was the first pharmacologist hired by the Bureau of Plant Industry. He appears to have been appointed in the summer of 1904 or not long afterward. Crawford took a medical degree at the College of Physicians and Surgeons of Baltimore before becoming an assistant in Abel's laboratory. He remained in the Bureau of Plant Industry until 1908, when he moved to the Department of Agriculture's Bureau of Animal Industry, apparently as their first pharmacologist. There he continued his investigations on the pharmacology of poisonous plants for another year until he left government service and joined the faculty at Stanford Uni-

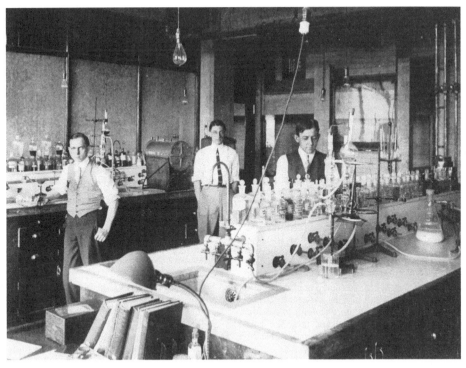

After the passage of the 1906 Act, the Drug Inspection Laboratory of the Bureau of Chemistry was busy testing drugs for purity. (c. 1910, courtesy of Kremers Reference Files).

versity. He was replaced in the Bureau of Plant Industry by Carl Alsberg.[35]

Conclusion

Pharmacology thus became established in Federal agencies such as the Hygienic Laboratory and the Bureau of Chemistry in the first decade of the twentieth century. A position in a Federal laboratory offered some pharmacologists an alternative to the more traditional academic career. There were still few opportunities for pharmacologists in industrial firms in this period, and working for a pharmaceutical company carried a certain stigma, as evidenced by the fact that the American Society for Pharmacology and Experimental Therapeutics would not admit industrial scientists to membership until 1941.[36] A job in a Federal agency, though still not as prestigious as a post at a respected university, at least did not suffer from this taint of "commercialism."

In addition, government salaries were competitive with those in academia, and research facilities in institutions such as the Hygienic Laboratory could rival or even exceed those in university laboratories. For example, assistant pharmacologists (the equivalent of junior faculty at a university) working under Hunt at the Hygienic Laboratory were earning about $1800 to $2000 per annum in 1909 and Salant tried to hire an assistant pharmacologist at the Bureau of Chemistry in 1912 for a salary of $1600 to $1800. By comparison, instructors and assistant professors in the basic sciences at the Harvard Medical School were earning between $800 and $1600 in 1907–1908 and pharmacology instructors were earning about $1000 a year at Michigan in 1917–18.[37] When Harvard was searching for someone to head their pharmacology department in 1912, Walter Cannon indicated that they could probably not secure a professor for less than $5000. He pointed out that to get their first choice, Reid Hunt (whom they eventually hired), they would probably have to match his Hygienic Laboratory salary of $6000, which would have been a generous sum for a university professor of pharmacology at the time. For example, Abel's salary in 1909–1910 was $5000, while the professor of pharmacology at Pennsylvania earned $5000 in 1912 and the professor of pharmacology at Michigan earned only $4000 in 1917.[38]

Cannon also noted that Hunt had an admirably equipped laboratory and ample funds for research in Washington. In 1914, Hunt's successor Voegtlin wrote to Abel that he often wished that Abel had "the same facilities and finances" that he himself enjoyed at the Hygienic Laboratory, adding that "Uncle Sam is pretty liberal." Although by 1920 Voegtlin was complaining to Abel about his salary ($4800) and about there being "too much politics in government work" to suit him, he apparently found his Federal career satisfying enough to remain at the Hygienic Laboratory and later the National Cancer Institute until his retirement in 1943.[39]

The new science of pharmacology found its way into government agencies largely as a result of public health concerns, especially about the nation's food and drug supply, but also at least in part as a result of increasing interest in scientific research in Federal laboratories. In her recent book, *Inventing the NIH*, Victoria Harden points out that it was during the Progressive Era that biomedical research began to assume a significant place in the Federal government, and that regulatory legislation enacted during this period helped to promote the expansion of scientific staffs in Federal agencies and their increasing involvement in research. The discipline of pharmacology was included in this broader trend. Pharmacology thus began to make its impact felt in the Federal government even while still in its American infancy.[40]

Notes and References

Acknowledgements: An earlier version of this paper was delivered at a joint meeting of the Society for History of the Federal Government and the National Council on Public History in Washington, D. C., April 25, 1987. I wish to thank James Cassedy and John Swann for their helpful comments on an earlier draft. The research for this paper was supported in part by NIH grant LM 03300 from the National Library of Medicine.

1. On the beginnings of experimental pharmacology, see, e.g., John E. Lesch, *Science and Medicine in France: The Emergence of Experimental Physiology, 1790–1855* (Cambridge, MA: Harvard University Press, 1984), pp. 145–165; B. Holmstedt and G. Liljestrand, eds., *Readings in Pharmacology* (Oxford: Pergamon Press, 1963), pp. 62–110; and Gustav Kuchinsky, "The Influence of Dorpat on the Emergence of Pharmacology as a Discipline," *Journal of the History of Medicine and the Allied Sciences*, 23 (1968): 258–271.

2. John Parascandola, "John J. Abel and the Early Development of Pharmacology at The Johns Hopkins University," *Bulletin of the History of Medicine*, 56 (1982): 512–527.

3. John Parascandola and John Swann, "Development of Pharmacology in American Schools of Pharmacy," *Pharmacy in History*, 25 (1983): 95–115.

4. Abraham Flexner, *Medical Education in the United States and Canada* (New York: Carnegie Foundation for the Advancement of Teaching, 1910), pp. 63–65.

5. On the early history of pharmacology in the United States, see Flexner, *Medical Education* (n. 4), and Elizabeth Keeney, *Sources in the History of American Pharmacology* (Madison, WI: American Institute of the History of Pharmacy, 1983).

6. K.K. Chen, "Meetings," in K.K. Chen, ed., *The American Society for Pharmacology and Experimental Therapeutics, Incorporated: The First Sixty Years, 1908–1969* (Bethesda, MD: American Society for Pharmacology and Experimental Therapeutics, 1969), pp. 1–119, especially pp. 6–7. The five individuals were W. Worth Hale and Reid Hunt of the Public Health Service's Hygienic Laboratory, and Carl Alsberg (Bureau of Plant Industry), Albert Crawford (Bureau of Animal Industry), and William Salant (Bureau of Chemistry) of the Department of Agriculture.

7. Victoria A. Harden, *Inventing the NIH: Federal Biomedical Research Policy, 1887–1937* (Baltimore: Johns Hopkins University Press, 1986), pp. 9–26.

8. Hunt to Surgeon General Walter Wyman, March 1, 1904, General File (1897–1923), Box 98, Record Group 90, National Archives, Washington, D.C.

9. For biographical information on Hunt, see Parascandola and Keeney, *American Pharmacology* (n. 5), pp. 38–40 and Eli Kennerly Marshall, "Reid Hunt, 1870–1948," *Biographical Memoires of the National Academy of Sciences*, 26 (1949): 25–49.

10. Reid Hunt, "Report of the Division of Pharmacology," in *Annual Report of the Surgeon-General of the Public Health and Marine-Hospital Service of the United States for the Fiscal Year 1905* (Washington, D.C.: Government Printing Office, 1906), pp. 226–227.

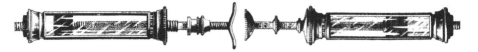

11. On the problems of patent medicine quackery and the passage of food and drug legislation, see James Harvey Young, *The Toadstool Millionaires: A Social History of Patent Medicines in America Before Federal Regulation* (Princeton, NJ: Princeton University Press, 1961). On the *United States Pharmacopoeia* and drug standards in America see Glenn Sonnedecker, "Drug Standards Become Official," in James Harvey Young, ed., *The Early Years of Federal Food and Drug Control* (Madison, WI: American Institute of the History of Pharmacy, 1982), pp. 28–39.

12. See the reports of the Division of Pharmacology in this period in *Annual Report of the Surgeon-General* (n. 10).

13. Milton Rosenau, "General Report of the Director," in *Annual Report of the Surgeon-General* (n. 10), 1906, page 231.

14. *Annual Report of the Surgeon-General* (n. 10), 1909, p. 71.

15. On the AMA's Council on Pharmacy and Chemistry, see Austin Smith, "The Council on Pharmacy and Chemistry and the Chemical Laboratory," in Morris Fishbein, ed., *A History of the American Medical Association, 1847–1947* (Philadelphia: W.B. Saunders, 1947), pp. 865–886. The *National Formulary* was first published by the American Pharmaceutical Association in 1888 to designate standards for drug preparations that were used by many physicians and pharmacists but did not qualify for inclusion in the *United States Pharmacopoeia*. See *Kremers and Urdang's History of Pharmacy*, fourth edition, revised by Glenn Sonnedecker (Philadelphia: J. B. Lippincott, 1976), pp. 275–278.

16. See the reports of the Division for this period in *Annual Report of the Surgeon-General* (n. 10).

17. See, e.g., the reports of the Division in *Annual Report of the Surgeon-General* (n. 10), 1906, p. 224; 1910, p. 55; 1911 p. 87; 1913, p. 55.

18. *Ibid.,* 1905, p. 226.

19. Rosenau to Surgeon General Walter Wyman, March 3, 1905, Public Health Service Records, RG 90, b. 515, file S423, National Archives, Washington, D. C. I am indebted to John Swann for calling my attention to this document.

20. See the reports of the Division in this period in *Annual Report of the Surgeon General* (n. 10) and the bibliography of Hunt's publications in Marshall, "Reid Hunt" (n. 9), pp. 38–41.

21. Reid Hunt and R. de M. Taveau, "On the Physiological Action of Certain Cholin Derivatives and New Methods for Detecting Cholin," *British Medical Journal*, 1906 (ii): 1788–1791.

22. On Hale, see Chen, "Meetings" (n. 6), p. 9.

23. See the reports of the Division in *Annual Report of the Surgeon General* (n. 10), pp. 85–86; 1910, p. 53; 1911, p. 84.

24. John Parascandola, "Carl Voegtlin and the 'Arsenic Receptor' in Chemotherapy," *J. Hist. Med.*, 32 (1977): 151–171. On Voegtlin, see also Parascandola and Keeney, *American Pharmacology* (n. 5), pp. 56–57.

25. Parascandola, "Carl Voegtlin" (n. 24), pp. 153–154 and Ramunas Kondratas, "The Biologics Control Act of 1902," in Young, ed., *Early Years* (n. 11), pp. 8–27.

26. Kebler to Abel, March 17, 1908, General Correspondence, Box 210, 3242, Record Group 97, National Archives, Washington, D.C.

27. Abel to Kebler, March 18, 1908, *ibid.*

28. Harvey Wiley, "1908 Report of Bureau of Chemistry," in *Federal Food, Drug and Cosmetic Law, Administrative Reports, 1907–1949* (Chicago: Commerce Clearing House, 1951), pp. 48–49; W.D. Bigelow to William Salant, General Correspondence, Box 249, 15444, Record Group 97, National Archives, Washington, D.C.

29. On Salant, see Parascandola and Keeney, *American Pharmacology* (n. 5), pp. 51–52.

30. See the annual reports of the Bureau in this period in *Administrative Reports* (n. 28).

31. For Wiley's efforts in these cases, see Oscar Anderson, *The Health of a Nation: Harvey W. Wiley and the Fight for Pure Food* (Chicago: University of Chicago Press, 1958), pp. 220–221, 235–237.

32. Harvey Wiley, "1911 Report of Bureau of Chemistry," in *Administrative Reports* (n. 28), p. 23.

33. See, e.g., W. Salant and J.B. Rieger, "The Elimination and Toxicity of Caffein in Nephrectomized Rabbits," *Proceedings of the Society for Experimental Biology and Medicine*, 9 (1912): 58–59 and W. Salant and J.K. Phelps, "The Influence of Caffein on Protein Metabolism in Dogs, with Some Remarks on Demethylation in the Body," *Journal of Pharmacology and Experimental Therapeutics*, 2 (1911): 401–402. Salant and his colleagues generally published only brief reports of their results in the "proceedings" of professional societies appearing in the journals associated with those bodies (as in the two cases cited here). They seem to have reserved fuller publication of their results for bulletins issued by the Bureau of Chemistry.

34. On Alsberg, see the biographical article by Mel Gorman in Wyndham Miles, ed., *American Chemists and Chemical Engineers* (Washington, D.C.: American Chemical Society, 1976), pp. 7–8.

35. U.G. Houck, *The Bureau of Animal Industry of the United States Department of Agriculture: Its Establishment, Achievements and Current Activities* (Washington, D.C.: privately printed, 1924), pp. 79–82. On Crawford, see the biographical sketch in Parascandola and Keeney, *American Pharmacology* (n. 5), p. 30.

36. See John Parascandola, "Industrial Research Comes of Age: The American Pharmaceutical Industry, 1920–1940," *Pharmacy in History*, 27 (1985): 12–21 and John Parascandola, "The 'Preposterous Provision': The American Society for Pharmacology and Experimental Therapeutics' Ban on Industrial Pharmacologists, 1908–1941," paper delivered at a symposium on "History of the Pharmaceutical Industry," Wellcome Institute for the History of Medicine, London, England, January 30, 1987 (publication forthcoming).

37. Report by Reid Hunt on Division of Pharmacology for January, 1909, February 2, 1909, Public Health Service Records, Record Group 90, b. 516, file 5423, National Archives (I am indebted to John Swann for calling this document to my attention); William Salant to John Abel, April 29, 1912, John J. Abel Papers, Alan Mason Chesney Archives, The Johns Hopkins Medical Institutions, Baltimore, Record Group 1; Kenneth Ludmerer, *Learning to Heal: The Development of American Medical Education* (New York: Basic Books, 1985), p. 126; Shirley Smith To C. W. Edmunds, July 14, 1917, Department of Pharmacology, University of Michigan, Ann Arbor (I am indebted to Dr. Henry Swain for a copy of this letter).

38. Walter Cannon to Edward Bradford, May 17, 1912, Dean's Office Subject Files, Harvard Medical School, Archives, Countway Library, Boston; Ira Remsen to John Abel, June 10, 1909, Abel Papers (n. 37), Record Group 1; Smith to Edmunds, July 14, 1917 (n. 37).

39. Cannon to Bradford, May 17, 1912 (n. 38); Carl Voegtlin to John Abel, April 15, 1920, Abel Papers (n. 37), Record Group 1. On Voegtlin, see Parascandola, "Carl Voegtlin" (n. 24) and Parascandola and Keeney, *American Pharmacology* (n. 5), pp. 56–57.

40. Harden, *Inventing the NIH* (n. 7), pp. 3, 27–32.

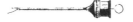
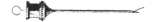

XII

The "Preposterous Provision": The American Society for Pharmacology and Experimental Therapeutics' Ban on Industrial Pharmacologists, 1908–1941

READERS familiar with Sinclair Lewis's classic novel *Arrowsmith*, published in 1925, will probably recall the character of Max Gottlieb, the idealistic immunologist who serves as a father figure to the young Martin Arrowsmith. At one point in the narrative, Gottlieb, who has always criticized the commercialism of certain large pharmaceutical firms, is forced for financial reasons to work for one of these companies. When the news of this situation reached the laboratories of great scientists around the world, ". . . sorrowing men wailed 'How could old Max have gone over to that damned pill-peddler?' "[1]

Although this incident is taken from a work of fiction, it reflects a real-life attitude on the part of many academic scientists towards their industrial colleagues in this period and beyond. Perhaps nowhere is this suspicion of scientific work carried out in industrial firms, and specifically in the pharmaceutical industry, better illustrated than in the case of American pharmacology. Industrial pharmacologists were actually banned from membership in the national society for American pharmacologists from its founding in 1908 until 1941.

The birth of modern experimental pharmacology, the science that deals with the investigation of the physiological action of drugs, dates back only to the nineteenth century. The discipline became institutionalized in German medical schools in the second half of the century, replacing the older didactic subject of materia medica, which emphasized the natural origin, composition, means of preparation and administration, and traditional therapeutic uses of drugs.

The Germanic model of experimental pharmacology was brought to the United States by John Jacob Abel, who assumed the chair of materia medica and therapeutics at the University of Michigan in 1891 after six and one-half years of studying biomedical science in Europe. Abel converted the traditional materia medica course at Michigan into a modern course in pharmacology. In 1893, he moved to The Johns Hopkins University, when its medical school opened, to occupy the chair of pharmacology there. He spent the rest of his career at Hopkins, where his laboratory served as the center of American pharmacology for decades.[2]

Other medical schools also began to make the transition from materia medica to pharmacology around the turn of the twentieth century, and by 1908 the American practitioners of this discipline had progressed far enough in their search for a professional identity that they felt the need for an organization of their own. In that year, eighteen men met in Abel's laboratory at Johns Hopkins to found the American Society for Pharmacology and Experimental Therapeutics (ASPET). Most American pharmacologists at the time were based in academia (in medical schools), as is reflected by the fact that eleven of the founders were employed by universities. Five others worked for the Federal government, in the Department of Agriculture or the Hygienic Laboratory of the Public Health Service, and two others were at the Rockefeller Institute for Medical Research.[3]

There were few pharmacologists associated with industry in the United States in 1908, yet the founders of the Society were apparently concerned enough about a potential threat from this quarter to insert the following two clauses into the new organization's constitution:

No one shall be admitted to membership who is in the permanent employ of any drug firm.

Entrance into the permanent employ of a drug firm shall constitute forfeiture of membership.[4]

These steps were taken, in the words of the Society's Council, "in order to avoid every external influence which would be inimical to the scientific interests of pharmacology."[5]

It is not clear who first proposed the ban on industrial pharmacologists. The committee which drafted the constitution consisted of Abel and three of his former associates at Johns Hopkins: Reid Hunt (Chairman), Arthur Loevenhart, and Albert Crawford.[6] Apparently, however, the above clauses were not contained in the first draft of the constitution circulated to the Council. A draft of the

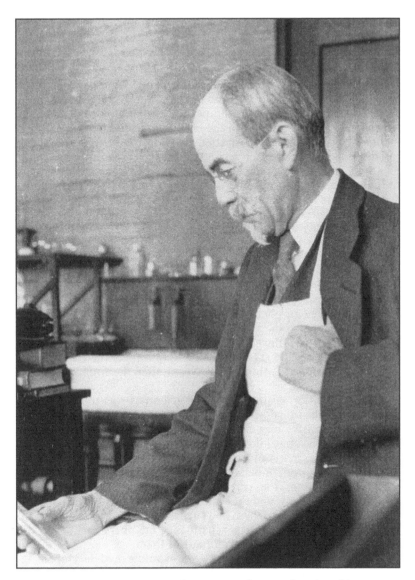

John Jacob Abel, the "Father of American Pharmacology," in his laboratory at The Johns Hopkins University (courtesy of the National Library of Medicine).

document from the files of C.W. Edmunds of the University of Michigan, a Council member, does not contain these clauses, but someone has penciled in the words "Employ by firm" in the section on membership.[7] Another (incomplete) version of the constitution, also from his files, contains changes in pencil which appear to be in Abel's hand. These include a new section in the article on membership, banning persons in the permanent employ of drug firms. It was inserted, however, with the notation "from Loevenhart."[8] Of course, even if Loevenhart drafted the wording of this clause, the original suggestion for such a ban could have come from any member of the committee or the Council. It would be ironic if Loevenhart initiated the idea, because he was later to become one of the most active leaders in the campaign to eliminate the membership restriction on industrial pharmacologists.

Whoever suggested the ban, it seems to have met with the general approval of the founders of the Society. There is no evidence in surviving correspondence and other records that there was any debate over adopting it. On the other hand, these documents do indicate that there was significant discussion about other membership matters, such as whether or not to admit clinicians who were not actually engaged in pharmacological research.[9] Apparently no one saw fit to challenge the prohibition against industrial pharmacologists, and a serious movement to change this rule did not begin for about another decade. The campaign to eliminate the ban was not successful until 1941, thirty-three years after the founding of the Society.

This prohibition against industrial scientists was unique among American professional scientific societies, so far as I can tell.[10] No doubt anti-industry bias existed on the part of academic scientists in other societies, but I do not know of any other case where it was carried to the extreme of explicitly singling out industry scientists for exclusion from membership. If we examine three related professional organizations, the American Chemical Society, the American Physiological Society, and the American Society of Biological Chemists, we find that none of them had such a clause in their constitution. In fact, all included industrial scientists as members long before the society of pharmacologists would admit them.

The American Chemical Society, for example, had developed significant ties with industry by the turn of this century. The first specialized division organized by the Society, in 1907, was the Division of Industrial and Engineering Chemistry, reflecting the large number of industrial chemists in the Society. Several of the Society's presidents in the period 1880–1920 were associated with the chemical industry.[11]

The other two societies are particularly relevant from a comparative point of view because of their close relationship with the pharmacology society. Both the American Society of Biological Chemists and the American Society for Pharmacology and Experimental Therapeutics were offshoots of the American Physiological Society, and the three societies held their meetings together for many years. There was significant overlap in membership between the societies. Abel, for example, was a member of all three.

The American Physiological Society admitted pharmacologist Elijah Houghton of Parke, Davis and Company as a member in 1901. Abel's associate at Johns Hopkins, Thomas Aldrich, was admitted to the physiologists' society in 1895, and did not have to relinquish his membership when he moved to Parke, Davis a few years later. In 1916, Aldrich, still at Parke, Davis, was admitted to membership in the American Society of Biological Chemists.[12]

Pharmacologists who could not be admitted to membership in their own professional society because of the restrictive clause were thus sometimes elected to membership in a sister organization. When Alfred Newton Richards of the University of Pennsylvania wrote to Abel in 1933 to ask him to second the nomination of industrial pharmacologist Hans Molitor of Merck for membership

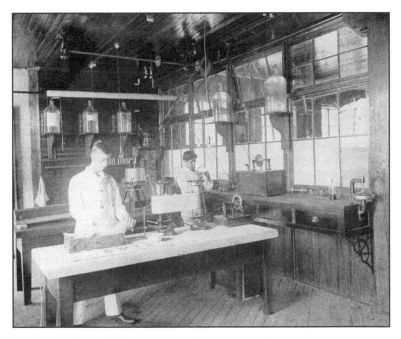

A pharmacological laboratory at Parke, Davis and Company in Detroit around the turn of the twentieth century (courtesy of the Kremers Reference Files, F. B. Power Pharmaceutical Library, University of Wisconsin-Madison).

34

in the physiological society, for example, he added: "I am not proposing him for membership in the Pharmacological Society because of the rule that people in the permanent employ of commercial firms are ineligible."[13] Evidence that the American Physiological Society may have even stretched their scope to accept pharmacologists who could not be admitted to ASPET because of their industrial employment is provided in the 1939 minutes of the Society. Action was deferred on the membership application of three pharmacologists from industry because "it was thought that the pharmacologists might revise their views regarding commercial pharmacologists," suggesting that the physiologists felt there might be no need to accept these scientists if they could become members of ASPET.[14]

Why then were the pharmacologists so much more concerned than their colleagues about admitting industrial scientists into their national society? What were the external influences "inimical to the scientific interests of pharmacology" that they were trying to avoid? Motivation is usually difficult to establish, and the early leaders of the Society did not leave a completely clear and neat record of justification for their action. The existing evidence allows us, however, to suggest at least some of the concerns which motivated American pharmacologists in this matter.

The industry that most concerned pharmacologists, and the one spelled out in the membership restriction clauses, was the pharmaceutical industry. During the first decade of the twentieth century, when the Society was founded, the American drug industry had a somewhat suspect reputation. Thousands of patent medicines of a dubious nature flooded the market, and patent medicine quackery, brought to public attention by muckraking journalists of the Progressive Era, was one of the factors that led to the passage of a national pure food and drug act in 1906. Although the more legitimate drug firms tried to distance themselves from the patent medicine promoters, they were not completely successful in lifting the cloud of suspicion that hung over the industry as a whole.[15]

Even the so-called "ethical" firms sometimes engaged in practices that pharmacologists considered objectionable. For example, Abel complained that his name had been used without his permission on occasion in drug advertisements or on drug labels. In a 1910 letter to a colleague, he warned: "Even reputable firms will do things that tend to damage men."[16] And five years later he expressed the following skeptical view about the advertising practices of drug manufacturers: "It is well known that the advertisers of drugs and medicines have often failed to confine their statements to actual facts and have yet to get the confidence of our profession."[17]

The traditional opposition of the medical community to patenting medical discoveries, reflected already in the Code of Ethics of the American Medical Association at its founding in 1847, probably influenced the views of many pharmacologists towards research in

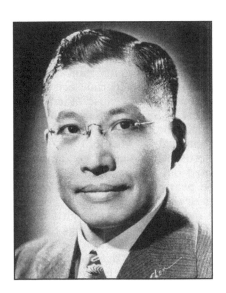

*Ko Kuei Chen of Eli Lilly
and Company, one of the
most prominent industrial
pharmacologists of the first
half of the twentieth century
(courtesy of the National
Library of Medicine).*

commercial firms.[18] Most of the first generation of American pharmacologists were trained as medical doctors, for there were no graduate programs in the subject in the United States. Even those who studied the subject abroad, like Abel, usually received the M.D. degree. Seventeen of the 18 founders of ASPET in 1908, for example, possessed medical degrees. By contrast, only 14 of the 29 founding members of the American Society of Biological Chemists in 1905 had M.D. degrees, and six of them were also founders of ASPET who in most cases considered their profession as pharmacology rather than biochemistry. Certainly only a relatively small proportion of the members of the American Chemical Society had M.D. degrees at the time. On the other hand, the American Physiological Society, which did not ban industry scientists, was also heavily medical in its membership.[19]

Pharmacologists may have been especially sensitive, relative to other scientists, about commercial influences on their work. It was the work of the pharmacologist, rather than that of the chemist or biochemist, that would decide at the experimental level the therapeutic potential and toxicity of a new drug. Academic pharmacologists were concerned that their industrial colleagues were subject to pressures from their employers to emphasize positive results and downplay negative results. Whether or not this was actually the case, it was certainly perceived to be so by many pharmacologists in academia and government. Robert Hatcher of Cornell, for example, expressed these concerns in a 1919 letter:

... nearly all workers in commercial houses deplore the limitations of their work due to the pressure for financially productive results, and to the ne-

36

cessity of avoiding publications that are inimical to financial interests . . . you need hardly ask proof that pressure is often put on investigators to supply desirable results.[20]

Torald Sollmann of Western Reserve University indicated that the founders of ASPET felt that a pharmacological society was "obliged to take these peculiar precautions, because otherwise it would be exposed to peculiar dangers."[21] Similarly, Samuel Meltzer of the Rockefeller Institute argued that the *Journal of Pharmacology and Experimental Therapeutics*, founded by Abel in 1909, had to be more careful about drug advertisements than, for example, a journal of morphology. He pointed out that many people would interpret an advertisement in the pharmacological journal as implying authoritative approval of a drug.[22]

Fears were also expressed that industrial pharmacologists might use the forum provided by the Society's annual meetings to extol the virtues of the products marketed by their employers. Reid Hunt, for example, expressed to Abel his concern that "the scientific meetings of the Society might become an opportunity for the reading of papers on drugs being exploited, or to be exploited, commercially."[23] The Society was so concerned about this potential problem that soon after it became a part of the newly-created Federation of American Societies for Experimental Biology in 1912, a motion was passed to ask that the Federation not transfer any paper to the ASPET program without the explicit consent of the Secretary of the Society. The main purpose of this resolution was to prevent the appearance on the program of papers of a "commercial nature."[24]

Abel was sensitive, as might be expected, about possible exploitation of the *Journal of Pharmacology and Experimental Therapeutics* for commercial purposes. The first paper from an industrial laboratory did not appear in the *Journal* until the sixth volume (1914), and there were few such papers before 1925. On the other hand, most American pharmaceutical firms were not carrying out much research that would have been suitable for publication in the *Journal* in the first quarter of the century. While there is thus no clear evidence that Abel actually discriminated against papers from industrial pharmacologists, he did express the view in 1926 that he had to be on his guard about criticism in publishing papers from manufacturing firms. He commented with respect to two of these papers submitted that year that they "might give the impression of not being sufficiently impartial from a scientific point of view" and that "some might get the impression that there is an advertising element in the papers." His main concern in the case of these two papers appears to have been the use of the trade names of the drugs involved. Abel felt that the trade names should be deleted entirely, or at most mentioned in brackets (following the chemical names) once or twice near the beginning of the paper, but not in the title or in any of the tables.[25]

One must also recall that in the early years of the Society, American pharmacology was still struggling to become a legitimate academic discipline. Pharmacologists were trying to escape the role assigned to materia medica, which was often viewed as essentially a handmaiden to therapeutics. Leaders such as John Abel emphasized that pharmacology was a basic biological science, related to but distinct from physiology.[26] Research carried out in pharmaceutical firms was considered to be largely of a practical or applied nature, and not contributing to the development of the fundamental science. Abel once explained to a colleague why he himself would not consider working on any problem suggested by a pharmaceutical firm:

Usually, problems of this nature could be worked out very well in the laboratories of the firms since they almost always concern questions of what I might call applied pharmacology. A pharmacologist of any training or ability should have so many problems of his own awaiting solution that he should not spend his time on matters of little theoretical importance for his science.[27]

Struggling to establish their discipline as an independent, basic science, the practitioners of pharmacology were especially anxious to avoid any taint of commercialism. Abel was so fastidious on this point that when he was elected as the Society's first president in 1908, he resigned from a special commission investigating the safety of saltpeter as a food additive. Although the commission was organized through the University of Illinois, it was funded in part by the American Packers Association. As the first president of an organization that banned industry pharmacologists from membership, Abel was concerned that his connection with the commission might be misunderstood, especially when he learned that rumors were circulating that he was "in the employ of the meat firms."[28]

In less than a decade, however, Abel began to soften his views on the question of industry pharmacologists. In early 1916, he wrote to a colleague in London that at the recent meeting (December, 1915) of ASPET in Boston he had sounded out some of the older members, such as Samuel Meltzer and Torald Sollmann, about the question of admitting pharmacologists in drug firms, such as Elijah Houghton, to membership in ASPET. He noted, however, that his colleagues were opposed to this step, believing that the time was not ripe for such an action. There was a feeling, he added, that "the drug house will not play 'fair' and will 'do us' at every opportunity."[29]

The issue was soon raised again, however, this time by Arthur Loevenhart of the University of Wisconsin. In 1918, Loevenhart discussed the question with Abel and, after receiving his support, submitted the following year an amendment to delete the membership restriction from the constitution. The amendment was originally scheduled to be discussed at a special meeting of the Society in April, 1919, but the issue was considered important and contro-

38

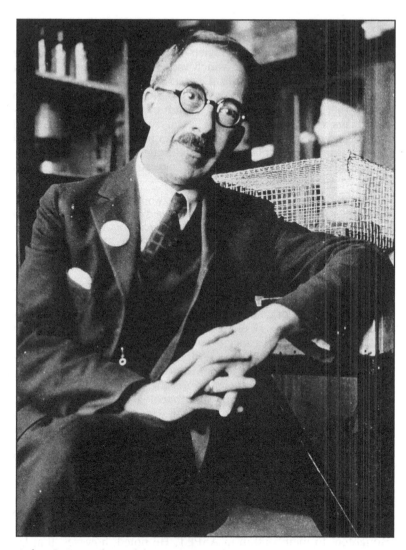

Arthur S. Loevenhart of the University of Wisconsin, who led the initial campaign to eliminate the American Society for Pharmacology and Experimental Therapeutics' membership ban on industrial pharmacologists (courtesy of the National Library of Medicine).

versial enough that it was decided to hold off consideration of it until the Society's regular meeting in Cincinnati the following December. Because of an unusually low attendance at that latter meeting however, no vote was taken on the amendment and it was referred to a special committee for evaluation. When a vote was finally taken at the 1920 meeting, the proposed amendment was unanimously defeated.[30] Abel was not in Chicago for the Society's meeting that year, and Loevenhart missed the business meeting due to a misunderstanding, so neither had an opportunity to speak on behalf of or vote for the amendment. Loevenhart vowed, however, to take up the fight again at some future date. Abel apparently still had mixed feelings about the issue, and admitted to a colleague after the meeting that he was less inclined to favor the amendment than he had been two years earlier.[31]

For the next two decades the issue remained a controversial one, periodically resurfacing to plague the Society. During this period, the proponents of changing the rule against industrial pharmacologists were unable to obtain the necessary four-fifths vote at an annual meeting to change the constitution on this point. There was, however, a growing sentiment to eliminate the restriction, culminating in the successful vote of 1941.

There were probably two major factors that contributed to the movement in the 1920s and 1930s to eliminate the ban against industrial pharmacologists. The first of these factors was the increase in the amount and quality of research being carried out by American pharmaceutical companies in the period between the two world wars. More and more pharmaceutical companies began to establish research facilities in the post World War I period, and some of the more prestigious companies began to become involved to some extent in basic research. As the image of research in the pharmaceutical industry improved, some of the stigma of being an industrial pharmacologist disappeared. A number of respected scientists, such as K. K. Chen at Lilly and Hans Molitor at Merck, followed in the footsteps of the fictional Max Gottlieb and joined the staff of pharmaceutical companies in the 1920s and 1930s. As pharmacologists of the stature of Chen and Molitor were excluded from membership in the Society, the pressure to change the constitution increased.[32]

In arguing the case for such a change, Abel wrote to Reid Hunt in 1927 that the large drug firms had a better attitude toward research than they did thirty years earlier.[33] In a letter to Sollmann in the same year, he noted that an increasing number of good pharmacologists were either not finding or not interested in academic positions and were pursuing careers with the larger pharmaceutical companies. Noting that he had originally been opposed to admitting industrial pharmacologists when the Society was founded, Abel added: "But times have changed and I wonder if we should not change with them."[34]

A second factor to be considered is the increasing involvement of academic pharmacologists with the drug industry in this period as consultants or in collaborative research agreements.[35] For example,

Loevenhart and later his successor at Wisconsin, Arthur Tatum, became involved in collaborative research on organic arsenical drugs with Parke, Davis and Company beginning in the 1920s.[36] In the early 1930s, University of Pennsylvania pharmacologist Alfred Newton Richards became a consultant to Merck on a regular basis and assisted them in developing an in-house program of pharmacological research.[37]

These consulting or collaborative arrangements were approached cautiously at first. Several colleagues, for example, wrote to Abel for counsel before undertaking such projects, seeking his opinion about the propriety of accepting payment from a pharmaceutical firm for performing some professional service.[38] Such arrangements became increasingly common and acceptable after World War I, and no doubt influenced the views of at least some pharmacologists about their industrial colleagues.

Even the traditional opposition on the part of many physicians and biomedical scientists to patenting medical discoveries began to erode in this period. By the mid-1930s at least a dozen universities were administering patents on medical discoveries by their faculty, further blurring the line between science and commerce.[39]

Those who supported changing the ASPET constitution to admit pharmacologists working for pharmaceutical firms argued that it was unnecessary to have a specific prohibition against these individuals. The Society's constitution and by-laws, it was claimed, provided adequate safeguards against the admission of unqualified members. Those who failed to meet the standards of the Society would be rejected, and any member who acted unethically or unprofessionally in some manner could be expelled under another provision of the constitution. Each applicant for membership should be judged individually on his or her merits, they argued, regardless of place of employment.[40]

Loevenhart complained that some, like Sollmann, criticized the low standards of pharmacological work in industry, but stood in the way of a major reform that might help to elevate these standards. Admitting industrial pharmacologists into ASPET would improve the chances of pharmaceutical firms to hire first-rate scientists, and company pharmacologists would benefit from their interaction with their academic colleagues within ASPET.[41]

Opponents of the change, however, were not satisfied with these arguments and continued to express concern that industrial pharmacologists might in time come to dominate the society and bend it to the needs of industry.[42] Robert Hatcher emphasized that the ideals of even the best scientists would gradually be broken down "by constant association with those who are in business with its insistent demand for financial success."[43] Some members tried to work out a compromise, whereby industry pharmacologists would be admitted as a new class of "associate members," but without the privilege of voting. But even this step went too far for some hard

core opponents of any change, and some of those who favored eliminating the membership restriction were concerned that this procedure would still mark their industrial colleagues as second class
citizens. The compromise effort never succeeded, and the issue remained unresolved.[44]

Some pharmacologists accepted the restriction on membership
gracefully. For example, when K. K. Chen joined the staff of Eli
Lilly and Company in 1929, he submitted his resignation to ASPET,
expressing "a desire to comply with the ethics of the Society and
leave it in good standing."[45]

Others employed by industrial firms were understandably dis-
turbed by the restriction on membership. When pharmacologist
David Macht, then at The Johns Hopkins University, contemplated
accepting an offer of a research position from the Baltimore drug
firm of Hynson, Westcott and Dunning in 1926, he wrote to Simon
Flexner of the Rockefeller Institute to seek his advice. Macht won-
dered whether accepting such a position would ruin his scientific
reputation and make it impossible for him to get back into academia.[46] Flexner replied, probably too optimistically:

Nowadays in this country it does not injure a man's reputation to go into
a pharmaceutical firm of good standing. Men like Clowes with the Lillys,
Anderson with Squibbs, and others, are in the scientific societies and are
respected.[47]

These men were indeed often members of scientific societies, but
were not, of course, admitted to ASPET. Macht did decide to accept
the job offer, but soon he began to write to Flexner complaining
about "the terrible and unjust discriminations made by other scientists more particularly medical men and pharmacologists against
anyone connected with a commercial concern."[48] He was especially
angered by what he called the "preposterous provision" in the constitution of the pharmacological society which excluded those employed in drug firms from membership.[49] British pharmacologist
Henry Dale, who had himself worked for a pharmaceutical firm
early in his career, would have sympathized with Macht on this
point, for in 1933 he wrote to an American colleague that he regarded the attitude of ASPET towards industrial pharmacologists
as "a piece of silly hypocrisy and pedantic snobbery."[50]

Although the rule remained in the constitution throughout the
1930s, one point at least was clarified during this decade. The question arose as to whether the phrase "in the permanent employ of a
drug firm" included a paid consultation arrangement with a pharmaceutical company on a long-term basis. Pharmacologists had
been consulting with drug firms before the 1930s, but the number
of such arrangements increased, and some of these involved extensive consultation over a long period of time. The matter seems to
have come to a head when A. N. Richards wrote to the Council of

ASPET on April 4, 1935, explaining that he had been acting as a paid consultant for Merck for three years, and that he felt it was his duty to bring this arrangement to the Council's attention because of the rule denying membership to those in the "permanent employ" of drug firms.[51]

The Council considered Richards' letter at its 1935 meeting, and agreed that the rule against industrial pharmacologists needed to be clarified with respect to consulting arrangements. A special committee was therefore established to study the problem, and in the meantime Richards was told that the Council did not feel that the arrangement he had with Merck violated the constitution.[52] It was recognized that by this time quite a few members were consulting with pharmaceutical firms.[53]

The committee, chaired by William deB. MacNider of the University of North Carolina, and including Abel as one of its members, recommended clarifying the two clauses in the constitution barring those "in the permanent employ of a drug firm" by adding the phrase "other than in the capacity of a consultant." Consulting arrangements would thus be explicitly excluded from the rule. They also proposed changing the term "drug firm" to "any organization concerned with the manufacture or sale of medicinal products." A majority of the members present at the 1936 annual meeting of ASPET (27 of 44) favored the amendment, but it did not receive the four-fifths majority needed for it to pass.[54] The same amendment was introduced again at the 1937 meeting, and this time it passed, although some members expressed concern about the advisability of passing an amendment "legalizing" consultation.[55] Meanwhile, there was no change in the status of pharmacologists whose sole or primary employer was a pharmaceutical company.

With the establishment of the Squibb Institute for Medical Research in 1938, its newly-appointed chief pharmacologist, Harry Van Dyke, tried a different approach to retaining his membership in the Society. Van Dyke pointed out that the Squibb Institute had been established for basic research, that it had its own board of scientific directors, and that it was relatively independent of the Squibb Company. He argued that he was therefore not really in the employ of a drug firm.[56] But the Society's Council refused to accept this argument. One officer commented:

Suppose Van Dyke would come out with a paper condemning, in no uncertain terms, one of E. R. Squibb and Sons' preparations. Van Dyke would lose his job. In other words, this means that Van Dyke is dependent upon E. R. Squibb and Sons for his livelihood.[57]

In any case, the Council felt that Van Dyke should not be treated differently from Chen, Molitor, and other industrial pharmacologists.[58]

The pressure to alter the constitution continued, however. In November of 1940, 24 distinguished members of the Society submitted another amendment to eliminate the ban on membership for industrial pharmacologists. The list of names included several who had been long-time opponents to amending the constitution for this purpose, such as Torald Sollmann and C. W. Edmunds.[59] It is not clear why these staunch foes of the amendment decided to change their position at this particular time, but certainly their switch played a key role in the eventual victory of the pro-amendment movement. On April 17, 1941, the 72 members present at the annual business meeting of ASPET unanimously approved amending the constitution to delete the restriction against industrial scientists, thus ending 33 years of a policy of discrimination against pharmacologists working for pharmaceutical firms.[60]

The improved image of industry science as pharmaceutical companies became more seriously involved in fundamental research, the entry of distinguished pharmacologists into the employ of industry, and the increasing involvement of academic scientists with industry as consultants all contributed to the eventual change in policy on the part of ASPET towards membership for industrial pharmacologists. The efforts of reputable drug firms to distance themselves from the manufacturers of quack patent medicines and increasing government regulation of the drug market may have also been factors in making the climate more favorable for the acceptance of industry pharmacologists by ASPET.

Over the past 40 years, the relationship between the Society and the pharmaceutical industry has become ever friendlier. In 1958, the Society established the membership category of corporate associates in an effort to secure financial support from industry.[61] There are currently some 40 to 50 corporate associates. It is not uncommon for an industrial scientist to be elected an officer, even President, of ASPET.[62] The situation is not significantly different from that of other scientific societies with significant industrial ties. The image of the pharmaceutical industry in the scientific community and the self-image of the pharmacology profession have improved to the point where a pharmacologist may accept a position in a pharmaceutical company without necessarily receiving the condemnation of his or her colleagues that the fictional Max Gottlieb did.

The concerns that motivated the founders of the American Society for Pharmacology and Experimental Therapeutics to institute their membership ban on industrial pharmacologists, however, have by no means disappeared. The increasing ties between industry and academia in recent times have caused renewed worries that the former may come to dominate the latter, and that science may become commercialized in the process. Some eighty years after the founding of ASPET, we are still searching for the appropriate balance of interaction between industrial and academic science. As John Swann noted in his recent book on the history of this inter-

44

action with respect to the pharmaceutical industry in the United States:

Universities, industry, and the public now have to decide how much collaboration is desirable for their needs; how much profit and impartiality they are willing to sacrifice; and which is the best possible course to satisfy the public good.[63]

Notes and References

The research for this paper was supported in part by NIH grant LM03300 from the National Library of Medicine.

1. Sinclair Lewis, *Arrowsmith* (New York: Harcourt Brace, 1925), p. 137.
2. See John Parascandola, "John J. Abel and the Early Development of Pharmacology at the Johns Hopkins University," *Bulletin of the History of Medicine* 56 (1982): 512–527.
3. K. K. Chen, "Meetings," in K. K. Chen, ed., *The American Society for Pharmacology and Experimental Therapeutics, Incorporated: The First Sixty Years, 1908–1969* (Bethesda, MD: American Society for Pharmacology and Experimental Therapeutics, 1969), pp. 5–11.
4. Ellsworth Cook, "Revisions of the Constitution and Bylaws," in Chen, *American Society* (n. 3), pp. 175–177, 184.
5. Undated draft of a letter from Reid Hunt to a committee of the council of the American Society for Pharmacology and Experimental Therapeutics appointed to draw up a constitution and bylaws, copy attached to a letter from Hunt to John Abel, January 2, 1909, John J. Abel Papers, Alan Mason Chesney Medical Archives, Johns Hopkins University, Baltimore, MD. The Abel Papers also contain a revised draft of this committee letter (also undated), and it includes the same statement.
6. Ibid. The initial draft named only Hunt, Crawford and Abel, but the revised draft added Loevenhart.
7. Typescript draft of constitution of the American Society for Pharmacology and Experimental Therapeutics, undated, in notebook on "Correspondence, ASPET Origins, C. W. Edmunds Files," American Society for Pharmacology and Experimental Therapeutics Archives, Bethesda, MD.
8. Incomplete typescript draft of ASPET constitution, undated, ibid.; Cook, "Revisions" (n. 4), p. 175.
9. See, for example, the correspondence in the Edmunds Files, ASPET Archives (n. 7); minutes of the organizational (1908) and first annual (1909) meeting of ASPET, Minutes and Records, volume 1 (1908–1916), ASPET Archives (n. 7); and the extensive correspondence in the founding of the Society in the Abel Papers (n. 5).
10. The Association of Official Agricultural Chemists did not admit industrial chemists, but there was no explicit ban in their constitution against such individuals. The Association accepted as active members only chemists associated with one of three types of institutions: the United States Department of Agriculture; any national, state or provincial experiment station or college engaged in agricultural chemistry research; and any national, state or provincial body charged with the official control of fertilizers, feeds and other agricultural products. In-

dustrial chemists were not singled out for exclusion. Chemists who worked for municipal laboratories or private research foundations, for example, were also ineligible to become active members. See Association of Official Agricultural Chemists, *Golden Anniversary of the Association of Official Agricultural Chemists, 1884–1934* (Washington, D.C.: 1934?), p. 19.

11. Charles Browne and Mary Weeks, *A History of the American Chemical Society: Seventy-five Eventful Years* (Washington, D.C.: American Chemical Society, 1952); Herman Skolnick and Kenneth Reese, eds., *A Century of Chemistry: The Role of Chemists and the American Chemical Society* (Washington, D.C.: American Chemical Society, 1976).

12. American Physiological Society, *History of the American Physiological Society, Semicentennial, 1887–1937* (Baltimore: 1938), John Brobeck, Orr Reynolds and Toby Appel, *History of the American Physiological Society: The First Century, 1887–1937* (Bethesda, MD: American Physiological Society, 1987); Russell H. Chittenden, *The First Twenty-five Years of the American Society for Biological Chemists* (New Haven, CT: American Society of Biological Chemists, 1945).

13. Letter from Richards to Abel, April 1, 1933, Abel Papers (n. 5).

14. Minutes of the Council, 1939, American Physiological Society Archives, Bethesda, MD. I am indebted to Toby Appel for calling my attention to these minutes and providing me with a copy.

15. On patent medicine quackery in this period, see James Harvey Young, *The Toadstool Millionaires: A Social History of Patent Medicines in America before Federal Regulation* (Princeton, NJ: Princeton University Press, 1961).

16. Abel to Robert Hatcher, January 31, 1910, Abel Papers (n. 5).

17. Abel to L. R. Hudson, December 7, 1915, Abel Papers (n. 5).

18. For a discussion of this point, see John Swann, *Academic Scientists and the Pharmaceutical Industry: Cooperative Research in Twentieth-Century America* (Baltimore: Johns Hopkins University Press, 1988), pp. 30–32.

19. For information on membership, see the society histories cited in notes 3, 11 and 12.

20. Hatcher to Arthur Loevenhart, December 26, 1919, Box 3, Arthur Loevenhart Papers, University of Wisconsin Archives, Madison, WI.

21. Sollman to Abel, February 9, 1927, Abel Papers (n. 5). Abel himself commented that ". . . for reasons evident to all medical men, it is the intention of the founders to impose unusual restrictions upon its members in respect to their connection with drug firms and other industrial concerns, a step that has my unqualified approval." Abel to Edmund James, January 5, 1909, Abel Papers (n. 5).

22. Meltzer to Abel, October 31, 1910, Abel Papers (n. 5).

23. Hunt to Abel, February 28, 1927, Abel Papers (n. 5).

24. Minutes of the fifth (1913) annual meeting of ASPET, Minutes and Records, volume 1 (1908–1916), ASPET Archives (n. 7).

25. Abel to Irvine Page, November 3, 1926, Abel Papers (n. 5).

26. John Abel, "The Methods of Pharmacology, with Experimental Illustration," *Pharmaceutical Era* 7 (1892): 105.

27. Abel to William De B. MacNider, April 5, 1935, Abel Papers (n. 5).

28. Abel to Edmund James, January 5, 1909 and Abel to A. P. Matthews, January 4, 1909, Abel Papers (n. 5).

46

29. Abel to Arthur Cushny, January 25, 1916, Abel Papers (n. 5).
30. Loevenhart to Abel, January 28, 1918, March 14, 1919, January 9, 1920, Abel Papers (n. 5); C. W. Edmunds to Abel, March 6, 1919, January 9, 1920, January 5, 1921, Abel Papers (n. 5); minutes of 11th (1919) and 12th (1920) annual meeting of ASPET, Minutes and Records, volume 2 (1917–1927), ASPET Archives (n. 7).
31. C. W. Edmunds to Abel, January 5, 1921, and Abel to Edmunds, January 10, 1921, Abel Papers (n. 5).
32. I have discussed the development of research in the American pharmaceutical industry during this period elsewhere. See John Parascandola, "Industrial Research Comes of Age: The American Pharmaceutical Industry, 1920–1940," *Pharmacy in History* 27 (1985): 12–21. See also Swann, *Scientists and the Pharmaceutical Industry* (n. 18), pp. 9–56, and Jonathan Liebenau, *Medical Science and Medical Industry: The Formation of the American Pharmaceutical Industry* (Baltimore: Johns Hopkins University Press, 1987).
33. Abel to Hunt, January 25, 1927, Abel Papers (n. 5).
34. Abel to Sollmann, February 2, 1927, Abel Papers (n. 5).
35. For a discussion of the growing interaction between academic scientists and the pharmaceutical industry in this period, see Swann, *Scientists and the Pharmaceutical Industry* (n. 18).
36. Ibid., pp. 93–117. See also John Swann, "Arthur Tatum, Parke-Davis, and the Discovery of Mapharsen as an Antisyphilitic Agent," *Journal of the History of Medicine and the Allied Sciences* 40 (1985): 167–187.
37. Swann, *Scientists and the Pharmaceutical Industry* (n. 18), pp. 65–86.
38. Robert Hatcher to Abel, January 28, 1910, A. N. Richards to Abel, August 30, 1930, William deB. MacNider to Abel, May 29, 1931, Abel Papers (n. 5).
39. Swann, *Scientists and the Pharmaceutical Industry* (n. 18), p. 75.
40. See, e.g., "Proposed Amendment to the Constitution of the American Society for Pharmacology and Experimental Therapeutics," undated printed document, minutes of 12th (1920) annual meeting of ASPET, Minutes and Records, volume 2 (1917–1927), ASPET Archives (n. 7). A copy of this proposed amendment from the 1920 meeting is also attached to a letter from Arthur Hirschfelder to Abel, January 20, 1927, Abel Papers (n. 5).
41. Loevenhart to Abel, March 14, 1919, Abel Papers (n. 5).
42. See, e.g., Robert Hatcher to Abel, February 4, 1927, Abel Papers (n. 5).
43. Ibid.
44. Sollmann to Abel, February 9, 1927, Abel to Arthur Loevenhart, February 16, 1927, Abel to David Macht, March 1, 1927, Macht to Abel, March 2, 1927, Abel to Chauncey Leake, March 22, 1932, Abel Papers (n. 5).
45. Minutes of the 20th (1929) annual meeting of ASPET, Minutes and Records, volume 3 (1928–1934), ASPET Archives (n. 7).
46. Macht to Flexner, April 5, 1926, Simon Flexner Papers, American Philosophical Society, Philadelphia, PA.
47. Flexner to Macht, April 5, 1926, Flexner Papers (n. 46). The name of Clowes is misspelled "Clawes" in the letter.
48. Macht to Flexner, October 25, 1928, Flexner Papers (n. 46).
49. Macht to Flexner, January 12, 1927, Flexner Papers (n. 46).
50. Dale to A. N. Richards, April 6, 1933, Box 32, A. N. Richards Papers, University of Pennsylvania Archives, Philadelphia, PA. I am grateful to John Swann for calling my attention to this letter.

51. Richards to ASPET Council, April 4, 1935, Richards Papers (n. 50).
52. E. M. K. Geiling to Richards, April 26, 1936, Box 10, Richards Papers (n. 50); minutes of the 26th (1935) annual meeting of the ASPET Council, Minutes and Records, volume 4 (1935–1937), ASPET Archives (n. 7).
53. E. M. K. Geiling to ASPET members, January 16, 1937, Minutes and Records, volume 4 (1935–1937), ASPET Archives (n. 7).
54. Minutes of the 27th (1936) annual meeting of ASPET, Minutes and Records, volume 4 (1935–1937), ASPET Archives (n. 7).
55. Minutes of the 28th (1937) annual meeting of ASPET, Minutes and Records, volume 4 (1935–1937), ASPET Archives (n. 7).
56. Van Dyke to Charles Gruber, July 14, 1938 and Van Dyke to G. Philip Grabfield, November 21, 1938, minutes of the 30th (1938) annual meeting of the ASPET Council, Minutes and Records, volume 5 (1938–1939), ASPET Archives (n. 7).
57. Arthur Tatum to G. Grabfield, July 22, 1938, Arthur Tatum Papers, Box 2, University of Wisconsin Archives, Madison, WI.
58. Minutes of the 30th (1939) annual meeting of the ASPET Council, Minutes and Records, volume 5 (1938–1939), ASPET Archives (n. 7).
59. Petition to G. Grabfield, November 6, 1940, Minutes and Records, volume 6 (1940–1941), ASPET Archives (n. 7).
60. Minutes of the 32nd (1941) annual meeting of the ASPET Council, Minutes and Records, volume 6 (1940–1941), ASPET Archives (n. 7).
61. K. K. Chen, "Membership," in Chen, *American Society* (n. 3), pp. 151–152. On the establishment of the corporate associates program, see also Otto Krayer to A. Weston, November 18, 1958, Box 13, Chauncey Leake Papers, National Library of Medicine, Bethesda, MD.
62. For information on the recent activities and policies of ASPET, see the periodical *The Pharmacologist*.
63. Swann, *Scientists and the Pharmaceutical Industry* (n. 18), pp. 170–181; the quotation is from p. 181.

The Search for the Active Oxytocic Principle of Ergot: Laboratory Science and Clinical Medicine in Conflict

As laboratory science began to make its impact felt on medicine in the late nineteenth and early twentieth centuries, the relationship between scientist and clinician was not always a harmonious one. Recent papers by Gerald Geison and Russell Maulitz have discussed the tensions that developed between laboratory science and clinical medicine with respect to physiology and bacteriology[1]. Even the titles of these papers stress the conflict between laboratory and clinic in the phrases "Divided We Stand" (Geison) and "Physician versus Bacteriologist" (Maulitz). Practicing physicians at times questioned the pragmatic value of basic research, while scientists in turn complained that clinicians were too short-sighted to appreciate the benefits that laboratory science would eventually bestow upon medical practice.

Like its sister sciences of physiology and bacteriology, pharmacology also sometimes came into conflict with clinical medicine[2]. Experimental pharmacology clearly emerged as a distinct discipline only in the second half of the nineteenth century. Geison has pointed out that physiologists claimed that their subject was a separate discipline and not a mere handmaiden of medicine, although the prospects of the new discipline remained intertwined with the destinies of medicine and medical educa-tion[3]. Similarly, pharmacologists argued that pharmacology was an inde-pendent science and not just a handmaiden of therapeutics, although they were usually quick to point out that pharmacological research would eventually yield results of practical value for medicine. John J. Abel, the most important figure in the early development of American pharmacology, reflected these views in the following quotation taken from an address delivered in 1891.

"Briefly, this science [pharmacology] tries to discover all the chemical and physical changes that go on in a living thing that has absorbed a substance capable of producing such changes, and it also attempts to discover the fate of the substance incorporated. It is not therefore an applied science, like therapeutics, but is one of the biological sciences, using that word in its widest sense, like its sister sciences, physiology, physiological chemistry, and pathology, it is making great progress along certain physical and chemical lines, which is pioneer work of a necessary kind toward an explanation of vital processes . . .

It was such experiments that led Buchheim and others to insist on the insufficiency of the mere bedside study of medicines, and led to the erection of special pharmacological laboratories in which experimenters can build up their science undisturbed by the intrusive demands of practical utility. But pharmacology once on a firm basis will yield valuable results for the practical man"[4].

In a 1910 address entitled "A Plea For Therapeutics," the eminent British pharmacologist Arthur Cushny appealed to pharmacologists and clinicians to work more closely together in the interest of improved therapeutics. According to Cushny, "pharmacologists abandoned the hospitals for the laboratory" because the foundations of their subject had to be laid on more definite observations than were possible in man. The subject thus came to be studied without any immediate bearing on its usefulness to medicine, and physicians were sometimes skeptical of its practical value. Although Cushny urged pharmacologists and physiologists to return to the problems of the sick bed, he also criticized practitioners for their failure to appreciate the ultimate value of experimental research. In addition, one of the causes cited by Cushny for the "slight antagonism which is sometimes observable between the experimental observer and the clinical exponent of therapeutics" was as follows:

"The laboratory-trained man expects accurate measurements; the clinician is unable to give them. He is unable or unwilling to devote the attention necessary to obtain accurate results, yet he is ready to express an opinion on the value of drugs, and is often to be heard expressing doubt as to the usefulness of experimental pharmacology. And the absence of accurate clinical records, such as we can use to substantiate our laboratory findings, is seriously hindering the advance of therapeutics"[5].

As an example of the lack of useful clinical data, Cushny cited the case of the use of ergot in obstetric practice. The drug was given to thousands of patients every year, yet he could not find in the literature any systematic, quantitative observations of the rate and duration of labor pains before and after the administration of the drug. Because of the lack of adequate data, clinicians argued about whether ergot should be given during labor to quicken childbirth, or whether its usefulness was limited to maintaining the tonic contraction of the uterus after birth (to reduce the incidence and extent of post-partum hemorrhage). Cushny also complained that laboratory scientists did not know what the obstetrician needed or wanted because they had no accurate clinical records of the action of ergot in labor nor any knowledge of what exact features the obstetrician desired to elicit. It was therefore not clear, for example, which of the active principles isolated from ergot up to that time might be most useful clinically[6].

The story of the search for the active oxytocic principle of ergot, which is the subject of this paper, can serve to illustrate the conflict between laboratory science and clinical medicine that we have been discussing up to this point.

Official ergot is the dried sclerotium (resting stage) of the fungus Claviceps purpurea developed on rye plants. The earliest known recorded reference to the use of ergot in childbirth is in a 1582 German herbal, but its use for this purpose may go back much earlier. European references in the seventeenth and eighteenth centuries suggest that the use of ergot to expedite labor, and sometimes in an attempt to induce abortion, was not uncommon, and not without controversy[7]. The drug seems to have received increased attention in medical circles, especially in the United States, as the result of the publication of a letter on the subject by Dr. John Stearns of Saratoga County, New York in 1808. Stearns described how he used a powder derived from "a spurious growth of rye" to "quicken" childbirth.

"In most cases you will be surprised by the suddenness of its operation; it is, therefore, necessary to be completely ready before you give the medicine, as the urgency of the pains will allow you but a short time afterwards. Since I have adopted the use of this powder I have seldom found a case that detained me more than three hours"[8].

Ergot was included in the first edition of the Pharmacopoeia of the United States of America in 1820 (in the list of secondary substances), and it also found its way into various European pharmacopoeias during the course of the nineteenth century[9]. In addition to its use in obstetrics, it was tried in the treatment of numerous diseases (e. g., pneumonia, bronchitis, whooping cough, gonorrhea, hemorrhoids and migraine)[10]. Ergot came to be administered in a variety of preparations: e. g., as a powder, an infusion, a decoction, a wine, an extract.

The extract became a common form in which to administer ergot, and the controversy that developed between pharmacologists and clinicians essentially concerned the best method for preparing such an extract in order to insure maximum therapeutic value. The sixth decennial revision (1880) of the Pharmacopoeia of the United States of America listed two extracts of ergot. Extractum Ergotae Fluidum (fluid extract of ergot) was prepared by subjecting ground ergot to percolation, using a 3:4 alcohol-water mixture as the menstruum (and later adding dilute hydrochloric acid). Extractum Ergotae (extract of ergot) was prepared by evaporating the fluid extract to one-fifth its original volume[11].

In addition to the alcoholic extract, an aqueous extract was also commonly employed. The French pharmacist Joseph Bonjean, for example, developed an aqueous extract of ergot (Bonjean's Ergotin) in the 1840s, and soon there were various commercial "ergotin" preparations on the market[12]. The first edition of the British Pharmacopoeia, published in 1864, included an aqueous extract under the name of Extractum Ergotae Liquidum (liquid extract of ergot). Powdered ergot was extracted with distilled water, and alcohol was then added to the extract to precipitate impurities[13]. In 1885, the British Pharmacopoeia added a second extract, Ergotinum (called Extractum Ergotae in later editions), prepared by evaporating the liquid extract to a "soft extract" (just as the U. S. P. included an ergot extract prepared by concentration of the fluid extract)[14].

It was the aqueous extraction procedure employed by the British Pharmacopoeia (as opposed to the alcoholic extraction method of the U. S. Pharmacopoeia) that was to become the center of the controversy that concerns us in this paper. Consequently our attention shall be focused primarily on the British scene.

Ergot contains a variety of physiologically active constituents, and relatively little progress was made in the nineteenth towards clarifying its chemical composition. In 1875, the French pharmacist Charles Tanret isolated the first crystalline substance, ergotinine, from ergot, but it proved to be pharmacologically inert. Various amorphous active materials, given different names, were obtained from ergot in the latter part of the century, but there was no success in isolating an active principle in a chemically pure form[15].

Shortly after the turn of the twentieth century, George Barger and Francis Carr in England and Fritz Kraft in Switzerland isolated what they believed to be a pure alkaloid, ergotoxine. Although the alkaloid itself was amorphous, it could be crystallized in the form of a salt[16]. Pharmacologist Henry Dale, Barger and Carr's colleague at the Wellcome Physiological Research Laboratories in London, investigated the pharmacology of the new ergot alkaloid. Dale's interest in ergot, and presumably that of his coworkers also, was stimulated by a request from his employer, Henry Wellcome, that he investigate the drug[17].

Dale's pharmacological experiments clearly showed that ergotoxine caused a toxic contraction of the uterus in pregnant cats. Barger and Dale recognized that, because of its relative insolubility in water, the official aqueous extract of the British Pharmacopoeia could not contain much ergotoxine. The stimulant effect of the liquid extract on involuntary muscle was too great to be accounted for by the amount of ergotoxine present, and hence they concluded that it was likely that pharmacopoeial extracts contained some other active prinicple[18].

The two Wellcome scientists were soon led to the discovery of other active substances in ergot extracts. A number of recent papers had shown that when materials like meat, or human placenta, were allowed to putrefy, substances (presumably bases) were produced which had pressor activity, i. e., they caused a rise in blood pressure. Ergot also exhibited pressor activity, presumably by causing contraction of the smooth muscle of the arterial walls. It occurred to Barger and Dale that the pressor substances produced by putrefaction might be similar to those in ergot extracts, expecially since they received information from manufacturers of the liquid extract that its preparation was inevitably accompanied by putrefaction. Barger and a colleague identified three bases with pressor properties from putrid meat, each of which they felt was derived from an amino acid by decarboxylation. One of these bases, p-hydroxyphenylethylamine, or tyramine, was also found to be present in significant quantities in watery extracts of ergot, and Barger and Dale concluded that it accounted for practically the whole of the pressor activity of these extracts[19]. In 1910, they reported the isolation of another physiologically active amine, histamine, from ergot extracts. Histamine produced marked contractions of the uterus, although its effect on blood pressure varied according to the species (e. g., it was raised in rodents but lowered in cats)[20].

The isolation of ergotoxine and several physiologically active amines from ergot opened the door for an attack on the therapeutic efficacy of the official aqueous extract of ergot in the British Pharmacopoeia. The opening salvo of what was to be a long, drawn-out battle was fired, appropriately enough, by Henry Dale (in a paper coauthored by F. H. Carr) at a 1913 British Pharmaceutical Conference in London. Dale's presentation was entitled "Ergot and Its Preparations: A Critical Review of the Requirements of the British Pharmacopoeia"[21]. He pointed out that until the last few years, the chemistry of ergot, particularly with regard to its active principles, was so obscure and confused that preparations in pharmacopoeias "necessarily had a traditional rather than a scientific sanction".

Various attempts had been made to standardize ergot physiologically, but there was a question as to which, if any, of the different physiological effects measured (cyanosis of a cock's comb, increase in blood pressure, contraction of isolated uterine muscle) served as a reliable index of therapeutic activity.

Now that the chief active principles of the drug had been isolated in a chemically pure state, Dale continued, it seemed an opportune time to submit the various preparations of the British Pharmacopoeia (1898 edition) to the test of this new knowledge. He reviewed for his audience the active principles that had been isolated from ergot, the alkaloid ergotoxine and various amines. In Dale's view, ergotoxine was largely responsible for the therapeutic activity of ergot, but the amines seemed to make an important contribution to the therapeutic value of ergot extracts. He regretted, however, that there was not more clinical, as opposed to experimental pharmacological, evidence on the relative importance of the different active principles in the therapeutic action of the drug.

On the basis of available evidence, Dale concluded that ergotoxine was the most important therapeutic principle, hence ergot extracts should be prepared in such a way as to maximize the amount of this substance[22]. Given the properties of ergotoxine (i. e., relatively soluble in alcohol-water mixtures but not in water or dry alcohol, unstable in alkaline solution), the ideal method for extracting it would be to use a moderately dilute alcohol acidified with a weak acid. Such an extract existed, Dale noted, in the fluidextract of the U. S. P. (although the U. S. P. method utilized dilute hydrochloric acid rather than a weak acid). On the other hand, he went on to state, "it would be difficult . . . to find worse methods than those laid down for the preparation of the extracts of the B. P." He recommended replacing the Extractum Ergotae Liquidum of the B. P. by the fluidextract of the U. S. P.

Dale conceded that the B. P. liquid extract contained active amines which had therapeutic value, but saw their chief importance as lying in their adjuvant and synergistic effect on the action of ergotoxine. In any case, if one desired the pharmacological effects of these amines, they were not unique to ergot and could easily be obtained pure from other sources[23]. In the discussion following his paper, Dale once again emphasized that pharmacologists did not have enough information on what medical men wanted. What was most needed to put the ergot question on a really satisfactory basis, be stressed, was more clinical experience[24].

Dale's recommendations went unheeded, however, by the compilers of the 1914 edition of the British Pharmacopoeia. Extractum Ergotae Liquidum remained official, the method of preparation essentially unchanged from the 1898 edition. Over the next two decades British pharmacologists continued to attack the aqueous extract, repeating Dale's arguments and offering new evidence to support the claim that the alcoholic extract was far superior to this preparation. The isolation of another active alkaloid from ergot, ergotamine, by Arthur Stoll of Switzerland in 1918 did not significantly alter the controversy over the extract. Ergotamine was shown to be pharmacologically very similar to ergotoxine, even if the two alkaloids differed chemically. In addition, its solubility characteristics were also similar to those of ergotoxine, so the aqueous extract contained very little of the new alkaloid[25]. Critics of the B. P. preparation thus continued to attack its therapeutic value.

These critics included some of Britain's most eminent pharmacologists. Dale himself, now Director of the National Institute for Medical Research, returned to the attack in 1922. At a joint meeting of the Sections of Obstetrics and Gynaecology and of Therapeutics and Pharmacology of the Royal Society of Medicine, he discussed the value of ergot in obstetrics and gynaecology, with special reference to its position in the British Pharmacopoeia. He again pointed out the shortcomings of the aqueous extract in terms of the relatively small quantity of specific ergot alkaloids (i. e., ergotoxine and ergotamine) that it contained. Dale admitted that his preparation, which apparently continued to find favor in obstetrical and gynaecological practice, might possess useful therapeutic activity. If so, however, this activity must be due to the amines produced by putrefaction during the extraction process. If these non-specific putrefactive bases were desired for use in obstetric and gynaecological treatment, however, then it would be easier and cheaper to obtain them by other methods from other sources, rather than "by casual and unregulated putrefaction of an obscure and expensive fungus", which was "not a scientific or even a sensible procedure". Dale also saw difficulties in "supposing that bases like these, which are undoubtedly present in many articles of diet, and which, further, are certainly produced by bacterial action in the intestine, could have any great therapeutic importance when administered by the mouth in relatively small quantities"[26].

In the ensuing discussion, Sir Nestor Tirard, one of the editors of the Bristish Pharmacopoeia, rose to the defense of the compilers of the book. He pointed out that various examining and licensing bodies, the

Therapeutic Committee of the British Medical Association, a committee of wholesale firms, and other sources had been solicited for suggestions for additions, ommissions or alterations in the B. P. In no single instance was a desire to omit ergot or its preparations expressed[27]. Dale countered that he felt that it was the function of the British Pharmacopoeia to lead rather than to follow the profession. Tirard then reminded Dale that the B. P. was controlled by international agreement requiring all liquid extracts to be watery extracts, with alcohol (if used) to be added subsequent to extraction, and that only in America had the alcoholic extract been retained in spite of this agreement. Undaunted, Dale replied that he wished the American disobedience had prevailed in his own country[28].

Other leaders of British pharmacology supported Dale's views. Walter Dixon of Cambridge University claimed that pharmacologists were clear that the American extract was superior to the British one[29]. A. J. Clark of University College, London, in a 1923 paper coauthored by W. A. Broom, charged that the B. P. method of preparation for the liquid extract of ergot appeared to be "frankly absurd". Clark and Broom introduced a new method of standardizing ergot, using the uterus of a rabbit, which became widely adopted, and an analysis of the B. P. liquid extract by their procedure convinced them of the inferiority of this product[30].

J. H. Burn, Director of the Pharmacological Laboratories of the Pharmaceutical Society of Great Britain, also became actively involved in the ergot controversy. Burn collaborated in 1927 with Aleck Bourne, an obstetric surgeon, on a clinical investigation of the action of pituitary extract and ergot preparations on the uterus in labor[31]. Dale and others had long been calling for more accurate clinical data on the use of ergot, and Burn and Bourne developed a method to allow them to measure the effects of drugs on the human uterus. It involved introducing a rubber bag, attached to the end of a catheter, into the uterus. The other end of the catheter was attached to a piece of rubber pressure tubing, which in turn was connected to a mercury manometer. In this manner, they were able to measure the force, frequency and duration of uterine contractions during labor[32].

Ergotamine was found to produce a powerful, prolonged contraction of the uterus. Burn and Bourne considered the condition of uterine spasm which it produced to be dangerous so long as the child and the placenta remained in utero, but they recommended ergotamine for the treatment of post-partum hemorrhage. They also examined the effects of histamine and tyramine, and concluded that the amounts of these amines present in the liquid extract of ergot would not be sufficient to exert any significant effect on the uterus[33]. It followed, they reasoned, that the B. P. liquid extract must be a "wholly inert preparation". Yet they recognized that it had been in clinical use in Britain for many years without any serious complaints arising against it from clinicians[34].

Burn and Bourne therefore decided to subject the liquid extract of ergot to a clinical test. For some reason, however, they chose not to use the method they had developed for directly measuring uterine contractions. Instead, they compared the effects of three different preparations on the rate of descent of the uterus and on the color and amount of lochial (post-labor) discharges during the first seven days after delivery. The three preparations employed were the U. S. P. alcoholic extract, the B. P. aqueous extract, and an extract of the proprietary article Marmite (a yeast extract) prepared so as to superficially resemble an extract of ergot. It is interesting to note that their study incorporated the use of a placebo (the Marmite extract) and a "double blind" procedure (neither the patients nor the person recording the observations were aware of which patients were receiving which preparations). The patients were divided into two groups of twelve and a third group of eight, each group receiving a different preparation.

Presumably the "active" preparation (or preparations) would affect the rate of descent of the uterus and the amount of blood in the discharge (and hence the color of the discharge). Examination of the results, however, showed that it was not possible to distinguish the changes in patients which received one extract from those in patients receiving either of the other extracts. Burn and Bourne concluded that this experiment might explain, at least in part, the lack of complaints from obstetricians regarding the efficacy of the B. P. extract, "for it appears that ordinary clinical methods do not suffice, in normal cases at least, even to demonstrate the presence in an extract of a considerable proportion of the highly potent specific alkaloid". (They were referring here to the U. S. P. extract, which had been shown to contain significant amounts of the active ergot alkaloids). They therefore concluded that "no serious attention can be paid to statements that the British Pharmacopoeial extract has a therapeutic action", and that the B. P. method of preparing the extract should be revised at the earliest opportunity[35].

Had they subjected the aqueous extract to the direct test that they had devised for measuring uterine contractions, they might well have come to a very different conclusion (as Chassar Moir did a few years later). The reason why they did not take this step was suggested by Burn after Moir's work in 1932. Burn pointed out that the measurement of intrauterine pressure can only be done when the mouth of the uterus is open, as in labor, and that the procedure was not without risk to the mother and to the child. Therefore, they were not anxious to multiply their observations using this method, and stopped after testing the known active constituents of ergot[36].

Burn thus joined the ranks of other distinguished British pharmacologists who attacked the therapeutic usefulness of the aqueous extract. He expressed his regret that the Pharmacopoeial Committee of the 1914 Pharmacopoeia had rejected the scientific evidence available to them at the time concerning this extract, "inasmuch as not one ounce of the thousands of gallons made since then can have been of the slightest medicinal value"[37]. One of the functions of the Pharmacological Laboratories of the Pharmaceutical Society, of which Burn was the Director, was to carry out biological assays of pharmaceutical preparations for manufacturers. The Pharmacological Laboratories, however, refused to accept samples of B. P. extracts, because it was a foregone conclusion that these samples would exhibit no activity when tested by the Broom-Clark assay procedure used by the laboratory[38]. Burn's critical attitude toward the individual clinician's ability to evaluate therapeutic agents is reflected in the following quotation.

"The recent demonstration of the uselessness of the watery extract is therefore, in addition, a demonstration that in many cases the clinician cannot form any opinion of the value of his remedies; the conditions of his work make it impossible for him to do so. The only trustworthy evidence he can offer is represented by a slow formation of opinion which takes many decades to complete"[39].

By now sufficient examples have been presented to document the British pharmacological community's militant criticism of the aqueous extract of ergot. It is not nearly so easy to find examples of clinicians defending the use of the preparation, at least in print[40]. Tirard's defense, cited earlier, was largely based on the absence of complaints from practitioners concerning the extract. This point was frequently stressed by those who supported the continued inclusion of the aqueous extract in the British Pharmacopoeia. For example, E. A. Lum, in a letter published in the Pharmaceutical Journal in 1932, argued that it appeared certain that the B. P. liquid extract had therapeutic value as hundreds of medical practitioners had used it with satisfaction for many years[41]. E. W. Mann of Southall Brothers and Barclay, Ltd., one of the manufacturers of the B. P. preparation, boasted that his firm had "not had a single complaint that the Ext. Ergotae Liq. sent out has failed to give the results expected by the medical practitioner prescribing it"[42].

Practicing obstetricians and gynaecologists, however, were no doubt much less likely to publish papers than were research pharmacologists, and hence it is more difficult to ascertain the view of the average clinician. A check of a number of obstetrics textbooks of the period by British authors indicated that the liquid extract was recommended in at least some of these works. Ergot was usually not discussed at length, however, and sometimes no clear recommendation was given as to which specific preparation to administer[43]. As previously noted, pharmacologists lamented the lack of published careful, systematic clinical observations on the effects of ergot.

At least one practitioner, J. Gordon Sharp, had published the results of clinical experiments measuring the effects of the liquid extract, the infusion, ergotoxine and tyramine on uterine contractions in 1911, before the controversy over the B. P. preparation had really gotten underway. Sharp did not measure intrauterine pressure directly, as Burn and Bourne were later to do, but attempted to quantify his observations by using a calibrated steel tape to record the changes in size of the abdomen during a labor pain. Sharp's observations led him to conclude that ergotoxine possessed no real advantage over the galenical preparations tested (i. e., the liquid extract and the infusion)[44]. Incidentally, Dale was present when the paper was delivered, and suggested in the ensuing discussion that the activity of the aqueous preparations was probably due to the histamine that they contained[45]. In the long run, however, Sharp's paper seems to have had little impact on the thinking of pharmacologists concerning the aqueous extract.

It is difficult to assess exactly how much use the B. P. extract found in therapeutics. There were various preparations of ergot and ergot alkaloids available during the period under discussion. In addition, pituitary extract was also beginning to come into use as an oxytocic agent by World War I. Obstetricians also disagreed about whether or not it was advisable to administer ergot to hasten labor, or whether it should just be used after delivery to control post-partum hemorrhage (apparently the more common use after the turn of the twentieth century).

The fact that the British Pharmacopoeia of 1914 continued to include the aqueous extract rather than the alcoholic extract is evidence of support for the former, although it does not tell us how frequently it was employed by practitioners. Although the United States Pharmacopoeia contained the alcoholic extract, the aqueous extract apparently was used by some American physicians since it was included in the National Formulary, at least in the fourth (1916) and fifth (1926) editions[46]. The British Pharmaceutical Codex, a dispensatory for medical practitioners and pharmacists published by the Pharmaceutical Society of Great Britain, underwent an interesting evolution of views about the liquid extract and the active principles of ergot. In 1907, just after ergotoxine had been isolated, the Codex touted it as the substance responsible for the whole action of ergot on the uterus, and argued that it should be preferred to the galenical preparations[47]. By 1911, ergotoxine had become "one of the active constituents of ergot", probably responsible for ,,only a small part of the action of ergot, since it is almost absent from the liquid extract". It now seemed "too early to decide" whether or not it had clinical value[48]. By 1923, the Codex concluded that: "Ergotoxine has been used clinically for its action on the uterus, but it is disappointing and gynaecologists are now generally agreed that it is not the active constituent of ergot they want"[49].

Evidence that the aqueous extract was actually used in significant quantities by British physicians was provided by the President of the Edinburgh Obstetrical Society. He reported that in 1926 thirteen Winchester quarts of pharmacopoeial liquid extract of ergot, and twelve dozen ampoules for hypodermic injection, had been used in the Royal Maternity Hospital[50]. Since the average dose of the liquid extract, according to the British Pharmacopoeia of 1914, was only 10 to 30 minims (approximately 0.6 to 1.8 cc), thousands of doses were apparently dispensed. If these figures are at all accurate, they would suggest that, at least at the Royal Maternity Hospital in Edinburgh, the B. P. extract was rather routinely used for obstetric patients.

Whatever the actual amount of the B. P. extract used, it is clear that there was a widespread impression that the preparation found favor amongst obstetricians and gynaecologists. The ergot question had become controversial enough for the British Pharmacopoeia Commission to appoint a special Sub-Committee on Ergot in 1931 to investigate the matter and make recommendations before a new British Pharmacopoeia was issued in 1932. The Committee was chaired by J. H. Burn, and included, among others, several other individuals who have been previously mentioned in this paper, namely F. H. Carr, H. H. Dale and W. A. Broom. The Sub-Committee issued its report in October of 1931, and the Commission decided, in light of the problems surrounding ergot, to publish and circulate the report and to solicit comments.

Much of the report was devoted to methods for standardizing ergot preparations. The report did contain a section, however, on the method for preparing a liquid extract. Although not specifically attacking the aqueous extract as worthless, the Sub-Committee clearly recommended that the procedure for the preparation of a liquid extract should in general follow the U.S.P. method (except that they suggested substituting tartaric acid for hydrochloric acid)[51]. When the new edition of the British Pharmacopoeia appeared in September of 1932, the pharmacologists at long last had their way and the traditional aqueous extract was replaced by the alcoholic extract recommended by the special Sub-Committee[52].

Ironically, just before the 1932 B. P. was published a paper appeared in the British Medical Journal providing strong clinical evidence for the therapeutic value of the old aqueous extract[53]. We must now turn our attention to this unexpected development. In 1931, the Therapeutic Trials Committee of the Medical Research Council, concerned about claims that ergotamine was clearly superior to ergotoxine, decided to arrange for a clinical test of the two drugs. The Committee approached Professor F. J. Browne of University College Hospital and proposed such a test. Browne invited Dr. J. Chassar Moir, a young obstetrician at the hospital, to undertake the investigation[54].

Moir decided to use a modification of the previously-discussed method of Burn and Bourne for measuring uterine contractions. He realized that since the mouth of the uterus remained open during the puerperium (the days following delivery), it should be possible to record the contractions during this period by the Burn-Bourne method. This procedure had several advantages over recording the intrauterine pressure of a woman in labor. First of all, it was a far safer procedure, involving less risk to the mother and none at all to the child. Secondly, the restlessness of a patient during labor could cause false and erratic recordings. Finally, since ergot was used at the time more for controlling post-partum hemorrhage than for inducing labor, it made more sense to test its action during the puerperium.

Moir soon settled the ergotamine-ergotoxine question, demonstrating that these two alkaloids were indistinguishable in their clinical action[55]. Having developed a successful method for studying the clinical effects of oxytocic agents, Moir decided to extend the scope of the investigation to include other constituents and preparations of ergot. One of these preparations was the much-criticized aqueous extract, which he expected to be largely inert. Much to his surprise, he found that it greatly surpassed the activity of the ergot alkaloids and amines that he had tried, and that the onset of action was extremely rapid[56]. Years later Moir recalled his first observation of the effects of the aqueous extract as follows:

"As I watched the needle mount higher and higher, my first reaction was that a fault had developed in the recording apparatus. My next was that the patient must be behaving in some unprecedented matter – but no, a quick inspection of the woman as she lay in the adjacent room showed that she was, in fact, calmly eating her lunch. My third and lasting impression was one of sheer astonishment . . .

Leaving my work, and with a mind still full of wonder, I made my way home. Then there flashed on me the true meaning of Dr. John Stearns' words. I realized that I had stumbled upon the long-forgotten 'Dr. John Stearns effect' "[57].

Here Moir was referring to Stearns' observation of the rapid onset of action of ergot. Stearns had administered the ergot orally, the way in which the liquid extract was also generally administered. When ergotamine or ergotoxine were administered orally, the onset of action was delayed for half an hour to an hour (although it took place much quicker when intravenous injection was employed). Histamine and tyramine were found by Moir to be inactive when given by mouth. The nature, frequency and onset of action of the contractions were so different from what he had observed with the known constituents of ergot that he had to conclude "that the oxytocic power of the liquid and solid extracts is due to a substance whose importance has hitherto been overlooked in the investigation of ergot"[58].

It is not irrelevant to the theme of this paper to quote Moir's recollection of the suspicion with which clinical research was viewed by some of his colleagues.

"As a recent-comer to the hospital I had sensed the need for caution in conducting clinical research. I knew that I had the support of my chief and of other senior members of the staff, but in some quarters there was undoubtedly an atmosphere of suspicion which sometimes even approached hostility. This opposition I largely overcame by placing my recording gear out of sight in a small room adjacent to the ward. From this room permanent communication had been established with the ward by means of a length of thin gas-piping which I had quietly placed between two convenient windows"[59].

Moir had discussed his work, as it progressed, with Henry Dale, who was a member of the Therapeutic Trials Committee, and had received the latter's encouragement to subject the various ergot constituents and preparations to clinical testing. Moir later recalled that Dale was delighted at the news that the liquid extract was active and appeared to contain some unknown oxytocic principle[60]. Dale himself admitted that he had to assume some responsibility for the view that the B. P. extract was inactive, but he immediately grasped the significance of Moir's work and became a strong supporter of his efforts[61]. In fact, he attached a note to Moir's paper in the British Medical Journal, praising the research as appearing "to open another chapter, and probably one of great importance, in the already complicated story of ergot and its active principles". Dale did not fail to point out, however, that Moir's results also indicated that the alcoholic extract appeared to be as active as the aqueous one, so that the unknown active principle must be satisfactorily extracted by alcohol as well as by water[62].

Dale arranged for Harold W. Dudley, a research chemist at the National Institute of Medical Research (which Dale directed), to work with Moir in an effort to isolate the unknown active principle. At first it was thought that the active principle was an amine, but later Dudley and Moir realized that it was an alkaloid. There was no known chemical or animal test by which the presence of the unknown principle could be detected, so each successive fraction in the isolation process had to be tested clinically[63]. It took nearly three years for Dudley and Moir to isolate the active substance in a relatively pure form. Dale sent their first published report on the new alkaloid, which they named "ergometrine", to the British Medical Journal on February 22, 1935, accompanied by a letter requesting prompt publication because a scientist in Baltimore was also in active pursuit of the active principle. "He seems to be getting rather warm, and it would be a grave disappointment to Moir, if he should have the end of the story anticipated, now that Dudley and he have really got there"[64]. The paper appeared in the March 16, 1935 issue of the Journal[65].

Actually there were two other groups, besides the scientist in Baltimore referred to above, that were also close to isolating the active oxytocic principle. Work on the problem had been proceeding simultaneously in four laboratories in three different countries, and each laboratory succeeded in independently isolating the new alkaloid at about the same time. As might be expected, the situation led to confusion and controversy over priority, a question which is too complex to explore in this paper[66].

The Baltimore scientist referred to by Dale was Marvin Thompson, Professor of Pharmacology at the School of Pharmacy of the University of Maryland. A group of clinicians and chemists from the Department of Obstetrics and Gynaecology and the Department of Chemistry at the

University of Chicago also succeeded in isolating the active oxytocic principle. Their work was carried out in cooperation with colleagues at Eli Lilly and Company. Finally, Arthur Stoll and Ernst Burckhardt of the Sandoz firm in Basle, Switzerland met with success as well.

Papers from each of the four laboratories were published in the early months of 1935[67]. Each group gave a different name to the alkaloid that they had isolated, and it was not immediately clear that these four substances (ergometrine, ergostetrine, ergotocin and ergobasine) were identical. Once again Henry Dale became involved in the ergot story. Dale gave a paper on the pharmacology of ergot at a medical congress in Montreux in September, 1935 and Stoll was present in the audience. In the ensuing discussion, Stoll expressed some doubt as to whether ergometrine was the same compound as his ergobasine. Dale suggested that the British and Swiss laboratories exchange specimens and compare the two alkaloids, and Stoll agreed[68]. Later Dale arranged to bring the Chicago and Baltimore researchers into the agreement, and a joint statement was eventually published by all four laboratories attesting to the identity of the four substances[69].

Dale, Dudley and Moir were annoyed at what they considered to be discourteous behavior on the part of their Baltimore and Chicago colleagues. The efforts of Dudley and Moir to isolate the active oxytocic principle were interrupted in late 1932 and early 1933 when Moir visited the United States for six months. Moir described his work on ergot and his method of measuring uterine contractions in both Baltimore and Chicago. He also indicated that he and Dudley were working to isolate the active principle. The British workers felt that their American colleagues, upon learning of Dudley and Moir's work, had immediately set out to try to anticipate them in the isolation of the new active principle. The Chicago group came in for particular criticism because it was felt that they had not been open about their competition with their British colleagues[70].

The assignment of four different names to the new alkaloid also led to confusion and controversy with respect to nomenclature. The arguments over what should be the official name of the new alkaloid were, of course, not unrelated to the question of priority of discovery. It surely did not escape the notice of the investigators involved that winning acceptance for their name for the new active principle would closely associate the discovery of this substance with their own work. Dale, in fact, suggested that attempts were being made "to use nomenclature in such a way as to obtain a spurious priority in the discovery"[71].

The Council on Pharmacy and Chemistry of the American Medical Association considered the question of nomenclature and rejected all four of the proposed names for the new alkaloid, adopting instead a name of its own for the substance, "ergonovine". The Council rejected the proposed names because either they were proprietary or they were "therapeutically suggestive". In the case of ergometrine, for example, Paul Leech, Secretary for the Council, pointed out to Dale that "metrine" (from the Greek metra, for uterus) clearly implied (as it was no doubt intended to) an action on the uterus. The Council's policy against therapeutically suggestive names was meant, Leech explained, as a protection not only against self-medication by the public, but also against "reflex" prescribing by physicians[72].

In Britain, however, the name ergometrine became official. Dale protested the decision of the Council on Pharmacy and Chemistry. He complained about the arrogance of the Council in ignoring the right of the discoverer of a substance to bestow upon it a name to be adopted for scientific use. In protest he resigned his position as a Corresponding Member of the Council[73].

Ergometrine, or ergonovine, was quickly recognized as the most important oxytocic principle in ergot. The British Medical Journal referred to the isolation of ergometrine as a "chemo-clinical discovery", and emphasized the importance of clinical experimentation in this development. In contrast, the Journal pointed out that ". . . experiments under the conditions of the pharmacological laboratory might never have led to the goal. Such experiments had, in fact, not succeeded even in recognizing the existence of the principle which combined chemical and clinical research has now succeeded in isolating"[74].

The faith of clinicians in the aqueous extract had at last been vindicated. The pharmacologists had been "wrong"; their experiments had failed to uncover the most important active oxytocic principle. In the presence of the other constituents in the liquid extract, the activity of ergometrine was not readily distinguishable by the pharmacological methods utilized.

Yet one might argue that while the clinicians won the battle, they lost the war. Laboratory science had come to play a major role in medical education, and laboratory research increasingly made its impact felt on medical practice. Even the discovery of ergometrine could be viewed not as the triumph of clinical medicine over laboratory science, but as an example of the value of applying the principles of scientific research to the clinical setting. On the other hand, it would be wrong to view the relationship between laboratory science and clinical medicine solely in terms of conflict.

As both Geison and Maulitz have pointed out, there was symbiosis as well as tension between the clinic and the laboratory[75]. The influence and prestige of the medical profession was enhanced by the perception of medicine as "scientific", and the biomedical sciences in turn benefited by the belief that the application of the results of their research would lead to advances in health care. The complex story of the search for the active oxytocic principle of ergot can serve to illustrate the cooperation, as well as the conflict, between the laboratory scientist and the clinician. For in the end it was the cooperation between laboratory scientists and clinicians that led to success.

Acknowledgement

Part of the research for this paper was carried out while the author was a visiting worker at the National Institute for Medical Research, London, England. I wish to thank the Director, A. V. Burgen, for the use of the Institute's facilities and for permission to utilize materials in the Institute's files, and the Librarian, R. D. Moore, for his assistance in the use of the library materials. I also wish to thank Lady Alison S. Todd and the Library of the Royal Society of London for permission to use the Henry Dale Papers. This research was supported in part by the National Science Foundation under Grant GS-14162.

Notes

1) Geison, Gerald: Divided We Stand: Physiologists and Clinicians in the American Context. In: The Therapeutic Revolution: Essays in the Social History of American Medicine (ed. by Morris Vogel and Charles Rosenberg). Philadelphia 1979, pp. 67–90. – Maulitz, Russell: "Physician Versus Bacteriologist": The Ideology of Science in Clinical Medicine. In: ibid., pp. 91–107.
2) For an example of a pharmacologist's view of the relationship between the two, see Clark, A. J.: Discussion on the Relation between Pharmacology and Clinical Medicine. In: Trans. Med.-Chir. Soc. Edinburgh, Edinburgh Med. J. N. S. *34*, II (1927), pp. 185–204. For a clinician's viewpoint, see Livingston, Alfred: Erroneous Deductions from Physiological Experimentation with Ergot. In: New York Med. J. *92* (1910), pp. 17–20.
3) Geison, Divided We Stand, pp. 67–68.
4) Abel, John: The Methods of Pharmacology, with Experimental Illustrations. In: Pharm. Era, *7* (1892), p. 105.
5) Cushny, A. R.: A Plea for Therapeutics. In: Proc. Roy. Soc. Med., Sect. Ther. Pharmacol., *4* (Oct. 18, 1892), pp. 3–5. The quotation is from p. 5.

6) Ibid. pp. 4—5.
7) On the early history of ergot in therapeutics, see Bove, Frank: The Story of Ergot. Basel 1970, pp. 271—276 and Barger, George: Ergot and Ergotism. London 1931, pp. 7—19.
8) Stearns, John: Letter to S. Akerly. In: The Medical Repository, second series, *5* (1808), pp. 308—309. The quotation is from p. 309.
9) On the inclusion of ergot in pharmacopoeias, see Barger, Ergot, p. 19.
10) Bove, Story of Ergot, pp. 276—278 and Haller, John, Jr.: Smut's Dark Poison: Ergot in History and Medicine. In: Trans. Stud. Coll. Phys. Philadelphia, series V, *3* (1981), p. 76—77.
11) The Pharmacopoeia of the United States of America, sixth decennial revision. New York 1880, pp. 116—117.
12) See, e. g., Bonjean, Joseph: Letter to P. A. Cap. In: J. Pharm. Chim. third series, *4* (1843), pp. 107—109.
13) British Pharmacopoeia, London 1864, pp. 224—225
14) British Pharmacopoeia, London 1885, p. 147.
15) Bove, Story of Ergot, pp. 87—96.
16) Barger, George and Carr, Francis: The Alkaloids of Ergot. In: J. Chem. Soc. *2* (1907), pp. 337—353; Kraft, Fritz: Ueber das Mutterkorn. In: Archiv Pharm. *244* (1906), pp. 336—359. It was later shown, in 1943, that "ergotoxine" was actually a mixture of three closely related alkaloids. During the period under consideration in this paper, however, it was believed to be a single substance.
17) Dale, Henry: Adventures in Physiology, with Excursions into Autopharmacology. London 1953, p. XI.
18) Barger, G. and Dale, H. H.: Ergotoxine and Some Other Constituents of Ergot. In: Biochem. J., *2* (1907), pp. 240—299. For their discussion of the preparations of the British Pharmacopoeia, see pp. 286—288.
19) Barger, G. and Dale, H. H.: The Water-Soluble Active Principles of Ergot. In: Proc. Physiol. Soc., J. Physiol., *38* (1909), pp. LXXVII—LXXIX; Dale, Adventures, p. XIII.
20) Barger, G. and Dale, H. H.: The Presence in Ergot and Physiological Activity of β-Imidazoylethylamine. In: Proc. Physiol. Soc., J. Physiol., *40* (1910), pp. XXXVIII—XL.
21) Carr, Francis and Dale, Henry: Ergot and Its Preparations: A Critical Review of the Requirements of the British Pharmacopoeia. In: Year Book of Pharmacy 1913, pp. 505—512.
22) Ibid., pp. 505—507. The quotation is from p. 505.
23) Ibid., pp. 509—511. The quotation is from p. 510.
24) Ibid., p. 515.
25) On the isolation and characterization of ergotamine, see Bove: Story of Ergot, pp. 105—106, 173—174, 260—261 and Barger: Ergot, pp. 134—138.
26) Dale, Henry: The Value of Ergot in Obstetrical and Gynaecological Practice; with Special Reference to Its Present Position in the British Pharmacopoeia. In: Proc. Roy. Soc. Med., Sect. Gyn. Obstet., *16* (Dec. 7, 1922), pp. 1—5. The quotations are from pp. 3—4.
27) Ibid., p. 5.

28) Ibid., p. 7. The meaning of Tirard's statement is unclear, especially since certain other pharmacopoeias also employed an alcoholic extraction process. See Barger: Ergot, pp. 181–187.

29) Dale, The Value of Ergot, p. 6.

30) Clark, A. J. and Broom, W. A.: The Activity of Pharmacopoeial Preparations of Ergot. In: Year Book of Pharmacy 1923, pp. 621–628. The quotation is from p. 628. Clark also attacked the B. P. extract before the Edinburgh Obstetrical Society. See Clark, A. J.: Do the Pharmacopoeial Preparations of Ergot Contain Any Active Principels? In: Trans. Edinburgh Obstet. Soc., Edinburgh Med. J., N. S. *34*, II (1927), pp. 109–116.

31) Bourne, Aleck and Burn, J. H.: The Dosage and Action of Pituitary Extract and of Ergot Alkaloids on the Uterus in Labor, with a Note on the Action of Adrenalin. In: J. Obstet. Gyn. British Emp. *34* (1927), pp. 249–272.

32) Ibid., pp. 251–252.

33) Ibid., pp. 259–264.

34) Ibid., p. 264.

35) Ibid., p. 265.

36) Burn, J. H.: Letter to editor. In: Pharm. J. *128* (1932), p. 510.

37) [J. H. Burn]: Extract from the Second Annual Report (1917) of the Pharmacological Laboratories of the Pharmaceutical Society of Great Britain. In: Pharm. J. *120* (1928), pp. 125–126.

38) Burn, J. H.: Some Methods of Biological Assay. In: Pharm. J. *117* (1926), p. 577.

39) [Burn], "Extract from Second Annual Report (1927)" p. 126.

40) After his lecture before the Edinburgh Obstetrical Society, A. J. Clark was surprised to find those who took part in the discussion agreeing with him that the official liquid extract was worthless. Those obstetricians who actively participated in the meetings of the Society, of course, were not necessarily representative of the average practitioner. Those who might have disagreed may also have been hesitant to engage in a public debate with one of Britain's most eminent pharmacologists. See Clark: Do the Pharmacopoeial Preparations of Ergot Contain Any Active Principles?, p. 121.

41) Lum, E. A.: Letter to editor. In: Pharm. J. *128* (1932), p. 139.

42) Mann, E. W.: Letter to editor. In: Pharm. J. *117* (1926), p. 633.

43) For examples of textbooks which recommend the aqueous extract, see Munro Kerr, J. M.; Ferguson, James H.; Young, James and Hendry, James: A Combined Textbook of Obstetrics and Gynaecology. Edinburgh 1923, p. 446 and Munro Kerr, J. M.: Operative Midwifery, third edition. New York 1916, pp. 11, 631–632. Henry Jellett and David Madill, in: A Manual of Midwifery, fourth edition, New York 1929, suggest the liquid extract of ergot as a therapeutic agent (pp. 154, 384–385, 975), but express some concern about the unreliability of pharmacopoeial preparations in terms of constancy of action and keeping powers (p. 154). They preferred a Burroughs Wellcome preparation called "Ernutin", which contained ergotoxine and synthetic histamine and tyramine. I did not find any textbooks which specifically discussed the controversy over the aqueous extract versus an alcoholic one, or which condemned the liquid extract as worthless.

44) Sharp, J. Gordon: A Clinical Experimental Study. In: Proc. Roy. Soc., Sect. Ther. Pharmacol. *4* (Apr. 11, 1911), p. 114−148. One cannot help but wonder whether Sharp's "clinical experimental study" was not a response to Arthur Cushny's lamentation about the lack of good clinical data on ergot in his previously-cited 1910 address, delivered before the same Therapeutical and Pharmacological Section of the Royal Society of Medicine. See Cushny: A Plea for Therapeutics, pp. 4−5. Cushny presided at the session at which Sharp's paper was delivered, and in the discussion following it praised the work as being of the character that the Section wished to encourage. See Sharp: Ergot, p. 150.

45) Sharp: Ergot, p. 149.

46) See, e. g., The National Formulary, fourth edition. 1916, p. 52.

47) The British Pharmaceutical Codex. London 1907, pp. 358−359.

48) The British Pharmaceutical Codex, 1911, pp. 384−385.

49) The British Pharmaceutical Codex, 1923, p. 412.

50) Discussion following Clark: Do Pharmacopoeial Preparations of Ergot Contain Any Active Principles?, p. 120.

51) Report of the Sub-Committee on Ergot, October, 1931. London: General Medical Council, Pharmacopoeial Commission. 1931, pp. 15−16.

52) The British Pharmacopoeia. London 1932, pp. 165−166.

53) Moir, Chassar: The Action of Ergot Preparations on the Puerperal Uterus: A Clinical Investigation with Special Reference to an Active Constituent of Ergot as yet Unidentified. In: British Med. J. 1932 (I), pp. 1119−1122.

54) Moir, J. Chassar: The History and Present-Day Use of Ergot. In: Canadian Med. Assoc. J. *72* (1955), p. 730.

55) Moir, Chassar: Clinical Comparison of Ergotoxine and Ergotamine: A Report to the Therapeutic Trials Committee of the Medical Research Council. In: British Med. J. 1932 (I), pp. 1022−1024. Moir's discussion of his choice of method appears on p. 1022.

56) Moir, Action of Ergot, pp. 1120−1121.

57) Moir, History and Present-Day Use of Ergot, p. 731.

58) Moir, Action of Ergot, p. 1121.

59) Moir, J. Chassar: The Obstetrician Bids, and the Uterus Contracts. In: British Med. J. 1964 (II), p. 1026. See also Moir, J. Chassar: Ergot: From "St. Anthony's Fire" to the Isolation of Its Active Principle, Ergometrine (Ergonovine). In: Amer. J. Obstet. Gyn. *120* (1974), p. 293.

60) Moir, J. Chassar: Letter to Henry Dale, July 24, 1957. In: Henry Dale Papers, Royal Society of London Library, box M1.

61) Dale, Henry: Letter to J. Chassar Moir, Dec. 21, 1954. In: Dale Papers, box M1.

62) Dale, H. H.: Note added to Moir, Action of Ergot, p. 1122.

63) Moir: History and Present-Day Use of Ergot, pp. 731−732; Moir: The Obstetrician Bids, pp. 1026−1027.

64) Dale, Henry: Letter to N. G. Horner, Feb. 22, 1935. In: Dale Papers, box B1.

65) Dudley, H. W. and Moir, Chassar: The Substance Responsible for the Traditional Clinical Effect of Ergot. In: British Med. J. 1935 (I), pp. 520−523.

66) For discussions of the literature, see Nelson, Erwin and Calvery, Herbert: Present Status of the Ergot Question. In: Physiol. Rev. *18* (1938), pp. 297–327 and Smith, Ralph D.: The Present Status of Ergonovine. In: J. Amer. Med. Assoc. *111* (1938), pp. 2201–2209.

67) See, e. g., Dudley and Moir: Substance Responsible. – Dudley, H. W.: Ergometrine. In: Proc. Roy. Soc. London, B, *118* (1935), pp. 478–484. – Thompson, Marvin: The Active Constituents of Ergot: A Pharmacological and Chemical Study. In: J. Amer. Pharm. Assoc. *24* (1935), pp. 24–38, 185–196. – Davis, M. E.; Adair, F. L.; Rogers, G.; Kharasch, M. S. and LeGault, R. R.: A New Active Principle in Ergot and Its Effects on Uterine Motility. In: Amer. J. Obstet. Gyn. *29* (1935), pp. 155–167. – Adair, F. L.; Davis, M. E.; Kharasch, M. S. and LeGault, R. R.: A Study of a New and Potent Ergot Derivative, Ergotocin. In: ibid., pp. 466–480. – Stoll, Arthur and Burckhardt, Ernst: L'ergobasine, un Nouvel alcoloide de l'ergot de seigle, soluble dans l'eau. In: Bull. Sci. Pharmacol. *42* (1935), pp. 257–266.

68) Henry Dale, letter to J. McKeen Cattell, Jan. 23, 1936, National Institute for Medical Research Files, London, (hereafter referred to as NIMR Files), Ergometrine .483/2. 1935–1936.

69) Kharasch, M. S.; King, H.; Stoll, A. and Thompson, Marvin R.: The New Ergot Alkaloid. In: Science *83* (1936), pp. 206–207. King acted in place of Dudley, who died on October 3, 1935.

70) See, e. g., the following letters from Henry Dale to G. H. A. Clowes, Aug. 28, 1935, to C. D. Leake, Aug. 21, 1935 and to G. Merck, Feb. 5, 1936, NIMR Files, Ergometrine .483/2. 1935–1936. Dale did not feel that Stoll had acted entirely fairly either. See also Dudley, H. W. and Moir, J. Chassar: The New Active Principle of Ergot. In: Science *81* (1935), pp. 559–560.

71) Henry Dale, letter to C. D. Leake, Aug. 21, 1935, NIMR Files, Ergometrine .483/2. 1935–1936.

72) The New Ergot Alkaloid: "Ergonovine". In: J. Amer. Med. Assoc. *106* (1936), p. 1008. See also the letters from Paul Leech to Henry Dale, May 22, 1936 and June 1, 1936, NIMR Files, Ergometrine .483/2. 1935–1936. Leech also expressed some concern that the name ergometrine might imply that this substance had some special or exclusive action on the uterus, when it was actually not the only oxytocic principle in ergot.

73) Henry Dale, letters to Paul N. Leech, March 16, 1936, Apr. 20, 1936, and Oct. 22, 1936, NIMR Files, Ergometrine .483/2. 1935–1936. The letter of Oct. 22 was published, at Dales's request, in J. Amer. Med. Assoc. *108* (1937), pp. 1969–1970. See also Dale, H. H.: The New Ergot Alkaloid. In: Science *82* (1935), pp. 99–101. Dale probably also played a role in drafting a critical editorial, entitled: The New Ergot Alkaloid: A Question of Nomenclature. In: Lancet 1936 (I), pp. 909–910. A draft typescript of this editorial appears in the same folder as Dale's correspondence with Paul Leech of the A. M. A. in the NIMR Files, Ergometrine .483/2. 1935–1936.

74) Ergometrine: A Chemo-Clinical Discovery. In: British Med. J. 1935 (I), pp. 532–533.

75) Geison: Divided We Stand, pp. 68, 85–87 and Maulitz: "Physician Versus Bacteriologist", pp. 103–104.

XIV

The Introduction of
Antibiotics into Therapeutics

A LTHOUGH the antibiotics only entered medical practice in a significant way less than half a century ago, these so-called "wonder
drugs" have already earned a secure place in the history of therapeutics. In fact, scholars discussing the history of penicillin and other
antibiotics have tended towards hyperbole in assessing the role of
these drugs in therapy. Thus, Gwyn Macfarlane has claimed that
"penicillin therapy is probably the greatest single medical advance of
all time."[1] James Whorton has called the antibiotics "the most spectacular therapeutic advance of medical history."[2] And Felix Marti-
Ibañez has stated that in medical history "there is perhaps no other
event as revolutionary as the discovery of antibiotics."[3]

While other writers on the history of medicine might dispute the
choice of antibiotics as the most significant medical advance in all of
history, it would probably be difficult to identify a class of therapeutic
agents which has had a greater impact on human health. It therefore
seems appropriate in a symposium on the history of therapeutics to
devote a paper to an examination of the development of these drugs
and their introduction into therapeutics. In this paper, I shall be using
the term"antibiotic," coined in the modern sense by Selman Waksman in 1942, to mean a chemical substance produced by a microorganism which destroys or inhibits the growth of other microorganisms.[4]

EARLY WORK ON ANTIBIOSIS

Although the antibiotics have only made their impact felt in therapeutics within the last four decades, the phenomenon of antibiosis itself has been known for more than a century. I shall leave aside here any speculations about whether certain folk remedies involving moldy bread and similar substances may have had therapeutic value due to the presence of antibiotics, and begin my story with scientific investigations of the phenomenon of microbial antagonism in the late nineteenth century. The first entry under antibiotics in the Garrison-Morton *Medical Bibliography* dates from 1876.[5] In a paper in the *Philosophical Transactions* that year, John Tyndall reported on the antagonism between certain bacteria and the *Penicillium* mold.[6] Tyndall was not the first to observe microbial antagonism, which was not uncommonly reported in the literature from the early 1870s on.[7]

Louis Pasteur may have been the first to clearly suggest that the antagonism between microbes might have therapeutic potential. In 1877, he noticed that urine, which is normally an excellent culture medium for the anthrax bacillus, would not support the growth of this organism if the urine were also inoculated with common aerobic bacteria. He interpreted this to mean that there was a struggle for existence between various kinds of microbes, just as between plants and higher animals, and that one microorganism might successfully prevent the multiplication of another. Pasteur went so far as to suggest that these facts perhaps justified the highest hopes for therapeutics.[8]

Several attempts were made over the next few decades to use "antibiosis," a term introduced by Vuillemin in 1889 to describe this phenomenon of "life against life,"[9] for therapeutic purposes, albeit without much success. Probably the antibiotic substance receiving the most extensive trial in this period was pyocyanase, an extract prepared from old cultures of the bacillus *Pseudomonas pyocyanea*. Pyocyanase was introduced by Emmerich and Löw in 1899 and seems to have received its most widespread use in the treatment of diphtheria, usually as a local spray. By 1914, however, pyocyanase had fallen into disuse. This was perhaps due to toxic side effects as well as to a greater interest in other therapeutic approaches such as antitoxin therapy and Ehrlich's synthetic chemotherapy.[10]

THE DISCOVERY OF PENICILLIN

When Alexander Fleming observed the antibacterial effects of a *Penicillium* mold in 1928, the phenomenon of antibiosis was thus already well known to microbiologists and medical researchers. The story of Fleming's discovery of penicillin is too well-known for me to discuss in detail here, hence I shall just briefly review the circumstances surrounding the event. While investigating the staphylococcus bacterium at St. Mary's Hospital in London, one of Fleming's culture plates was accidentally contaminated by a *Penicillium* mold. Upon observing that no colonies of the bacterium were growing for some distance around the mold, he decided to further investigate the antibacterial properties of the mold. Fleming proceeded to culture the mold on the surface of a broth and to test the filtrate of the broth culture, which he called penicillin, for antibacterial activity. He found that on culture plates penicillin inhibited the growth of such pathogenic organisms as hemolytic streptococcus and pneumoccus. He also tested the toxicity of the substance towards animals and found it to be exceptionally low. In a paper published in 1929, he reported these results and suggested that penicillin might prove useful as an antiseptic for local application to infected areas. He apparently did not envision its use, however, as an internal or systemic chemotherapeutic agent.[11]

Some attempts were made to isolate the active agent of the mold, by Craddock and Ridley in Fleming's laboratory and by Raistrick, Lovell and Clutterbuck at the Lodon School of Tropical Medicine, but without success. There were even a few isolated attempts to use the mold juice clinically as an external agent in infections in the early 1930s (e.g., by Fleming himself and by C. G. Paine at the Sheffield Royal Infirmary), but they did not lead anywhere.[12] Neither Fleming nor anyone else seems to have taken the step of testing the substance by injection into experimentally-diseased animals. Penicillin thus remained essentially a laboratory curiosity for about a decade after the publication of Fleming's paper.

The introduction of penicillin into therapeutics was a result of the work of scientists at the William Dunn School of Pathology at Oxford University. Australian-born Howard Florey was appointed to the chair of pathology at Oxford in 1935. Ironically the subject which eventually led Florey and his colleagues to an interest in penicillin was another discovery of Alexander Fleming's — lysozyme. In 1922, while studying a culture of his own nasal secretion, Fleming discovered a new bacterium, *Micrococcus lysodeikticus*, which was readily lysed by a substance present in the nasal secretion. He later found that this same substance, which he called lysozyme, was also present in other bodily secretions such as tears and saliva, as well as in egg white and certain plant tissues. Although he was never able to isolate lysozyme, Fleming concluded that it must be an enzyme. It seemed likely to Fleming that this natural substance played a role in the defenses of the organism against bacteria, but since common pathogenic bacteria such as streptococci and staphylococci proved to be resistant to lysozyme, it did not arouse much interest in the medical community.[13]

Howard Florey became interested in lysozyme through his own work on mucus. Florey set out with a colleague in 1929 to test the hypothesis that mucus has an antibacterial action and that any such action was related to its lysozyme content. They examined various animal preparations and eventually had to conclude that the presence or absence of lysozyme seemed to have little to do with natural immunity. An appendix to their paper in the *British Journal of Experimental Pathology* in 1930 discussed inhibition of one bacterium by another. This appendix described the inhibition of the growth of one of their lysozyme test organisms in the vicinity of *B. Coli* on a culture plate, and pointed out that this type of bacterial antagonism was a well-known phenomenon, citing a 1928 review article on the subject. No mention was made, however, of Fleming's 1929 paper on penicillin which was published in the same journal as their own paper.[14]

Florey's interest in lysozyme continued over the years. Soon after

XIV

going to Oxford, Florey began to look around for a biochemist for his laboratory. At the recommendation of F. Gowland Hopkins, he hired a young Jewish refugee from Nazi Germany, Ernst Boris Chain. Once lysozyme was isolated in crystalline form by E. P. Abraham and Robert Robinson in 1937, Chain began to investigate its mode of action on bacteria. He and L. A. Epstein showed that lysozyme was a polysaccharidase and that it attacked a glucosamine in the bacterial cell wall.[15]

During the course of his review of the literature on lysozyme, Chain apparently became interested in the whole subject of antibacterial substances produced by microorganisms, a subject which, as we have seen, had earlier attracted Florey's attention. Among the papers which Chain came across in his literature search was Fleming's paper on penicillin. Penicillin attracted his attention because it was presumed to be an enzyme with lytic powers, such as lysozyme. Florey and Chain decided to investigate the antibacterial action of several products of microbial origin, originally focusing on penicillin, pyocyanase, and actinomycetin. The latter was a bacteriolytic filtrate from a species of actinomycetes which had been studied extensively by Gratia and Dath in the 1920s and by Welsch in the 1930s. Although they mentioned the therapeutic potential of these substances in grant applications at the time, both Florey and Chain later stated that it was a scientific interest in the problem rather than a therapeutic goal which initially motivated their researches.[16]

In 1939, when Florey and Chain were still in the early stages of this work, another development occurred which stimulated further interest in the therapeutic potential of antibiosis. Rene Dubos isolated an organism from soil, later identified as *Bacillus brevis*, which was capable of attacking gram positive microorganisms. From this bacillus he obtained a substance which he called tyrothricin, which was later shown to consist of two polypeptide components, gramicidin and tyrocidine. Unfortunately, these antibiotic substances proved to be too toxic for internal use in humans, although gramicidin found some use for topical applications. More importantly, Dubos' work encouraged research on antibiotics. One of those influenced to undertake work in this area was Dubos' former teacher, Selman Waksman, about whom I shall have more to say later.[17]

Meanwhile the Oxford group, which had come to include several other scientists such as Norman Heatley and E. P. Abraham, made significant progress in their work on penicillin. They managed to isolate a brown powder that exhibited such extraordinarily high antibacterial properties that they assumed it was relatively pure. Actually, penicillin was so much more effective as an antibacterial agent than any other drug known at the time, including the then recently introduced sulfonamides, that the Oxford team at first greatly underestimated its potency. The crude brown powder that they initially isolated was later shown to contain less than 1% penicillin.

Toxicity tests yielded no evidence that penicillin was harmful to the experimental animals used. Then in May of 1940 came the first test of penicillin's activity against pathogenic organisms *in vitro*. Eight mice were injected with a virulent strain of streptococci, with four left untreated as controls and four treated with penicillin. The results were sufficiently promising to convince Florey, Chain and coworkers of penicillin's promise as a therapeutic agent. By the next morning, all four of the untreated mice were dead. All of the mice treated with penicillin were alive and three were in perfectly normal health, although the fourth died two days later.

In the early work at Oxford, the penicillin was produced by growing the mold on the surface of a broth in an Erlenmeyer flask, essentially as Fleming had done. The conical flasks took up a lot of space and were not available in sufficient numbers to produce the large amounts of penicillin that would be needed for further testing of the drug. It was felt that a flat vessel with a large surface area would be more advantageous, and the Oxford group began to experiment with various kinds of common objects such as dishes, trays, pans and biscuit tins.

The old-style urinal or bed pan was found to be a very satisfactory vessel. It provided a relatively large surface area over a shallow fluid and had a side arm for inoculation and withdrawal of the fluid. But the demand for these in military hospitals made it impossible to obtain them in large quantities for penicillin production. Britain was being subjected to heavy bombing, and it was not easy to obtain many types of supplies. The Oxford laboratory managed to arrange, however, for a manufacturer to produce a similar type of container for use in the penicillin work, a rather flat rectangular ceramic vessel. These vessels could be stacked horizontally for greater economy of space, provided relatively more surface area than an Erlenmeyer flask, and had a side arm for ease of inoculation.[18]

As more penicillin was produced, further animal studies were carried out, and in August of 1940 the Oxford team published a brief account of their work on "Penicillin as a chemotherapeutic agent" in *The Lancet.*[19] This first publication on penicillin from Oxford attracted the attention of Alexander Fleming, who immediately contacted Florey and went to visit the laboratory to see what was being done with his "old penicillin."[20]

Eventually Florey and his colleagues were prepared to undertake their first trials of the drug in human patients. First, the drug was given to a volunteer dying of cancer, as a test of its toxicity in humans. The first patient to receive penicillin produced at Oxford in an effort to treat an infection was a policeman suffering a severe case of staphylococcal and streptococcal infection resulting from a cut on his face. He was near death when penicillin therapy was begun in February of 1941, and within a few days he was making a striking recovery. Unfortunately, the supply of available penicillin soon ran out, and the patient relapsed and died. Florey was disappointed, and he decided that it was necessary to accumulate a larger supply of the drug before treating future cases and to work with children, if possible, so that the dose required would be smaller.[21]

Actually, the policeman treated in Oxford was not the first human patient to receive the drug internally in an effort to treat an infection. Some four months earlier a patient at Presbyterian Hospital in New York had been treated for subacute bacterial endocarditis with penicillin, although without success. Martin Henry Dawson, a clinician at the College of Physicians and Surgeons of Columbia University, recognized on reading the first publication of the Oxford group on their animal experiments that penicillin had therapeutic potential in the treatment of streptococcal and pneumococcal infections. He obtained cultures of the penicillin-producing strain of *Penicillium notatum* from Chain in England and from Roger Reid of the Johns Hopkins Hospital, who had obtained the mold from Fleming several years earlier. Dawson and coworkers Gladys Hobby and Karl Meyer managed to obtain penicillin extracts from Reid's sample with which they treated four patients with subacute bacterial endocarditis and eight patients with chronic staphylococcal blepharitis. Sufficient penicillin was not available for adequate therapy in the case of the former group of patients, but those with the staphylococcal eye infection responded well to the treatment. The Columbia researchers reported their results on penicillin at a meeting of the American Society for Clinical Investigation in May, 1941. Although this work was published only in abstract form, it was reported on in newspapers such as *The New York Times* which helped bring penicillin to the attention of Americans, including officials at Charles Pfizer and Company.[22]

Clinical trials in Oxford continued and a report on the first ten cases was published in *The Lancet* in August of 1941.[23] Although the results were encouraging, they were hardly statistically significant. Florey recognized that much greater quantities of penicillin would be needed to carry out the large-scale clinical trials that were necessary to establish the therapeutic value of penicillin.

DEVELOPMENT OF LARGE-SCALE PRODUCTION OF PENICILLIN

Unable to generate as much interest in penicillin as he had hoped to on the part of the pharmaceutical industry in wartime Britain, Florey traveled to the United States with Norman Heatley in July, 1941 in an effort to stimulate American interest in the drug. One of the first places that they visited was the Northern Regional Research Laboratory of the United States Department of Agriculture in Peoria, Illinois. The Peoria group agreed to tackle the problem of trying to improve the yield of penicillin produced by the mold, and did manage, over a period of time, to increase penicillin production dramatically through a variety of innovations.

One avenue of attack undertaken in Peoria was to find strains of the *Penicillium* mold that produced greater quantities of penicillin than the original Fleming strain. Of all the samples of mold collected and tested, many of them sent in from great distances, it is ironic that the most productive strain discovered came from a moldy cantaloupe melon from a Peoria fruit stand. The "cantaloupe strain" was later further improved in academic laboratories by producing mutant strains through the use of chemicals or irradiation. The Peoria group also played a key role in the development of deep-tank fermentation which was much more efficient than surface-culture fermentation of the mold.[24]

While Florey was in the United States, he visited several pharmaceutical companies and tried to interest them in penicillin, with some success. In fact, a few such firms had already begun work on the antibiotic before Florey arrived. For example, Randolph Major, director of research at Merck, developed an interest in penicillin. He was encouraged by microbiologist Selman Waksman of Rutgers University, who had become a consultant to the firm in 1938. Merck chemists were struggling to isolate penicillin at the time of Florey's visit.[25]

Perhaps more important was Florey's success in creating interest in the drug on the part of the Office of Scientific Research and Development (OSRD), recently established by the Federal government, and its Committee on Medical Research (CMR), chaired by University of Pennsylvania pharmacologist A. N. Richards. The OSRD and CMR set about to organize a concerted program of penicillin research involving the pooling of information and results. With the encouragement of the CMR, several pharmaceutical companies agreed to undertake collaborative efforts in penicillin research and development. Industrial cooperation also occurred in Britain where, in 1942, the Therapeutic Research Corporation of Great Britain was established by five pharmaceutical firms for the purpose of sharing research results. Later that year a sixth company joined the group, and a committee was established, at the request of the Ministry of Supply, to coordinate work on the production and purification of penicillin.

With the entry of the United States into the war, the American pharmaceutical industry became accountable to the War Production Board (WPB). The WPB soon established a formal penicillin program with Albert Elder as coordinator. The Board was concerned not just with research in industry, as the CMR had been, but also with productivity. Its penicillin program involved some twenty commercial firms as well as government and academic research laboratories. The Board also controlled the supply of penicillin in the United States with most of it going to the military. A prime goal of the government was to have adequate supplies of the drug available for the planned invasion of Europe, scheduled for the spring of 1944.[26]

Feelings of wartime patriotism greatly stimulated work on penicillin in Britain and the United States. The coordinator of the American penicillin program, for example, wrote to manufacturers in 1943: "You are urged to impress upon every worker in your plant that penicillin produced *today* will be saving the life of someone in a few days or curing the disease of someone now incapacitated. Put up slogans in your plant! Place notices in the pay envelopes! Create an enthusiasm for the job down to the lowest worker in your plant."[27]

Meanwhile penicillin was being tested clinically on a large scale for its effectiveness on a number of pathological conditions. The drug was shown to be effective in the treatment of a wide variety of infections, including various pneumococcal, streptococcal, staphylococcal and gonococcal infections. The United States Army established the value of penicillin in the treatment of surgical and wound infections. Clinical studies demonstrated its effectiveness against syphilis, and by 1944, it was the primary treatment for this disease in the armed forces of Britain and the United States.[28]

As publicity concerning this new "miracle drug" began to reach the public, the demand for penicillin increased. But supplies were at first very limited, and as noted earlier, priority was given to military use. In the United States, Dr. Chester S. Keefer of Boston, Chairman of the National Research Council's Committee on Chemotherapy, had the unenviable task of rationing supplies of the drug for civilian use. Keefer had to restrict the use of the drug to cases where it was fairly clear that penicillin would be helpful and where other methods of treatment had failed. Part of his job was also to collect detailed clinical information about the use of the drug so that a fuller understanding of its potential and its limitations could be developed. Not surprisingly, Keefer was beseiged with pleas for penicillin.[29] As one newspaper account noted, "Many laymen — husbands, wives, parents, brothers, sisters, friends — beg Dr. Keefer for penicillin. In every case the petitioner is told to arrange that a full dossier on the patient's condition be sent in by the doctor in charge. When this is received, the decision is made on a medical, not an emotional basis."[30]

Fortunately, penicillin production began to increase dramatically by early 1944. Production of the drug in the United States jumped from 21 billion units in 1943 to 1,663 billion units in 1944.[31] The American government was eventually able to remove all restrictions on its availability, and as of March 15, 1945, penicillin was distributed through the usual channels and made available to the consumer in his or her corner pharmacy. By 1949, the annual production of penicillin in the United States was 133,229 billion units, and the price had dropped from twenty dollars per 100,000 units in 1943 to less than ten cents.[32]

PENICILLIN OUTSIDE
THE ANGLO-AMERICAN COMMUNITY

Knowledge of the therapeutic potential of penicillin soon began to spread to other countries, arousing interest in the production of the drug. Research on penicillin began at the Swiss Federal Institute of Technology in 1942, but did not yield spectacular results.[33] There were also efforts to produce the drug in Germany as early as 1942, but relatively little was accomplished during the war years.[34]

Work on penicillin was carried out in several German-occupied countries during the war. A Dutch fermentation firm, the Gistfabriek (or "yeast factory"), first learned of penicillin through British radio broadcasts and pamphlets dropped by British planes. The company then obtained the August 7, 1943 issue of *Klinische Wochenschrift* containing an article by Manfred Kiese which abstracted various English-language papers on penicillin published in the period 1940–1943. Papers on other antibiotic substances were also cited in this review. Gistfabriek began to produce small amounts of penicillin in 1944. In occupied France, penicillin was being produced at the Pasteur Institute and at the Rhone-Poulenc firm in 1943, with the monthly output reaching 765,000 units by December of 1944.[35] Rumors of the promise of penicillin reached occupied Czechoslovakia late in 1942, and work on the drug was begun at the Fragner Company. Enough penicillin was eventually produced to carry out clinical trials during the war.[36]

Research on penicillin was initiated in Japan in February, 1944, when the first meeting of the Penicillin Committee was held at the Military Medical College in Tokyo. The Japanese first became aware of penicillin through the review article by Kiese in *Klinische Wochenschrift* mentioned earlier. A copy of this journal had been sent from Germany by submarine. A plan to organize a penicillin group, drafted by surgeon major Katsuhiko Inagaki and his colleagues, was approved by the War Minister. By the end of the war, the Japanese were producing relatively small amounts of penicillin and treating patients with it. In the post-war era, Japan has emerged as a major contributor to antibiotics research and production.[37]

Although a laboratory of antibiotics was established by the Ministry of Health in Moscow as early as 1942, penicillin does not seem to have received extensive attention in the Soviet Union during the war years. Dubos's work on tyrothricin would appear to have had more impact, and a new antibiotic, gramicidin S (Soviet gramicidin) was isolated from *Bacillus brevis* in the summer of 1942. The drug received widespread use for topical application to control local infections.[38] At the close of the war, a project was organized in the United States to raise funds to give the Soviet people a penicillin plant and research laboratory. The effort did not succeed, however, but fell prey to the cold war mentality that soon developed between the two former allies.[39]

ANTIBIOTICS AFTER PENICILLIN

The tremendous success of penicillin as a systemic chemotherapeutic agent opened up the "era of antibiotics." Even before the end of the war, several other antibiotic substances had been discovered. The work of Dubos and the discovery of gramicidin S have already been mentioned above. One of the most active and productive wartime antibiotics research laboratories was that of Selman Waksman at Rutgers University. Trained as a soil microbiologist, Waksman had long been aware of the phenomenon of antibiosis. It was only after the work of his former student Dubos on tyrothricin, however, that he began a systematic search for antibiotic substances produced by soil microorganisms.

Waksman focused his researches on a group of microorganisms known as actinomycetes, which had interested him from early in his career. These organisms display some of the characteristics of bacteria and some of the characteristics of fungi. In retrospect this choice of organisms was a fortunate one, since they have turned out to be producers of some of the most important antibiotics introduced into therapy. In 1940, Waksman and his colleagues isolated their first antibiotic substance from actinomycetes, and called it actinomycin. Although it was active against a large number of bacteria, it was too toxic for use as a therapeutic agent. Streptothricin was isolated in 1942 and seemed at first to have therapeutic promise, but it was later shown to have a delayed toxicity in the animal body.

The real breakthrough in Waksman's laboratory came with the isolation of streptomycin in 1943. The name was derived from *Streptomyces*, the name assigned by Waksman to the particular group of actinomycetes from which the antibiotic was isolated. Streptomycin's greatest value proved to be in the treatment of tuberculosis. Because of the development of resistant strains of the tubercle bacillus and because of the drug's adverse side effects, it was later found that tuberculosis could be treated more effectively by using streptomycin in combination with another drug, such as para-aminosalicylic acid or isoniazid.[40]

Within a few years after the end of the war, three more important antibiotics had been added to the list of such drugs; chloramphenicol (1947), chlortetracycline (1948), and oxytetracycline (1950). These drugs were the first so-called "broad spectrum antibiotics," characterized by their ability to inhibit a variety of different types of bacteria (both gram-negative and gram-positive) and some rickettsia. All were isolated from *Streptomyces* in the laboratories of American pharmaceutical companies. Their discovery was the result of large-scale screening programs aimed at identifying antibiotic substances produced by soil microorganisms. The discovery of oxytetracycline, for example, represented the culmination of an extremely intensive screening program involving more than 100,000 samples of soil from many different parts of the world.[41]

Over the past three decades hundreds more antibiotic substances have been discovered, although only a relatively small proportion of these have found significant therapeutic use. Among the more important of these therapeutically are erythromycin, tetracycline, the cephalosporins, and the semisynthetic penicillins. With very few exceptions, these drugs are produced by microbial fermentation rather than by chemical synthesis. It may be noted in passing that most antibiotics have been named on a subjective basis, sometimes leading to interesting results. Antibiotics have been named, for example, after the discoverer's laboratory (nystatin, for the New York State Board of Health Laboratories), his wife (helenine), his secretary (vernamycin), and his mother-in-law (saramycetin). Bacitracin was named after a girl named Tracy, from whose wound the bacillus that produced it was isolated. One antibiotic was even named after a movie (rifomycin, from *Rififi*).[42]

IMPACT OF ANTIBIOTICS ON THERAPEUTICS

Antibiotics were found to be effective in the treatment of a host of infectious diseases: pneumococcal pneumonia, rheumatic fever, bacterial endocarditis, syphilis, gonorrhea, tuberculosis, meningococcal meningitis, diphtheria, typhus, Rocky Mountain spotted fever, etc. Within a decade after penicillin was first made freely available for civilian use in the United States in 1945, the antibiotics had become the most important class of drugs in the treatment of infectious disease. In 1948, antibiotics prescriptions accounted for only 1.5% of the total number written in the United States; by 1952, that figure had risen to 13.7%.[43]

A Federal Trade Commission report issued in 1958 attempted to analyze the effect of the introduction of antibiotics on American public health. Although admitting that antibiotic use was only one factor contributing to declining rates of incidence and mortality in many infectious diseases over the previous decade or so, the report pointed to evidence suggesting that the antibiotics made a significant contribution to this decline. In examining the occurrence of reportable diseases, for example, it was found that over the period 1946–1955 there was a 42% drop for diseases in which antibiotics were effective and only a 20% drop for diseases in which antibiotics were not regarded as effective. The Commission concluded that "it appears that the use of antibiotics, early diagnosis and other factors have limited the epidemic spread and thus the number of these diseases which occurred."[44]

More convincing evidence for the impact of antibiotics was provided in the Commission's analysis of mortality statistics for certain infectious diseases. The Commission examined mortality statistics for eight important diseases for which antibiotics offered effective therapy: tuberculosis, syphilis, dysentery, scarlet fever, diphtheria, whooping cough, meningococcal infections, and pneumonia. They found a 56.4% decrease in the total number of deaths for these diseases combined in the period 1945–1955. The decline for all other causes of death over this same period was only 8.1%. The figures were also dramatic for certain diseases where antibiotics offered a significant new therapy. For example, the decrease in tuberculosis mortality over this period was 75.2%, as compared with a decrease of 28.6% during the previous ten years.[45]

In another 1958 publication, C. C. Dauer, Medical Adviser, National Office of Vital Health Statistics, United States Public Health Service, reported that mortality rates from infectious diseases had declined at a more rapid rate since sulfonamides and antibiotics came into use as therapeutic agents. He estimated that 1.5 million lives had been saved over the previous fifteen years as a result of this accelerated decline in mortality, recognizing, however, that other factors in addition to sulfonamide and antibiotic therapy contributed to the saving of these lives.[46]

Whatever the exact number of lives saved by the antibiotics since their introduction into therapeutics, it would be difficult to deny that they have played an important role in the declining mortality due to infectious disease. The past few decades have seen a significant change in the patterns of disease and death in industrialized nations. One study of changes in causes of deaths in Graz, Austria, for example, showed that deaths due to infections decreased 56% over the period 1930–1970. By contrast, deaths from malignancies over those same four decades increased 27% and deaths from degenerative diseases increased 44%.[47] It has been estimated that four out of five of the leading causes of deaths in children were microbially related at about the time that the sulfonamides and antibiotics were first introduced, whereas twenty years later four out of five were non-microbial.[48]

Antibiotics have also expanded what surgeons can do by helping to control infections. Walsh McDermott has argued that: "There are several areas of surgery today that would hardly be possible were it not for the antimicrobial technology. The arena of cardiac surgery, organ transplantation and the management of severe burns can serve as examples."[49]

The introduction of antibiotics also served as a stimulus to the growth of the pharmaceutical industry and to the expansion of research in this industry in countries such as the United States and Japan. The total number of pounds of antibiotics produced by American pharmaceutical firms increased from 240,332 in 1948 to 3,081,373 in 1956. Twenty-nine new antibiotic substances were introduced from

1949 through 1956 by these firms, although all of them did not remain in production. Typically these products were protected by patents and, consequently, were produced exclusively by one company. The ethical drug idustry in the United States became much more dependent on the development of patentable new drugs for generating profits in the post-World War II period, with antibiotics leading the way at first. By 1956, sales of antibiotics represented 17% to 39% of the total sales of major producers such as Lilly, Parke Davis and Pfizer.[50]

On the negative side, concern has been expressed about the misuse and overuse of antibiotics. Evidence about the adverse side effects of antibiotics began to surface, and it was recognized that frequent exposure to antibiotic drugs could increase the proportion of antibiotic-resistant strains in a given population of microorganisms. Antibiotics were frequently prescribed in conditions where they were not effective, such as virus-induced respiratory tract infections. These negative developments also had a positive side, in that they helped to increase awareness of the problem of iatrogenic disease and to stimulate efforts towards a more rational therapeutics.[51]

The evidence suggests, however, that the "golden age" of antibiotics is over. In 1979, Philip Paterson pointed out that all of the major classes of clinically significant antibiotics had been discovered by 1959, and that subsequently introduced antibiotics largely represented molecular rearrangements or semisynthetic modifications of previously discovered drugs. In addition, he noted, strains of pathogenic microorganisms which were resistant to antibiotics seemed to be appearing more often. In Paterson's view, the "bug-drug" perspective that had come to dominate therapeutics in the antibiotic era had deflected much attention from other promising lines of research, such as host immune defense systems and the development of new vaccines. He felt, however, that the balance was shifting as the limitations of antibiotic therapy were increasingly realized.[52]

Antibiotics will no doubt continue to play a significant role in therapeutics, and new antibiotics will probably continue to be discovered, although probably not at the same pace and with the same dramatic results as in the "golden age" of the 1940s and 1950s. As with other new drug discoveries, however, there was too much of a tendency at first to see antibiotic therapy as a panacea. In time, we have begun to recognize the limitations of these "wonder drugs." Historians a generation or two in the future will be able to look back on the "antibiotic era" with greater perspective than we can do today, and to more fully assess the role of antibiotics in twentieth-century therapeutics.

ACKNOWLEDGEMENTS

I would like to acknowledge the assistance of Margaret Kaiser, reference librarian in the History of Medicine Division, National Library of Medicine, in locating some of the source materials used in preparing this paper. I would also like to thank John Swann and my fellow participants at the 10th International Symposium on the Comparative History of Medicine — East and West for their helpful comments on earlier drafts of this paper.

NOTES & REFERENCES

1) Gwyn Macfarlane, *Alexander Fleming: the man and the myth* (Cambridge, MA: Harvard University Press, 1984), p. 268.

2) James Whorton, "'Antibiotic abandon': The resurgence of therapeutic rationalism," in J. Parascandola, ed., *The history of antibiotics: a symposium* (Madison, WI: American Institute of the History of Pharmacy, 1980), p. 126.

3) Felix Marti-Ibañez, *Men, molds, and history* (New York: MD Publications, 1958), p. 1.

4) Selman Waksman, "History of the word 'antibiotic,'" *J. Hist. Med.*, 1973, **28**: 284–286.

5) Leslie T. Morton, *A medical bibliography (Garrison and Morton): an annotated check-list of texts illustrating the history of medicine*, 4th edition (Aldershot: Gower, 1983), p. 248.

6) John Tyndall, "The optical deportment of the atmosphere in relation to the phenomenon of putrefaction and infection,"*Phil. Trans.*, 1876, **166**: 27–74.

7) For discussions of early observations of microbial antagonism, see J. Brunel, "Antibiosis from Pasteur to Fleming," *J. Hist. Med.*, 1951, **6**: 287–301; J. K. Crellin, "Antibiosis in the 19th Century," in Parascandola, ed., *Antibiotics*, pp. 5–13; H. W. Florey, E. Chain, N. G. Heatley, M. A. Jennings, A. G. Sand-

ers, E. P. Abraham and M. E. Florey, *Antibiotics*, vol. 1 (London: Oxford University Press, 1949), pp. 1–73.

8) Louis Pasteur and Jules F. Joubert, "Charbon et septicémie," *C. R. Acad. Sci. (Paris)*, 1877, **85**: 101–115.

9) Paul Vuillemin, "Antibioses et symbiose," *C. R. Assoc. Francaise Avance. Sci.*, Pt. 2, 1889 (publ. 1890), **18**: 525–543.

10) On pyocyanase, see Florey, *et al.*, *Antibiotics*, vol. 1, pp. 19–26; Rudolf Emmerich and Oscar Löw, "Bacteriolytische Enzyme als Ursache der erworbenen Immunität und die Heilung von Infectionskrankheiten durch dieselben," *Z. Hyg. Infectionskr.*, 1889, **31**: 1–65.

11) Alexander Fleming, "On the antibacterial action of cultures of a penicillium, with special reference to their use in the isolation of *B. Influenzae*," *Brit. J. Exp. Path.*, 1929, **10**: 226–236. See also Macfarlane, *Fleming*, pp. 117–138.

12) Gladys Hobby, *Penicillin: meeting the challenge* (New Haven, CT: Yale University Press, 1985), pp. 48–50. For a discussion of the work of C. G. Paine, whose claim to have used penicillin therapeutically at this time has been substantiated by documented clinical notes, see Milton Wainwright and Harold T. Swan, "C. G. Paine and the earliest surviving clinical records of penicillin therapy," *Med. Hist.*, 1986, **30**: 42–56. I am grateful to Vivian Nutton for calling my attention to this paper.

13) Macfarlane, *Fleming*, pp. 98–111; Gwyn Macfarlane, *Howard Florey: the making of a great scientist* (Oxford: Oxford University Press, 1979), pp. 177–179.

14) N. E. Goldsworthy and H. W. Florey, "Some properties of mucus, with special reference to its antibacterial functions," *Brit. J. Exp. Path.*, 1930, **9**: 192–208; Macfarlane, *Florey*, pp. 179–182.

15) L. A. Epstein and E. B. Chain, "Some observations on the preparation and properties of the substrate of lysozyme," *Brit. J. Exp. Path.*, 1940, **21**: 339–355; Macfarlane, *Florey*, pp. 276–279.

16) Macfarlane, *Florey*, pp. 279–286; Florey, *et al.*, *Antibiotics*, vol. 1, pp. 50–52; Trevor Williams, *Howard Florey: Penicillin and after* (Oxford: Oxford University Press, 1984), pp. 86–92.

17) Rene Dubos, "Studies on a bactericidal agent extracted from a soil bacillus. I. Preparation of the agent. Its *in vitro* activity," *J. Exp. Med.*, 1939, **70**: 1–10; Rene Dubos, "Studies on a bactericidal agent extracted from a soil bacillus. II. Protective effect of the bactericidal agent against experimental pneumococcal infections in man," *J. Exp. Med.*, 1939, **70**: 11–17; Florey, *et al.*, *Antibiotics*, vol. I, pp. 422–442.

18) This discussion of the efforts to culture and isolate penicillin at Oxford is based on Florey, *et al.*, *Antibiotics*, vol. II, pp. 635–647; H. W. Florey and E. P. Abraham, "The work on penicillin at Oxford" *J. Hist. Med.*, 1951, **6**: 302–317; E. Chain, "A short history of the penicillin discovery from Fleming's early observations in 1929 to the present time," in Parascandola, ed., *Antibiotics*, pp. 15–29.

19) E. Chain, H. W. Florey, A. D. Gardner, N. G Heatley, M. A. Jennings, J. Om-Ewing and A. G. Sanders, "Penicillin as a chemotherapeutic agent," *Lancet*,

1940(2): 226–228.

20) Macfarlane, *Florey*, p. 323.

21) *Ibid.*, pp. 330–331; Lennard Bickel, *Rise up to life: a biography of Howard Walter Florey who gave penicillin to the world* (London: Angus and Robertson, 1972), pp. 121–123.

22) Bickel, *Rise up*, pp. 124–129; Hobby, *Penicillin*, pp. 69–79: "Giant' germicide yielded by mold," *N. Y. Times*, May 6, 1941, p. 23. I am indebted to my colleague Peter Hirtle and to Donald Shay of the Center for the History of Microbiology, University of Maryland, Baltimore-County for a copy of the N. Y. Times article.

23) E. P. Abraham, E. Chain, C. M. Fletcher, A. D. Gardner, N. G. Heatley, M. A. Jennings and H. W. Florey, "Further observations on penicillin," *Lancet*, 1941(2): 177–188.

24) On the Peoria research, see Robert Coghill, "The development of penicillin strains," in Albert Elder, ed., *The history of penicillin production* (New York: American Institute of Chemical Engineers, 1970), pp. 15–21; Emerson Lyons, "Deep-tank fermentation," in *ibid.*, pp. 33–36; Hobby, *Penicillin*, pp. 94–103.

25) W. H. Helfand, H. B. Woodruff, K. M. H. Coleman and D. L. Cowen, "Wartime industrial development of penicillin in the United States, " in Parascandola, ed., *Antibiotics*, pp. 31–33.

26) On the CMR and WPB involvement with penicillin, see *ibid.*, pp. 38–50; Albert Elder, "The role of the government in the penicillin program," in Elder, ed., *Penicillin Production*, pp. 3–11; A. N. Richards, "Production of penicillin in the United States (1941–1946)," *Nature*, 1964, **201**: 441–445; John Swann, "The search for synthetic penicillin during World War II, "*Brit. J. Hist. Sci.*, 1983, **16**: 154–190.

27) Elder, "role of the government," p. 7.

28) On the use of penicillin in treating various diseases, see Hobby, *Penicillin*, pp. 115–124, 141–170; Harry Dowling, *Fighting infection: conquests of the twentieth century* (Cambridge, MA: Harvard University Press), pp. 136–157.

29) On Keefer and the allocation of penicillin, see Dowling, *Infection*, pp. 132–133; Hobby, *Penicillin*, pp. 141–143.

30) J. G. Rogers, *N. Y. Herald Tribune*, Oct. 17, 1943.

31) Hobby, *Penicillin*, p. 197.

32) George Urdang, "The antibiotics and pharmacy," *J. Hist. Med.*, 1951, **6**: 388–405. The figures are from p. 403.

33) L. Ettlinger, "Wartime research on penicillin in Switzerland and antibiotic screening," in Parascandola, ed., *Antibiotics*, pp. 57–67.

34) Hobby, *Penicillin*, pp. 207–208.

35) *Ibid.*, pp. 202–206.

36) Letter from K. Wiesner to David Perlman, November 29, 1976 (copy in possession of author).

37) Yukimasa Yagisawa, "Early history of antibiotics in Japan," in Parascandola, ed., *Antibiotics*, pp. 69–90.

38) G. F. Gause, "Gramicidin S and early antibiotic research in the Soviet Union,"

in Parascandola, ed., *Antibiotics*, pp. 91–95.

39) Patricia Spain Ward, "Antibiotics and international relations at the close of World War II," in Parascandola, ed., *Antibiotics*, pp. 101–112.

40) Hubert Lechevalier, "The search for antibiotics at Rutgers University," in Parascandola, ed., *Antibiotics*, pp. 113–123; Dowling, *Infection*, pp. 158–173.

41) On the "broad-spectrum" antibiotics, see Dowling, *Infection*, pp. 174–192.

42) On the naming of antibiotics, see David Perlman, *Antibiotics* (Chicago: Rand McNally, 1970), p. 10.

43) Federal Trade Commission, *Economic Report on Antibiotics Manufacture, June 1958* (Washington, D.C.: United States Government Printing Office, 1958), p. 270.

44) *Ibid.*, p. 277.

45) *Ibid.*, p. 279.

46) C. C. Dauer, "A demographic analysis of recent changes in mortality, morbidity, and age group distribution in our population," in Iago Galdston, ed., *The impact of antibiotics on medicine and society* (New York: International Universities Press, 1958), pp. 98–120.

47) Broda Barnes, Max Ratzenhofer, and Richard Gisi, "The role of natural consequences in the changing death patterns," *J. Amer. Ger. Soc.*, 1974, **22**: 176–179.

48) Walsh McDermott (with David Rogers), "Social ramifications of control of microbial disease," *Johns Hopkins Med. J.*, 1982, **151**: 302–312. The figures are from p. 308.

49) *Ibid.*, p. 308.

50) See Federal Trade Commission, *Economic Report*, pp. 65–109, 199–224 for information on antibiotics production and sales.

51) See Whorton, "'Antibiotic abandon,'" pp. 125–136.

52) Philip Paterson, "Infectious diseases — Into the 1980's and beyond," *J. Infect. Dis.*, 1979, **140**: 125–126. See also Guenter Risse and John Parascandola, "From bug and drug to human host: The control of infectious disease," unpublished paper delivered at a symposium on "Science in medicine, 1906–1981," Emory University, Atlanta, 1981.

Miracle at Carville:

The Introduction of the Sulfones for the Treatment of Leprosy

U NTIL the 1940s, patients suffering from leprosy, or Hansen's disease, had little hope for significant and sustained improvement in their medical condition. In the United States in the twentieth century, many victims of the disease were hospitalized in the national leprosarium operated by the Public Health Service in Carville, Louisiana (commonly referred to simply as Carville). Although patients at Carville received the best available care, the stigma associated with the disease, and consequently with the hospital, led many a patient to feel as if he or she were, in the words of one patient, "an exile in my own country."[1] Another patient described the hospital as "the place of isolation."[2] Patients frequently spent many years, sometimes the rest of their lives, at the hospital. It was at Carville that an event occurred in the 1940s that was dramatically to change the fortunes of those suffering from leprosy. The purpose of this paper is to examine this important breakthrough, the introduction of the sulfones

for the treatment of leprosy by Dr. Guy Faget and his colleagues.

The Development of the Leprosy Hospital at Carville

Towards the end of the nineteenth century, concerns over leprosy as a contagious disease led to the passage of an act by the state legislature of Louisiana in 1892 mandating that all persons with leprosy be confined "in an institution isolated and used for the treatment of said disease." Louisiana is one of the states where leprosy is most common in the United States. At the time, the only housing for lepers in the city of New Orleans was described by dermatologist Isadore Dyer as a "pest-house" where lepers were housed "under conditions of almost neglect." In a presentation to the Orleans Parish Medical Society in 1894, Dyer called for the creation of an institution for lepers that was based on humanitarian principles. He asked that it be made "an asylum of refuge, rather than one of horror and reproach."

On the recommendation of the Orleans Parish Medical Society, the state legislature of

A version of this paper was presented at the AIHP meeting in Nashville, TN, March, 1996.

Louisiana passed an act that set up the "Board of Control for the Louisiana Leper Home" in September of 1894, with Dr. Isadore Dyer as its President. Because of community opposition, Dyer was unable to find a site for the facility in New Orleans, and he finally leased an abandoned sugar plantation situated on the banks of the Mississippi River between Baton Rogue and New Orleans. He was able to obtain this property only under the pretext that it would be used as an ostrich farm. The plantation, called Indian Camp, was located near the hamlet of Carville, and the leprosarium came to be referred to simply as Carville. On 30 November 1894, the first patients, five men and two women, arrived by barge at Indian Camp.

Dyer soon arranged a contract with the Daughters of Charity of St. Vincent De Paul, who had served at the New Orleans Charity Hospital for sixty years, to provide the new facility with nursing services and domestic management. In 1896, the first four sisters arrived to take up their duties at Carville, beginning a tradition that continues up to the present.[3]

Carville remained a state institution until 1921, when it was taken over by the Federal government. For years Dyer promoted the concept of Carville as a center for leprosy research and treatment, but the state seemed content to operate it essentially as an asylum. Finally in 1917, Congress authorized the Public Health Service (PHS) to establish a national leprosarium, with Dyer (by then Dean of the Tulane University Medical School) testifying on behalf of a bill introduced by Senator Joseph E. Ransdell of Louisiana. After several other potential sites for such a hospital were abandoned due to resistance from local communities, it was decided to purchase the Louisiana Leper Home, which the state was quite willing to sell. Given the active roles played by Dyer and Ransdell in the movement to create a national leprosy hospital, it was not surprising that Louisiana should become the home for the new facility. In 1921, Carville became U. S. Marine Hospital Number 66 of the PHS. The hospital officially became the National Hansen's Disease Center in 1980, and was renamed the Gillis W.

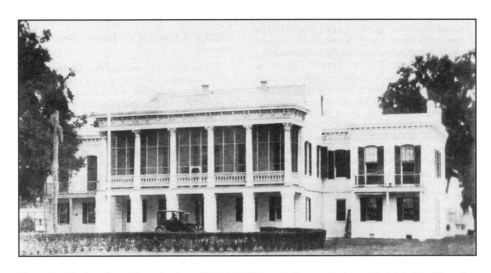

The original Indian Camp Plantation home (built in 1857) eventually served to house administrative offices of the Public Health Service leprosy hospital at Carville, Louisiana, now known as the Gillis W. Long Hansen's Disease Center. (Courtesy of the National Library of Medicine)

Long Hansen's Disease Center in honor of Congressman Long of Louisiana after his death in 1985.

As soon as the PHS took over Carville, it assigned to the hospital its first full-time, resident physicians and medical support staff, in addition to the nurses already there. Dr. Oswald Denney, who had served as director of the hospital for leprosy patients in the Philippines, was appointed as the first Chief Medical Officer. Under the 1917 law that authorized a national leprosarium, the PHS Surgeon General was authorized, upon the request of local health officials, to compel those suffering from leprosy to go to Carville even against their will. Patients at Carville were not free to leave of their own volition, and it was not until about 1960 that Carville became a voluntary hospital.[4]

Chaulmoogra Oil in the Treatment of Leprosy

Numerous remedies had been tried against leprosy over the years, without significant success. By 1940, however, chaulmoogra oil and its derivatives had become the most widely accepted treatment for the disease at Carville and elsewhere. The oil was a remedy from the Orient that had found its way into Western medicine in the nineteenth century. It is extracted from the seeds of a tropical tree of the genus *Hydnocarpus*, and is also known as Hydnocarpus oil. Although many physicians were convinced that this drug was effective against leprosy, others were extremely skeptical about the claims that were made for it. George McCoy, who had served for many years as director of the National Institute (later Institutes) of Health, published an attack on chaulmoogra oil in 1942. McCoy noted that many experienced students of the disease expressed serious doubts about the value of the oil in treating leprosy, especially when discussing the subject in private. He quoted (anonymously) the views of four experts in leprosy whom he had consulted, all of them critical about the effectiveness of the oil.[5]

Whether or not one believed that chaulmoogra oil was of any value in treating leprosy, it would have been difficult to argue that it was an ideal therapeutic agent. Patient Stanley Stein, who took the oil for many years without being cured of the disease (although he believed that it had once cleared up a cluster of nodules on his temple), wrote of his experiences with the drug at Carville:

Whether I was to take the oil externally, internally, or—as someone once said—eternally, was up to me. The oral doses were nauseously given out in the cafeteria at mealtime. The injections were administered in what to me was a distressingly public manner . . . the after effects were sometimes frightful—painful suppurating abscesses which the chaulmoogra oil would generate in the patient's backside. . . . I was hospitalized several times with chaulmoogra-induced, rear-end ulceration.[6]

Stein, who came from a pharmacy background, was familiar with chaulmoogra oil before going to Carville. He was born Sidney Maurice Levyson on 10 June 1899 in Gonzales, Texas, but he changed his name upon entering the leprosy hospital, as did many of the patients, to spare his family from the stigma associated with the disease. His father was a registered pharmacist, but left the practice to manage the family general store. When the family moved to Boerne, Texas, Stein's father purchased a drugstore and resumed his old occupation. The family lived in an apartment behind the drugstore and young Stanley frequently assisted his father's drug clerk in his duties.

Stein remembers being both frightened and fascinated by one particular customer, a mysterious lady who always wore a heavy black veil. It was rumored that she had been a famous and beautiful actress or singer, but that her features had been ravaged by some horrible disease. One day Stein was helping the clerk to fill a prescription, and he felt nauseated by a foul-smelling oily liquid. The clerk explained that the substance was chaulmoogra oil, and that the prescription was for the lady with the veil, who had leprosy. Stein, who associated the disease with the Middle Ages, was stunned to learn of its existence in twentieth-century Texas. He was unaware at the time, of course, that he would one day fall victim to the disease himself.

Stein graduated from the University of Texas School of Pharmacy in Galveston, and, after receiving his license, began to practice at the family drugstore in Boerne in 1919. That summer he began to notice that he sometimes woke up in the morning with his face swollen and red, but neither he nor his doctor thought it

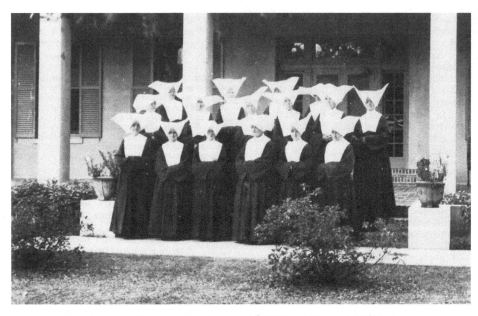

Daughters of Charity nurses at Carville, 1947. (Courtesy of the National Library of Medicine)

was anything serious. By this time, Stein was anxious to move to a bigger city, so he persuaded his father, who was in poor health, to sell the drugstore. The family moved to San Antonio, where Stanley went to work in Wagner's Drugstore. Late in 1920, he consulted a physician about a dermatological condition, and was shocked to learn that he had leprosy. He struggled with the disease for years, trying his best to hide it, but finally decided to admit himself into Carville in 1931.[7]

At Carville Stein was reintroduced to chaulmoogra oil, this time as a patient. After a time, he obtained the job of dispensing medications to patients, for which he was paid a small stipend. As Stein recalled:

My duties consisted of sitting at a table in the cafeteria, and handing out chaulmoogra oil capsules from four large ointment jars. The capsules were graded from five to twenty-five drops, and as I placed them on butter chips and set one on each patient's tray, I came to know the patients as ten-droppers or fifteen-droppers even before I knew their names.[8]

Having been trained as a pharmacist, Stein kept meticulous records, and was surprised by the amount of the nauseating oil consumed by some of the patients. One patient, for example, requested twelve 25-drop capsules at each meal, and Stein found it hard to believe that the man could possibly absorb this much of the drug. Later he learned that some patients were requesting more of the medication than they actually used, and were sending the extra capsules home to other family members afflicted with the disease. In this way, they hoped to spare their relatives from confinement at Carville.[9]

Other medications that Stein dispensed included Fowler's Solution and strychnine sulfate, which were among the substances used to supplement the chaulmoogra oil therapy. Periodically other drugs would be tried against the disease. Stein volunteered, for example, to participate in a clinical trial of the dye trypan blue in 1933. Stein also reported that Carville residents secretly tried various substances, such as willow bark tea, on a self-medication basis. This was the state of therapy for leprosy at the time that Dr. Guy Faget arrived at Carville.

Faget and the Introduction of the Sulfones

Guy Faget was born in New Orleans in 1891 and obtained his M.D. degree at Tulane University in 1914. He spent the next year as an intern in the Public Health Service's marine hospital in New Orleans. After holding several positions for short periods, he enlisted in the British Colonial Medical Service, where he spent over five years in British Honduras. Faget returned to the United States and joined the Public Health Service (PHS) in 1922. For the next eighteen years, he served in various PHS hospitals in different parts of the country before being assigned to be Medical Officer in Charge of the hospital at Carville in July of 1940.[10]

Before coming to Carville, Faget had carried out research on malaria, a disease which he himself suffered from during his stay in British

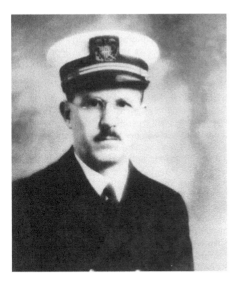

Guy Faget, who directed the clinical tests of the sulfone drug Promin at the Carville hospital. (Courtesy of the National Library of Medicine)

Honduras, and on tuberculosis. These studies were relevant to his later work on leprosy. Tuberculosis and leprosy are both caused by acid-fast bacteria, so Faget had already acquired some experience with a disease caused by this type of organism in his tuberculosis research. In the course of his work on malaria, Faget had experimented with the use of sulfonamides (or sulfa drugs) against the disease relatively soon after this class of drugs had been introduced as therapeutic agents in the 1930s. Although the sulfonamides did not prove to be effective against malaria, other investigators were carrying out studies at about the same time which suggested that these compounds might have some activity against the tubercle bacillus. Faget was aware of this work, and shortly after his arrival at Carville he began investigating the promise of the sulfa drugs in leprosy.[11]

At the time, no one had successfully cultured the causative organism of human leprosy in an artificial culture medium or in any animal model. New potential treatments for the disease thus tended to be tested directly on human patients. Aware of the experimental use of the sulfonamides in tuberculosis, Faget began trying sulfa drugs such as sulfanilamide and sulfathiazole on volunteer patients at Carville. Soon, however, his interest turned to another sulfa compound, Promin, produced by Parke Davis and Company. Promin belongs to a class of drugs called sulfones, which are chemically related to the sulfonamides and have a somewhat similar bacteriostatic spectrum. Scientists at the Mayo Clinic reported in a paper published in October of 1940 that Promin was effective in suppressing tuberculosis infections in guinea pigs, and attention was soon focused on the potential use of the sulfones in treating the disease. Although the sulfones did not prove to be successful therapeutic agents against tuberculosis, this research stimulated Faget's interest in their potential use against leprosy.[12]

On 9 December 1940, Faget wrote to Dr. E.A. Sharp, Director of Clinical Investigation for Parke Davis. Faget noted that he was greatly interested in the work at the Mayo Clinic on tuberculosis in guinea pigs. The Mayo researchers had obtained their best results with the Parke Davis compound Promin, and Faget asked whether Sharp was aware of any other experimental work with this drug in acid-fast diseases. Sharp informed Faget that Dr. E.V. Cowdry of Washington University in St. Louis was conducting experiments with Promin on rat leprosy under a grant from the Public Health Service. Although rat leprosy was not the same as human leprosy, Cowdry believed that the diseases were similar enough "to justify the hope that experiments on rat leprosy may yield clues to the treatment of human leprosy."[13]

Cowdry reported to Faget that the survival time of the leprous rats treated with Promin was somewhat longer than that of the controls, and that the treated animals were definitely in better condition than the controls as the experiment progressed. Encouraged by these results, Faget and his colleagues decided to go ahead with clinical trials of Promin at Carville. On 10 March 1941, the first six volunteer patients were injected with the drug. At first the drug had been tried orally, but that proved to be too toxic, and a switch was made to intravenous injection. Even this route of administration had side effects, the most important of which was a slow destruction of red blood cells leading in some cases to anemia, which had to be counteracted by antianemic therapy such as iron salts or liver extract.[14]

In November of 1943, the Carville team published the first results of the Promin study. Of 22 patients who had been receiving the drug for at least 12 months, 15 showed improvement, and five tested negative for the presence of the leprosy bacillus. Preliminary results with another 46 patients who had been receiving the drug for less than a year also showed improvement in 26 out of 46 in the group, and seven of them became bacteriologically negative.

Experiments with another Promin-like compound (referred to as Internal Antiseptic 307), also from Parke Davis, led to significant improvements in 20 patients when compared to 20 controls who received a placebo. This compound was chosen over Promin for the control study because it could be given orally, and the Carville researchers believed that "it would have been more difficult to manage a control series of patients on intravenous injections [of placebo] without arousing their suspicions." Faget and his co-authors cautiously concluded that "promin appears to be capable of inhibiting the

progress of leprosy in a considerable percentage of cases," but called for further studies before more definitive conclusions could be drawn about the therapeutic value of the drug.[15]

In addition to continuing the study of Promin, Faget and his colleagues also began experimenting with other sulfone drugs at Carville. They began using Diasone (manufactured by Abbott) in July, 1943 and Promizole (manufactured by Parke Davis) in March, 1945. Both of these drugs could be given by oral administration (making it easier for patients to treat themselves on an outpatient basis) and showed promise in the treatment of leprosy.[16]

Clinical trials of the sulfones against the disease were also being carried out by other investigators by this time. For example, Ernest Muir, who was in touch with the Carville researchers, began treating patients at the Chacachacara Leprosarium in Trinidad with diasone in 1944. Concerned about the toxicity exhibited by Promin when given orally, Muir administered Diasone intravenously at first. In later work carried out after he left Trinidad, he switched to the oral route used by the Carville group with this drug.[17] Another sulfone drug, Sulphetrone (manufactured by Burroughs Wellcome), was also tried against leprosy with encouraging results by several investigators in the late 1940s.[18]

The studies of Faget and others firmly established the value of Promin and other sulfones in the treatment of leprosy. In 1947, chaulmoogra oil therapy was officially abandoned and the sulfones became the treatment of choice at Carville. The sulfones also eventually led to a change of policy from one of isolation of leprosy victims to one of outpatient treatment with drugs. As early as 1948, the hospital began to allow, under certain conditions, the medical discharge of patients who were still in the so-called "communicable state" (i.e., who were not bacteriologically negative). Patient morale and optimism increased as the evidence of the efficacy of the sulfones accumulated.[19] One of the early patients to receive Promin, Betty Martin, entitled her autobiography *Miracle at Carville* in recognition of the dramatic improvement in the situation of leprosy patients brought about by the sulfones.[20]

Conclusion

There have been further improvements in the therapy of leprosy since the 1940s. The sulfones are derivatives of the compound diaminodiphenylsulfone (DDS), also known as dapsone, first synthesized in 1908. Although the so-called mother substance of the sulfones was shown to have activity against leprosy in the 1940s, it did not come into widespread clinical use until the 1950s because at first it was believed to be too toxic. Eventually it was shown that because it had a higher therapeutic efficacy than the other sulfones, dapsone could be given in lower doses, thus reducing the toxic effect. It was also absorbed very well from the gut, hence was effective when administered orally (e.g., in the form of tablets). Dapsone was also relatively inexpensive, presumably because of the low dosage required and because, unlike the other sulfones used in the treatment of leprosy, it was not a proprietary drug. At first it was not even being produced commercially in most countries, but the rising demand for the drug changed that situation.[21]

Over time there was an increasing problem of patients who failed to respond to sulfone therapy because of microbial resistance to the drugs. Fortunately, other drugs, such as clofazimine and rifampin, were discovered to be effective against leprosy. Multi-drug therapy is now always used to circumvent the problem of resistance to particular drugs. Such treatment renders the patient noninfectious within a few days and relapse is uncommon in patients completing a standard course of multi-drug therapy.[22]

As for Guy Faget, whose clinical studies ushered in the era of the sulfones, he met an untimely end at the age of 56. On 23 December 1945, Faget suffered a heart attack from which he recovered. He returned to work at Carville in April of 1946, but after a second heart attack he gave up his position as Medical Officer in Charge of the leprosy hospital. In the spring of 1947, he was transferred to the Public Health Service hospital in New Orleans, where he was to continue his research on the treatment of leprosy. On 17 July 1947, Faget died from multiple injuries received in a fall from the window of a fifth-floor bathroom of the New Orleans hospital. The death was ruled accidental. There was speculation that Faget may have felt the symptoms of another potential heart attack coming on, opened and leaned out of the window for air, then lost his balance and fell to his death.[23]

But Faget left behind a legacy of hope for those suffering from leprosy, now preferably called Hansen's disease. These individuals no longer are forced to live in institutional confinement. The work of Faget and his colleagues on sulfones had indeed initiated a miracle at Carville.

Notes and References

1. Stanley Stein (with Lawrence G. Blochman), *Alone No Longer: The Story of a Man Who Refused to be One of the Living Dead* (New York: Funk and Wagnalls, 1963), p. 4.

2. Betty Martin, *Miracle at Carville*, edited by Evelyn Wells (Garden City, NY: Doubleday, 1950), p. 14.

3. On the history of the Louisiana Leper Home, see Isadore Dyer, "The History of the Louisiana Leper Home," *New Orleans Med. Surg. J.* 54 (1902): 714-737; Sally K. Reeves and William D. Reeves, *National Register Evaluation Gillis W. Long Hansen's Disease Center: The Final Report* (Carville, LA: U.S. Department of Health and Human Services, 1991), pp. 27-31; Charles Calandro, "From Disgrace to Dignity—The Louisiana Leper Home, 1894-1921," M.A. Thesis, Louisiana State University, 1980.

4. On the 1917 law and the assumption by PHS of responsibility for the hospital, see Reeves and Reeves, *National Register* (n. 3), pp. 31-39; Calandro, "Disgrace to Dignity" (n. 3); Bess Furman, *A Profile of the United States Public Health Service 1798-1948* (Washington, D.C.: U.S. Department of Health and Human Services, 1973), pp. 311-312, 347-349. For more detailed discussion of the confinement of patients at Carville, see John Parascandola, "'An Exile in My Own Country:' The Confinement of Leprosy Patients at the United States National Leprosarium," *Medicina nei Secoli* NS 10(1988):111-125; Zachary Gussow, *Leprosy, Racism, and Public Health: Social Policy in Chronic Disease Control* (Boulder, CO: Westview Press, 1989); Zachary Gussow and George S. Tracy, "Stigma and the Leprosy Phenomenon: The Social History of a Disease in the Nineteenth and Twentieth Centuries," *Bull. Hist. Med.* 44 (1970): 425-449.

5. G.W. McCoy, "Chaulmoogra Oil in the Treatment of Leprosy," *Pub. Health Rep.* 57 (1942): 1727-1733.

6. Stein, *Alone No Longer* (n. 1), pp. 38-39.

7. On Stein's early life and pharmacy experience, see Stein, *Alone No Longer* (n. 1), pp. 1-38.

8. Stein, *Alone No Longer* (n. 1), p. 56.

9. Stein, *Alone No Longer* (n. 1), pp. 56-57.

10. Biographical information on Faget is taken from "Dr. Guy H. Faget 'Pioneer Sulfone Therapist' (1891 to 1947)," *The Star* (published by the patients at Carville) 6 [12] (August, 1947): 8-9; "Dr. Guy Henry Faget 1891-1947," *Internat. J. Leprosy* 15 (1947): 338; and from documents in his official

personnel file, Federal Records Center, National Archives and Records Administration, St. Louis.

11 . See the references in note 10. See also Arnold R. Rich and Richard H. Follis, Jr., "The Inhibitory Effect of Sulfanilamide on the Development of Experimental Tuberculosis in the Guinea Pig," *Bull. Johns Hopkins Hosp.* 62 (1938): 77-84; G.H. Faget, "History Taking in the Early Diagnosis of Pulmonary Tuberculosis," *Pub. Health Rep.* 45 (1930): 323-326; and G.H. Faget, M.R. Palmer, and R.O. Sherwood, "Unsuccessful Treatment of Malaria with Sulfonamide Compounds," *Pub. Health Rep.* 53 (1938): 1364-1367.

12 . G.H. Faget, F.A. Johansen, and Sister Hilary Ross, "Sulfanilamide in the Treatment of Leprosy," *Pub. Health Rep.* 57 (1942): 1892-1899; W.H. Feldman, H.C. Hinshaw, and H.E. Moses, "The Effect of Promin (Sodium Salt of P,P'-Diaminodiphenylsulfone-N,N'-Dextrose Sulfonate) on Experimental Tuberculosis: A Preliminary Report," *Proc. Staff Meet. Mayo Clinic* 15 (1940): 695-699; Stein, *Alone No Longer* (n. 1), pp. 219-221.

13 . Stein, *Alone No Longer* (n. 1), p. 220; E.V. Cowdry and C. Ruangsiri, "Influence of Promin, Starch and Heptaldehyde on Experimental Leprosy in Rats," *Arch. Path.* 32 (1941): 632-640 (the quotation is from p. 632).

14 . Stein, *Alone No Longer* (n. 1), pp. 221-222; G.H. Faget, R.C. Pogge, F.A. Johansen, J.F. Dinan, B.M. Prejean, and C.G. Eccles, "The Promin Treatment of Leprosy. A Progress Report," *Pub. Health Rep.* 58 (1943): 1729-1741.

15 . Faget, et al, "Promin" (n. 14). The quotations are from pp. 1740-1741.

16 . G.H. Faget, R.C. Pogge, and F.A. Johansen, "Promizole Treatment of Leprosy," *Pub. Health Rep.* 61 (1946): 957-960; G.H. Faget, R.C. Pogge, and F.A. Johansen, "Present Status of Diasone in the Treatment of Leprosy," *ibid.*, pp. 960-963; G.H. Faget and Paul T. Erickson, "Chemotherapy of Leprosy," *J. Amer. Med. Assoc.* 136 (1948): 451-457.

17 . Ernest Muir, "Diasone in the Treatment of Leprosy," *Leprosy Rev.* 17 (1946): 87-95; O.C. Wenger to Thomas Parran, 7 June 1944 and G.H. Faget to the Surgeon General, 26 May 1944, Record Group 90 (Public Health Service), National Archives, Washington, D.C., General Classified Records, 1936-1944, Group IX, 0425 (leprosy). The Public Health Service records are now housed in the Archives II facility in College Park, MD.

18 . See, for example, Dharmendra, "The Results of Sulphetrone Treatment of Leprosy in the Gobra Hospital, Calcutta," *Leprosy in India* 22 (April, 1950): 46-59.

19 . Stein, *Alone No Longer* (n. 1), p. 242; memorandum by Watson B. Miller, February 19, 1951, Public Health Service Hospitals Historical Collection, MS C 471, National Library of Medicine, Bethesda, MD, box 14, folder 7.

20 . Stein, *Alone No Longer* (n. 1), p. 222; Martin, *Miracle at Carville* (n. 2).

21 . A.T. Roy, "Diaminodiphenylsulphone in Leprosy: Its Oral and Parenteral Use, A Comparison," *Leprosy Review* 25 (1954): 77-80; H.W. Wade, "The Trend to DDS," *Internat. J. Leprosy* 19 (1951): 344-349; C.J. Austin, "Modern Leprosy Treatment," *Leprosy Rev.* 25 (1954): 174-178; Louis S. Goodman and Alfred Gilman, *The Pharmacological Basis of Therapeutics*, second edition (New York: Macmillan, 1955), pp. 1251-1255, 1271-1275; Ernest Muir, *Manual of Leprosy*, supplement to the first edition (Edinburgh: E. and S. Livingston, 1952), pp. 1-4.

22 . Robert R. Jacobson, "Hansen's Disease Drugs in Use: Current Recommendations for Treatment," *The Star* 51 [4] (March-April, 1990): 1-4.

23 . "Dr. Faget Returns," *The Star* 5 [8] (April, 1946): 10; letters and documents in Faget's official personnel file (n. 10), e.g., James G. Terrill, Jr. to Director of Insurance, Veterans Administration, August 15, 1947.

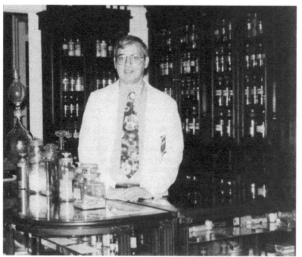

AIHP Council Chair John Parascandola visited the New Orleans Pharmacy Museum at the opening reception of the Blue Cross and Blue Shield Association conference on "Managing the Prescription Drug Benefit," last fall. Dr. Parascandola delivered a lecture on the history of the pharmaceutical profession at the conference.

John Mahoney and the Introduction of Penicillin to Treat Syphilis

W HEN the German scientist Paul Ehrlich introduced Salvarsan for the treatment of syphilis in 1910, it was hailed as a wonder drug. For centuries physicians had used mercury and a variety of other compounds to treat syphilis without great success. Salvarsan and other arsenical drugs indeed represented a significant advance in syphilis therapy and became the standard treatment for the disease.[1] But although the arsenicals could produce a cure, at least in the early stages of syphilis, there were significant drawbacks to their use. The drugs were complicated to administer and could have toxic side effects.[2] In addition, success depended upon prolonged treatment. A standard course of therapy might involve the patient visiting his or her doctor weekly for a year or more to receive injections of arsenic and bismuth drugs. Under these circumstances, it is not surprising that there was a high rate of noncompliance. By the early 1940s, so-called rapid treatment methods requiring from five days to several weeks had been developed, with the drug being administered by intravenous drip or multiple injections. This intense treatment had to be carefully monitored and involved an increased risk of untoward reactions. The intravenous drip method required hospitalization of the patient. Clearly a better

An earlier, abridged version of this paper was given at the 34th International Congress of the History of Pharmacy, Florence, Italy, October 20-23, 1999. I wish to thank Gary Gernhart for assistance in locating some of the sources used in this paper.

therapeutic agent was needed, and that agent turned out to be penicillin.[3]

Penicillin Enters Therapeutics

As is well known, penicillin was discovered by Alexander Fleming, whose paper on the subject was published in 1929. It was not until penicillin was taken up by Howard Florey, Ernst Chain, and their colleagues at Oxford University a decade later, however, that it was developed into a successful therapeutic agent. In animal studies and some ten clinical cases conducted by the Oxford team, penicillin showed extraordinary promise as an antimicrobial drug.[4]

Substantial amounts of penicillin were needed for the extensive clinical trials required to confirm the promise of these early results, and to provide adequate supplies of the drug for therapeutic use if it did live up to its potential. Florey recognized that large-scale production of penicillin was probably out of the question in Britain, whose chemical industry was fully absorbed in the war effort. So Florey and his colleague Norman Heatley traveled to the United States in the summer of 1941 to see if they could interest the Americans in the effort to produce penicillin on a large scale.[5]

Most important among the institutions visited by Florey and Heatley was the Department of Agriculture's Northern Regional Research Laboratory (NRRL) in Peoria, Illinois, of interest largely because of the expertise of its

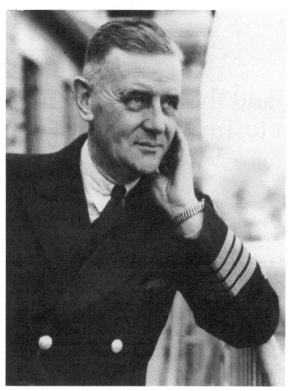

John Mahoney in his Public Health Service uniform (courtesy of the National Library of Medicine).

Fermentation Division. This contact proved to be crucial to the success of the project, as the NRRL contributed innovations that made large-scale production of penicillin possible.

Orville May, Director of the NRRL, agreed to have the Laboratory undertake a vigorous program to increase penicillin yields. Within a few weeks, Andrew Moyer found that he could significantly increase the yield of penicillin by substituting lactose for the sucrose used by the Oxford team in their culture medium. Shortly thereafter, Moyer made the even more important discovery that the addition of corn-steep liquor to the fermentation medium produced a ten-fold increase in yield. Corn-steep liquor was a by-product of the corn wet-milling process, and the NRRL, in an attempt to find a use for it, tried it in essentially all of their fermentation work. Later, the Peoria labo-

ratory increased the yield of penicillin still further by the addition of penicillin precursors, such as phenylacetic acid, to the fermentation medium.

It was recognized that the Oxford group's method of growing the mold on the surface of a nutrient medium was inefficient, and that growth in submerged culture would be a superior process. Florey's *Penicillium* culture, however, produced only traces of penicillin when grown in submerged culture. Under the direction of Kenneth Raper, staff at the NRRL screened various *Penicillium* strains and found one that produced acceptable yields of penicillin in submerged culture. Soon a global search was underway for better penicillin-producing strains, with soil samples being sent to the NRRL from around the world. Ironically, the most productive strain came from a moldy cantaloupe from a Peoria fruit market. A more productive mutant of the so-called cantaloupe strain was produced with the use of X-rays at the Carnegie Institution. When this strain was exposed to ultraviolet radiation at the University of Wisconsin, its productivity was increased still further.[6]

While Heatley remained in Peoria helping the NRRL staff get the penicillin work started, Florey visited various pharmaceutical companies to try to interest them in the drug. Although Florey was disappointed in the immediate results of his trip, three companies (Merck, Squibb, and Lilly) had actually conducted some penicillin research before Florey's arrival, and Pfizer seemed on the verge of investigating the drug as well. At this time, however, the promise of penicillin was still based on only limited clinical trials.

Florey next visited his old friend Alfred Newton Richards, then vice president for medical affairs at the University of Pennsylvania. More importantly, Richards was chair of the Committee on Medical Research (CMR) of the Office of Scientific Research and Development (OSRD). The OSRD had been created in June 1941, to assure that adequate attention was given to research on scientific and medical problems relating to national defense. Richards had great respect for Florey and trusted his judgement about the potential value of penicillin. He approached the four drug firms that Florey indicated had shown some interest in the drug (Merck, Squibb, Lilly, and Pfizer) and informed them that they would be serving the national interest if they undertook penicillin production and that there might be support from the federal government. It was agreed that although the companies would pursue their research activities independently, they would keep the CMR apprised of developments, and the Committee could make the information more widely available (with the permission of the company involved) if that were deemed in the public interest.

Although there was some concern that investments in fermentation processes might be wasted if a commercially-viable synthesis of penicillin were developed, other companies also began to show an interest in the drug. Some firms worked out collaborative agreements of their own (e.g., Merck and Squibb, later joined by Pfizer). Pharmaceutical and chemical companies played an especially important role in solving the engineering and scientific problems inherent in scaling up submerged fermentation from a pilot plant to a manufacturing scale. On 1 March 1944, Pfizer opened the first commercial plant for large-scale production of penicillin by submerged culture in Brooklyn, New York.

Meanwhile, clinical studies in the military and civilian sectors were confirming the therapeutic promise of penicillin. The drug was shown to be effective in the treatment of a wide variety of infections, including streptococcal and staphylococcal infections. The United States Army established the value of penicillin in the treatment of surgical and wound infections.

The increasingly obvious value of penicillin in the war effort led the War Production Board (WPB) in 1943 to take responsibility for increased production of the drug. The WPB investigated more than 175 companies before selecting 21 to participate in a penicillin program under the direction of Albert Elder. These firms received top priority on construction materials and other supplies necessary to meet the production goals. The WPB controlled the disposition of all of the penicillin produced. One of the major goals was to have an adequate supply of the drug on hand for the proposed D-Day invasion of Europe.[7]

Venereal Disease in Wartime

Venereal disease has typically been a cause of concern in wartime, and the Second World War was no exception. Governments feared that soldiers indulging in sex with prostitutes or so-called "promiscuous" women were in danger of contracting a venereal disease and becoming incapacitated. The concern over the rate of venereal disease infection in American military recruits in the First World War I had in fact been a major factor in the establishment of a Division of Venereal Diseases in the United States Public Health Service through the Chamberlain-Kahn Act in 1918.

Although the support for venereal disease work waned after the war ended, the Public Health Service (PHS) initiated a reinvigorated campaign against venereal disease after Thomas Parran became Surgeon General of the PHS in 1936. Parran had earlier been head of the Venereal Disease Division, and was strongly committed to fighting venereal diseases. Through his speeches and publications, he helped to break the taboo on discussing syphilis and other venereal diseases in the popular press. He also played a key role in the passage of the National Venereal Disease Control Act in 1938. The act provided federal funding through the PHS to the states for venereal disease control programs, as well as supporting research into the treatment and prevention of venereal disease.[8]

With the outbreak of the Second World War in Europe, Parran's educational campaign against venereal disease was intensified. As a part of its efforts to combat venereal disease, the PHS issued posters, brochures, and other publications on the subject. Motion picture films were also a part of the campaign to educate the military and the public about syphilis and gonorrhea. The PHS even collaborated with Warner Brothers Studios in 1943 to produce a 30-minute version, known as "Magic Bullets," of the 1940 feature film "Dr. Ehrlich's Magic Bullet." (On the negative side, PHS was also conducting the now-infamous Tuskegee syphilis experiment in Alabama at this time.)[9]

It should also be noted that the PHS viewed pharmacists as important players in venereal disease education and control. In 1942, the Surgeon General sent a letter to the editors of pharmaceutical and medical journals, enclosing a press release on "The Pharmacist and VD Control." The release pointed out that pharmacists were in a good position to educate the public about venereal disease because people with such infections often go to them for advice and medicine. Using their personal influence, pharmacists can direct patients who have not sought medical attention for their condition to see a doctor, and steer them away from patent medicines advertised to cure syphilis and gonorrhea. Ppharmacists could also distribute pamphlets and display posters on the subject in the pharmacy. As good citizens, pharmacists should also support community efforts to control venereal disease. The press release concluded:

By participating actively in the venereal disease control program being promoted by the United States Public Health Service and State health authorities, and by the Joint Committee of the American Social Hygiene Association and the American Pharmaceutical Association, pharmacists of the country will strengthen public confidence in their profession. At the same time they will know personally that their best efforts are being given toward the elimination of the venereal disease scourge, both for the best interests of the civilian population and for the greater fighting efficiency of the armed forces of the Nation.[10]

John Mahoney and the Venereal Disease Research Laboratory

In addition to its prevention and treatment programs, the Public Health Service also contributed to research efforts on venereal disease. One of the responsibilities assigned to the Division of Venereal Diseases by the 1918 Chamberlain-Kahn Act was "to study and investigate the cause, treatment, and prevention of venereal diseases."[11] Over the following years, the Division provided funding to universities such as the University of Pennsylvania and Johns Hopkins University to support research on venereal disease. In addition, the Division itself carried out its own research, especially clinical studies at the clinic at Hot Springs, Arkansas, maintained by the PHS in cooperation with the National Park Service and the Arkansas State Board of Health, which was intended primarily for the treatment of indigent cases of venereal disease. In addition, investigations of rabbit syphilis were carried out at the PHS Hygienic Laboratory (forerunner of the National Institutes of Health) in the 1920s.[12]

In 1927, while Thomas Parran headed the Division of Venereal Diseases, arrangements were made for an experienced PHS commissioned officer to be detailed for venereal disease work to the marine hospital operated by the PHS in Staten Island, New York. One of the primary functions of the PHS, dating back to its origins, had been the operation of hospitals for the care of merchant seamen. The physician-officer assigned to the Staten Island facility in 1927 was asked to study methods of treating syphilis and gonorrhea, with a special emphasis on efforts to shorten the period necessary for cure of these diseases. The *Annual Report* of the PHS for 1927 commented: "Since a considerable percentage of the work in the marine hospitals is on account of venereal diseases, any success in the prevention and improved treatment of these diseases would effect a very direct saving to the Government."[13]

A small research laboratory was set up, and additional staff were soon assigned to the work. In addition to the laboratory experiments, clinical studies were also undertaken with the cooperation of hospital staff. In 1929, Dr. John F. Mahoney assumed direction of this laboratory, which was later named the Venereal Disease Research Laboratory.[14]

John Mahoney was born on 1 August 1889, in Fond du Lac, Wisconsin. He graduated from Marquette Medical College in Milwaukee in 1914, and then undertook internships at the Milwaukee County Hospital and the Chicago Lying-in Hospital. In October 1917, he joined the Public Health Service as a scientific assistant. The following March he was commissioned as an Assistant Surgeon in the Public Health Service Commissioned Corps.

Mahoney followed a pattern that was typical of many young officers of the Service at that time, serving for relatively short periods of time at various quarantine stations and marine hospitals. He also served for a time at the Ellis Island Immigration Station. From late 1925 to early 1929, Mahoney was assigned to work abroad on the medical aspects of immigration in Ireland, England, and Germany. He took advantage of his service in Europe to visit laboratories and clinics to study syphilis, a disease that interested him. When Mahoney returned to the United States in 1929, he was assigned to the Staten Island Marine Hospital.[15]

Mahoney and his colleagues at the Venereal Disease Research Laboratory carried out both laboratory and clinical studies on venereal disease. Their studies led to an enhanced knowledge of the mechanism and rate of penetration into tissues by the spirochete, the microorganism that causes syphilis. Mahoney's group also

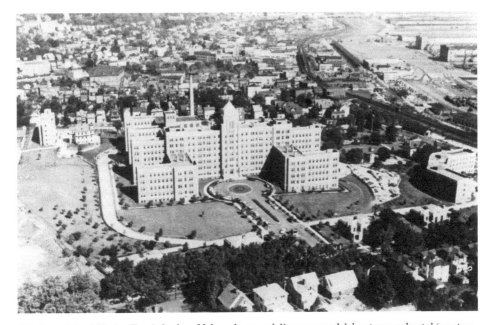

The Staten Island Marine Hospital, where Mahoney's venereal disease research laboratory was located (courtesy of the Program Support Center, Department of Health and Human Services).

significantly improved the serologic tests used in diagnosing the disease. When the sulfonamides were introduced in the 1930s, the Venereal Disease Research Laboratory investigated and helped to demonstrate the efficiency of these drugs in the treatment of gonorrhea.[16]

Penicillin and Syphilis

Thus when penicillin was introduced as a therapeutic agent during World War II, Mahoney already had substantial experience with syphilis and its treatment. He also became aware of a paper by Wallace Herrell and his colleagues at the Mayo Clinic, published in the *Journal of the American Medical Association* in May 1943, which showed that penicillin was effective against sulfonamide-resistant gonorrhea.[17] In a paper published in 1956, Mahoney recalled that he received his initial supply of penicillin through the National Research Council, and that the drug was earmarked for further development of a therapy for male gonorrhea (presumably as a follow-up to the initial observations of the Mayo Clinic investigators).[18] The emphasis on male gonorrhea no doubt reflected the priority of the military with respect to the supply of penicillin. Mahoney's recollections are supported by a note in the first paper from his laboratory on penicillin, which credits the federal program, involving the National Research Council and the Office of Scientific Research and Development, as the source of the penicillin.[19] Two other accounts of the initial source of Mahoney's penicillin exist, but I have not been able to corroborate either one. Ralph Williams, who undoubtedly knew Mahoney, stated in his history of the PHS that at first Mahoney and his colleagues actually grew the *Penicillium* mold themselves to produce penicillin for their work because it was in such short supply.[20] In his history of venereal disease in America, historian Allan Brandt states that Mahoney received his first penicillin in early 1943 from investigators in Oxford, England.[21]

However Mahoney came by his initial supply of penicillin, he and his coworkers did confirm the observations of the Mayo Clinic researchers on the efficacy of penicillin in the treatment of sulfonamide-resistant gonorrhea.[22] But Mahoney also decided to divert a small

amount of the drug from the gonorrhea research to test it against syphilis. He later noted that it had long been a rule in the Venereal Disease Research Laboratory to test any preparation that it worked with for therapeutic activity against experimental syphilis in rabbits.[23] According to Mahoney's coworker R. C. Arnold, the drug was first tried against spirochetes (the microorganisms that cause the disease) *in vitro*, and failed to show any activity.[24] Fortunately, the Staten Island investigators proceeded to the next step of trying the drug *in vivo* in syphilitic rabbits. The results of limited animal tests were so encouraging that Mahoney decided to move ahead quickly to clinical experiments. He justified this early move to human use because penicillin appeared to be generally non-toxic and no harm would be done to the patients if the drug did not work and he had to return to arsenic therapy.[25] In 1943, it had not yet been recognized that penicillin could produce serious toxic effects in some patients.[26]

On the basis of their initial animal results, Mahoney and his colleagues were provided with additional penicillin through the government program so that they could try the drug in humans as well as expand the animal studies. In June 1943, Mahoney, Arnold, and serologist Ad Harris began their study with four patients. A preliminary report on these first four cases was presented at the meeting of the American Public Health Association in New York on 14 October 1943 and published in December of that year.[27] The four syphilis patients were given six intramuscular injections of penicillin a day for eight days, for a total of 1,200,000 units of the drug. No significant toxic side effects were observed. The investigators reported that: "The results of the blood studies indicate that the therapy was responsible for a more or less rapid and complete disappearance from the blood stream of the reacting substance which is measured by the various tests and which is usually associated with activity in early syphilis."[28]

Four cases, of course, were not enough to base any definitive conclusions on, and there was always a danger that the patients might relapse after a time. Mahoney therefore intended to continue observation of the patients for as long as possible. The Staten Island researchers were willing to make only a rather cautious statement about the effectiveness of penicillin against syphilis in this preliminary paper.

Should the more extensive and prolonged experience confirm the impression which is to be gained by the pilot study, a rebuilding of the structure of syphilis therapy may become necessary. This development of an optimal therapy will require carefully controlled studies designed to determine the most effective relationship between the amount of the drug and the duration of the treatment period. Also, the role of the treatment in latent disease and visceral and central nervous system syphilis will require careful scrutiny before the reasonably effective measures which are available at present may be replaced by a therapy based upon penicillin. Because of the long post treatment period of observation which is a requisite for the evaluation of a syphilis therapy, the progress toward the adoption of a new mode of treatment must, of necessity, be deliberate.[29]

Microbiologist Gladys Hobby later recalled the excitement created by Mahoney's presentation of the penicillin paper at the American Public Health Association meeting.

I have a mental image of the room where I first heard Mahoney and his associates describe their results on the use of penicillin in the treatment of syphilis. The room was crowded. Loudspeakers and projection equipment were not as sophisticated then as now. Everyone strained to hear what was said, and the impact was electrifying. By then much had been written on penicillin, but no one had expected that an antibacterial agent would be active against spirochetes as well. Hearing John Mahoney describe the effect of penicillin on the course of syphilitic lesions was overwhelming.[30]

The paper delivered at the meeting was reported on in the popular press as well. In a story headed "New Magic Bullet," *Time* discussed how Mahoney, in a "jam-packed session" of the meeting, announced that "penicillin had apparently cured four cases of early syphilis." Dr. Mahoney, according to the magazine, was "stunned" by the results. *Time* also reported Mahoney's cautious statement that penicillin would have to be tested in a large number of cases over a long period of time before it could be considered a cure for syphilis, along with his admission that it was possible that a "reconstruction" of syphilis therapy might be necessary. One doctor who took the floor to comment on the paper was carried away by his enthusiasm to exult: "This is probably the most significant paper ever presented in the medical field."[31]

A month later, PHS physician John Heller, Jr. discussed syphilis control at the annual meeting of the Southern Medical Association in Cincinnati. He referred to the work of Mahoney and his colleagues on the use of penicillin as "overshadowing anything that has happened in syphilis control since the days of Ehrlich."[32]

The results of the clinical tests at the Staten Island hospital, limited as they were, were sufficient to convince Alfred Newton Richards, Chairman of the Medical Research Committee, of the need to move forward with more extensive clinical trials. He later said of the work of Mahoney and colleagues on penicillin and syphilis: "This discovery gave a new and highly important turn to the examination and treatment of that disease."[33]

Under the auspices of the Committee on Medical Research, chaired by Richards, a cooperative clinical trial of penicillin in the treatment of syphilis was organized in the fall of 1943. The project was under the specific direction of the Subcommittee on Venereal Diseases of the National Research Council. The subcommittee appointed a Penicillin Panel, with Mahoney serving as one of the members, to oversee the study.[34]

In October 1943, the subcommittee organized a conference with representatives from the Public Health Service, the Committee on Medical Research, eight civilian venereal disease clinics, the British Central Scientific Service, and the Canadian Army Medical Corps. At this meeting, which Richards called "the beginning of a revolution in the treatment of syphilis," it was agreed that the eight civilian venereal disease clinics, along with one each from the Army, the Navy, and the Public Health Service, would participate in the study. It was anticipated that a sufficient supply of penicillin to treat 350 patients a month could be made available for the purposes of the study. The study was later expanded to include other facilities. It remained under the direction of the Penicillin Panel of the Subcommittee on Venereal Disease until the PHS assumed responsibility for its continuation at the beginning of 1946.[35]

As would be expected, the Staten Island Marine Hospital was one of the original sites chosen for the clinical study with Mahoney of course directing the work there. In a paper published in the *Journal of the American Medical Association* in September, 1944 Mahoney and his coworkers reported on the further progress of the original four patients treated, as well as providing some preliminary observations on their results with an additional one hundred patients with early syphilis. Although the results continued to be positive, Mahoney knew that it was too early to be sure that cures had been effected, and he concluded the paper with the following cautious statement:

"It is desired to recall that the disease syphilis is one which is characterized by chronicity, with long periods of latency and a distinct tendency to clinical and serologic recurrence. The evaluation of any therapy will require a prolonged trial utilizing a wide variety of treatment schedules and a carefully controlled follow-up system. The combined experience available at this time has served to illuminate only a few of the important aspects. The remainder must await the passage of time."[36]

Immediately following this paper in the *Journal* was another paper by Mahoney, Joseph Earle Moore of Johns Hopkins, W. Barry Wood of Washington University, and Walter Schwartz and Thomas Sternberg of the Army Medical Corps. This paper provided a preliminary report of 1,418 cases involving the penicillin treatment of early syphilis from all of the clinics in the cooperative study. Although the authors continued to exhibit caution, they were able to demonstrate that penicillin treatment led to the disappearance of the spirochete from open lesions, the healing of these lesions, and a reversal of the blood serologic response from positive to negative (presumably due to the elimination of the spirochetes from the blood).[37]

While the scientific investigators enjoyed the luxury of withholding their final verdict on the effectiveness of penicillin against syphilis, waiting for a definitive answer was not an option for those charged with the medical care of the troops in a wartime situation. By April 1944, the Chief of the Army's Preventive Medicine Service was requesting advice about the earliest possible time that penicillin treatment of syphilis might be applied in the Army. Just three months later, on June 26, the Army adopted penicillin as the routine treatment for syphilis. Fortunately by that time the supply of penicillin had increased significantly. The British armed forces soon followed their American colleagues in adopting penicillin as the standard treatment for the disease.[38]

Penicillin allowed military physicians to get men suffering from venereal disease back on their feet and available for combat quickly. Raymond Vonderlehr and John Heller of the PHS, summarizing the remarks made by Army Colonel Donald M. Pillsbury at a 1944 conference in St. Louis, reported that:

Colonel Pillsbury pointed out that treatment with penicillin makes this possible because most of the patients remained ambulatory and began to convalesce almost immediately after treatment was begun. This arrangement made it possible to keep the infected men close to the front lines. As soon as penicillin treatment was completed the men were returned to active duty.[39]

As penicillin first became available to military physicians, there was not necessarily enough of the drug to treat all of the cases that might potentially benefit from it. Penicillin of course had therapeutic value in the treatment of war wounds and various infections, as well as in the treatment of syphilis and gonorrhea. Physician-ethicist Henry Beecher called attention to the problem facing military surgeons in a paper published in 1969:

Allocation of penicillin within the Military was not without its troubles: When the first sizable shipment arrived at the North African Theatre of Operations, U.S.A., in 1943, a decision had to be made between using it for 'sulfa fast' gonorrhea or for infected war wounds. Colonel Edward D. Churchill, Chief Surgical Consultant for that Theatre, opted for use in those wounded in battle. The Theatre Surgeon made the decision to use the available penicillin for those 'wounded' in brothels. Before indignation takes over, one must recall the military manpower shortage of those days. In a week or less, those overcrowding the military hospitals with venereal disease could be restored to health and returned to the battle line.[40]

A moral issue of a different sort was raised by those concerned about the impact of penicillin on sexual mores. As it became more and more obvious that syphilis and gonorrhea could be cured relatively quickly and painlessly with penicillin, some feared that this situation would encourage sexual promiscuity and immorality. One historian has cited a theologian of the period who worried that venereal disease would come to be regarded as strictly a medical problem, with its sociological and moral implications ignored.[41] A graduate

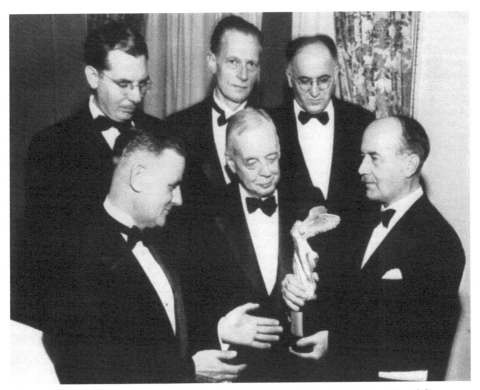

John Mahoney (lower left) receiving the Albert Lasker Clinical Research Award in 1946 (courtesy of the National Library of Medicine).

student in social work, who completed a project in a venereal disease rapid treatment center for her M.S. degree in 1947, admitted in her dissertation that she could not answer the question of "whether penicillin will be a help or a hindrance to the control of venereal disease; whether by making the treatment so short and effective patients will lose the fear of contracting the disease and will show more laxness in their sex behavior."[42] A number of public health officials suggested that it was possible that the quicker and less arduous penicillin treatment could actually lead to an increase in venereal disease.[43] It should be noted that similar concerns about the undermining of standards of morality had been voiced when Ehrlich's Salvarsan was introduced to treat syphilis.[44]

Concerns about the impact that penicillin might have on sexual behavior did not materially slow the adoption of the drug for the treatment of syphilis and gonorrhea. Nor, however, has effective drug therapy for sexually-transmitted diseases eliminated the social and moral issues surrounding these diseases.

Conclusion

Further clinical trials with penicillin by Mahoney and others confirmed its place as the treatment of choice for syphilis.[45] Not only did the drug cure the disease, but it quickly rendered patients non-infectious, thereby preventing them from spreading it to others. As Brandt and Jones have noted in their historical chapter in *Sexually Transmitted Diseases*, penicillin led to a dramatic decline in the incidence of syphilis. By the late 1950s, rates of infection in the United States reached an all-time low. Any illusion that the disease was on its way to being eliminated, however, was shattered by the fact that rates began to climb again in the early 1960s. Changes in sexual mores due to the increasing availability of contraceptives and a decline in funding for public venereal disease programs are two of the factors that may have contributed to this reversal of the downward trend.[46] If penicillin has not eliminated syphilis, however, it has at least provided a safe, quick, easy, and effective treatment for this disease.

In recognition of his contribution to this discovery, John Mahoney received the prestigious Albert Lasker Award for Clinical Research in 1946 for "distinguished service as a pioneer in the treatment of syphilis with penicillin."[47] In December 1949, he retired from the Public Health Service. That was not to be the end of his career, however, for he went on to become the Health Commissioner of the City of New York, and then the Director of the City Health Department's Bureau of Laboratories until his death in 1957.[48] Although he had a long and distinguished career in public health, during which time he made a number of significant contributions to the field, he will no doubt always be remembered best for his part in revolutionizing the treatment of syphilis.

Notes and Reference

1. John Parascandola, "The Theoretical Basis of Paul Ehrlich's Chemotherapy," *Journal of the History of Medicine and Allied Sciences* 36 (1981): 19-43.

2. Patricia Spain Ward, "The American Reception of Salvarsan," *Journal of the History of Medicine and Allied Sciences* 36 (1981): 44-62; Janice Dickin McGinnis, "From Salvarsan to Penicillin: Medical Science and VD Control in Canada," in Wendy Mitchinson and Janice Dickin McGinnis, eds., *Essays in the History of Canadian Medicine* (Toronto: McClelland and Stewart, 1988), pp. 126-147, pp. 132-137.

3. Rudolph Kampmeier, "The Introduction of Penicillin for the Treatment of Syphilis," *Sexually Transmitted Diseases* 8 (1981): 260-265, p. 260; Rudolph Kampmeier, "Syphilis Therapy: An Historical Perspective," *Journal of the American Venereal Disease Association* 3 (1976): 99-108, p. 105; Harry Arnold, "Penicillin and Early Syphilis," *JAMA* 251 (1984): 2011-2012; Louis Chargin and William Leifer, "Massive-Dose Arsenotherapy of Early Syphilis by Intravenous

'Drip" Method," *A. M. A. Archives of Dermatology* 73 (1956): 482-484.

4. On the history of penicillin, see Ronald Hare, *The Birth of Penicillin and the Disarming of Microbes* (London: George Allen and Unwin, 1970); Gladys Hobby, *Penicillin: Meeting the Challenge* (New Haven, CT: Yale University Press, 1985); H. W. Florey, E. Chain, N. G. Heatley, M. A. Jennings, A. G. Sanders, E. P. Abraham, and M.E. Florey, *Antibiotics*, volume II (London: Oxford University Press, 1949), pp. 631-671.

5. Florey, *et al.*, *Antibiotics* (n. 4), p. 649.

6. On the contributions of the Northern Regional Research Laboratory to penicillin production, see Percy A. Wells, "Some Aspects of the Early History of Penicillin in the United States," *Journal of the Washington Academy of Sciences* 65 (1975): 96-101; George Kaufmann, "The Penicillin Project: From Petri Dish to Fermentation Vat," *Chemistry* 51[7] (September 1978): 11-17; Robert D. Coghill, "The Development of Penicillin Strains," in Albert L. Elder, ed., *The History of Penicillin Production* (New York: American Institute of Chemical Engineers, 1970), pp. 15-21.

7. On the wartime penicillin production program in the United States and the contributions of government and industry, see Hobby, *Penicillin* (n. 4); W. H. Helfand, H. B. Woodruff, K. M .H. Coleman, and D. L. Cowen, "Wartime Industrial Development of Penicillin in the United States," in John Parascandola, ed., *The History of Antibiotics: A Symposium* (Madison, WI: American Institute of the History of Pharmacy, 1980), pp. 31- 56; Albert L. Elder, "The Role of the Government in the Penicillin Program," in Elder, ed., *History* (n. 6), pp. 3-11.

8. On efforts to control venereal disease in the United States, see Allan M. Brandt, *No Magic Bullet: A Social History of Venereal Disease in the United States Since 1880* (New York: Oxford University Press, 1985, revised edition 1987). For biographical information on Parran, see Lynne Page Snyder, "Thomas J. Parran, Jr.," in Lois N. Magner, *Doctors, Nurses, and Medical Practitioners: A Bio-Bibliographical Sourcebook* (Westport, CT: Greenwood Press, 1997), pp. 209-215.

9. On the use of films in the PHS educational program, see Susan E. Lederer and John Parascandola, "Screening Syphilis: Dr. Ehrlich's Magic Bullet Meets the Public Health Service," *Journal of the History of Medicine and Allied Sciences* 53 (1998): 345-370 ; John Parascandola, "VD at the Movies: PHS Films of the 1930s and 1940s," *Public Health Reports* 111 (1996): 173-175. On the Tuskegee study, see James H. Jones, *Bad Blood: The Tuskegee Syphilis Experiment*, new and expanded edition (New York: Maxwell McMillan International, 1993) and Susan M. Reverby, *Tuskegee's Truths: Rethinking the Tuskegee Syphilis Study* (Chapel Hill, NC: University of North Carolina Press, 2000).

10. Surgeon General to Editor, October 12, 1942, 1942 folder, General Classified Records, 1936-1944, Group IX, General Files, 0425, Records of the Public Health Service, Record Group 90, National Archives, Washington, D.C.

11. *Annual Report of the Surgeon General of the Public Health Service of the United States* (hereafter referred to as *PHS Annual Report*), 1919, p. 234.

12. See *PHS Annual Report* (n. 11) for the 1920s. On the Hot Springs clinic, see Edwina Walls, "Hot Springs Waters and the Treatment of Venereal Diseases: The U.S. Public Health Service Clinic and Camp Garraday," *Journal of the Arkansas Medical Society* 91(1995): 430-437.

13. *PHS Annual Report* (n. 11), 1927, p. 285.

14. *PHS Annual Report* (n. 11), 1929, p. 268; Ralph Chester Williams, *The United States Public Health Service, 1798-1950* (Washington, D.C.: Commissioned Officers Association of the United States Public Health Service, 1951), p. 387.
15. Biographical information on Mahoney was obtained from Williams, *Public Health Service* (n. 14), pp. 387-390; David E. Price, "John Friend Mahoney," *Dictionary of American Biography*, Supplement Six (New York: Charles Scribner's Sons, 1980), pp. 423-424; official personnel folder of John F. Mahoney, Federal Records Center, National Archives and Records Administration, St. Louis.
16. See, for example, J. F. Mahoney, C. J. Van Slyke, and J. Durward Thayer, "Sulfanilamide Therapy in Hospitalized Gonorrhea," *American Journal of Syphilis Gonorrhea and Venereal Diseases* 22 (1938): 691-698. See also Williams, *Public Health Service* (n. 14), p. 388; Price, "Mahoney"(n. 15), p. 424.
17. Wallace E. Herrell, Edward N. Cook, and Luther Thompson, "Use of Penicillin in Sulfonamide Resistant Gonorrheal Infections," *Journal of the American Medical Association* 122 (1943): 289-292.
18. John F. Mahoney, "Some of the Early Phases of Penicillin Therapy of Syphilis," *A. M. A. Archives of Dermatology* 73 (1956): 485-488. Mahoney refers (p. 485) to penicillin first being made available to him by the National Research Council in 1942, but I think it more likely in 1943. First of all, Mahoney seems to indicate that he was given the supply after Herrell and his colleagues at the Mayo Clinic had reported their results, which were published in May, 1943 (n. 17), although Mahoney could conceivably have learned of the results before publication. He does, however, cite their published paper. In addition, penicillin supplies were extremely limited throughout 1942. For example, it was apparently not until April 1, 1943 that the first American military casualties were treated by penicillin. Finally, Mahoney indicates that he moved fairly quickly from gonorrhea to syphilis, and the syphilis work was not reported until well into 1943.
19. J. F. Mahoney, Charles Ferguson, M. Bucholtz, and C. J. Van Slyke, "The Use of Penicillin Sodium in the Treatment of Sulfonamide-Resistant Gonorrhea in Men," *American Journal of Syphilis, Gonorrhea, and Venereal Diseases* 27 (1943): 525-528, p. 525.
20. Williams, *Public Health Service* (n. 14), p. 388.
21. Brandt, *No Magic Bullet* (n. 8), p. 170.
22. Mahoney, *et al.*, "Use of Penicillin" (n. 19).
23. Mahoney, "Early Phases" (n. 18), p. 486.
24. Arnold is quoted in Hobby, *Penicillin* (n. 4), p. 152. Hobby also notes on the same page that Harry Eagle of the Johns Hopkins University School of Medicine had also observed that penicillin had no effect on spirochetes *in vitro*.
25. J. F. Mahoney, R. C. Arnold, and Ad Harris, "Penicillin Treatment of Early Syphilis: A Preliminary Report," *Venereal Disease Information* 24 (1943): 355-357, p. 355. The same paper was published in the same month in *American Journal of Public Health* 33 (1943): 1387-1391 (see p. 1387). This paper also indicates that the penicillin was obtained through the National Research Council and the Office of Scientific Research and Development.
26. On the development of a recognition of the side effects that penicillin could cause in some patients, see James C. Whorton, "'Antibiotic Abandon': The Resurgence of Therapeutic Rationalism," in Parascandola, ed., *History of Antibiotics* (n. 7), pp. 125-136.

27. Mahoney, *et al.*, "Penicillin Treatment" (n. 25).
28. *Ibid.*, p. 356 (in *VDI* paper) and p. 1390 (in *AJPH* paper).
29. *Ibid.*, p 356 (in *VDI* paper) and pp. 1390-1391 (in *AJPH* paper).
30. Hobby, *Penicillin* (n. 4), pp. 155-156.
31. "New Magic Bullet," *Time* 42 (October 25, 1943): 38, 40.
32. J. R. Heller, Jr., "Syphilis Control in Wartime," *Southern Medical Journal* 37 (1944): 219-223, p. 222.
33. A. N. Richards, "Production of Penicillin in the United States (1941-1946)," *Nature* 201 (1964): 441-445, p. 444.
34. Joseph Earle Moore, J. F. Mahoney, Walter Schwartz, Thomas Sternberg, and W. Barry Wood, "The Treatment of Early Syphilis With Penicillin: A Preliminary Report of 1,418 Cases," *Journal of the American Medical Association* 126 (1944): 67-72, pp. 67-68; Kampmeier, "Introduction" (n. 3), pp. 260-261; Joseph Earle Moore, *Penicillin in Syphilis* (Springfield, IL: Charles C. Thomas, 1947), p. 4.
35. Richards, "Production" (n. 33), p. 444; J. E. Moore, "Preliminary Statement," in National Research Council - U. S. Public Health Service, *Meeting of Penicillin Investigators*, February 7 and 8, 1946, p. 1 (a copy of this document is at the National Library of Medicine).
36. J. F. Mahoney, R. C. Arnold, Burton L. Sterner, Ad Harris, and M. R. Zwally, "Penicillin Treatment of Early Syphilis: II," *Journal of the American Medical Association* 126 (1944): 63-67, p. 67. This paper was reprinted as a "Landmark Article" in *ibid.*, 251 (1984): 2005-2010.
37. Moore, *et al.*, "Treatment" (n. 34).
38. Richards, "Production" (n. 33), p. 444; Alexander Fleming, *Penicillin: Its Practical Application* (Blakiston: Philadelphia, 1946), p. 283; Odin W. Anderson, *Syphilis and Society: Problems of Control in the United States, 1912-1964* (Chicago: Center for Health Administration Studies, Research Series 22, 1965), pp. 20-21.
39. R. A. Vonderlehr and J. R. Heller, Jr., *The Control of Venereal Disease* (New York: Reynal and Hitchcock, 1946), p.3.
40. Henry K. Beecher, "Scarce Resources and Medical Advancement," *Daedalus* 98 (1969): 275-313, pp. 280-281.
41. McGinnis, "Salvarsan" (n. 2), p. 145.
42. Judith Torregrosa, "A Study of Forty-Four Syphilitic Patients Under Treatment at the Louisville Rapid Treatment Center from March 1, 1947 to April 15, 1947," M.S. in Social Work dissertation, University of Louisville, 1947, p. v.
43. See, for example, Richard A. Koch and Ray Lyman Wilbur, "Promiscuity as a Factor in the Spread of Venereal Disease," *Journal of Social Hygiene* 30 (1944): 517-529; Vonderlehr and Heller, *Control* (n. 39), p. 65.
44. McGinnis, "Salvarsan"(n. 2), p. 146; Brandt, *No Magic Bullet* (n. 8), p. 46.
45. See, for example, R. C. Arnold, J. F. Mahoney, John C. Cutler, and Sacha Levitan, "Penicillin Therapy in Early Syphilis: III," *Journal of Venereal Disease Information* 28 (1947): 241-244.
46. Allan M. Brandt and David Shumway Jones, "Historical Perspectives on Sexually Transmitted Diseases: Challenges for Prevention and Control," in King K. Holmes, Per-Anders Mardh, P. Frederick Sparling, Stanley M. Lemon, Walter E. Stamm, Peter Piot, and Judith N. Wasserheit, eds., *Sexually Transmitted Diseases*, third edition (New York: McGraw-Hill, 1999), pp. 15-21, p. 18.
47. *Albert Lasker Awards Fortieth Anniversary* (New York: Albert and Mary Lasker Foundation, 1985), p. 23.
48. Price, "Mahoney" (n. 15), p. 424.

From Germs to Genes:

Trends in Drug Therapy, 1852-2002

Delivered at the AIHP-APhA symposium on "Trends and Events in American Pharmacy, 1852–2002" at the Sesquicentennial meeting of the American Pharmaceutical Association in Philadelphia, 17 March 2002.

Less than a decade after the founding of the American Pharmaceutical Association, the noted American physician Oliver Wendell Holmes, addressing the Massachusetts Medical Society in 1860, made his oft-quoted statement that " if the whole materia medica, as now used, could be sunk to the bottom of the sea, it would be all the better for mankind—and all the worse for the fishes."[1]

The pharmaceutical armamentarium of the middle of the nineteenth century was not quite so useless as the skeptic Holmes suggested. Even he qualified his condemnation by admitting that there were exceptions to his generalization, such as opium. Yet it is a striking fact that the drug therapy of the period around 1850 was in many ways more similar to that of antiquity and the Middle Ages than to that of the early twenty-first century. As historian Charles Rosenberg has noted: "Medical therapeutics changed remarkably little in the two millennia preceding 1800."[2]

This point can be illustrated by comparing the drug therapy of today to that of the middle of the nineteenth century. A useful starting point is an examination of a list of the ten most prescribed drugs of the year 2000 in the United States and their therapeutic uses (Table I).[3]

TABLE I

Ten Most Prescribed Drugs (U.S., 2000)

Drug	Use
Vicodin	Pain Killer
Lipitor	Lower Cholesterol
Premarin	Treat Menopausal Problems & Some Cancers
Synthroid	Treat Thyroid Problems
Atenolol	Treat High Blood Pressure
Lasix	Diuretic
Prilosec	Treat GERD
Albuterol	Treat Asthma
Norvasc	Treat High Blood Pressure
Alprazolam	Treat Anxiety Disorder

It is not surprising that none of these drugs were available in 1852. More importantly, however, there were no truly effective medicines available to American physicians of that period to treat most of the conditions noted in Table I, for example, cancer and thyroid problems. The physician of 1852 would not have even recognized the existence of conditions such as gastroesophageal reflux disease (GERD), high cholesterol levels, and anxiety disorder. In fact, their whole way of viewing disease and drug therapy was very different from the way we understand these subjects today.

Unfortunately, to my knowledge there are no lists of the most prescribed drugs of 1852 for the purposes of comparison. In order to give you some idea of the drug therapy of that day, however, we can examine one of the textbooks of materia medica and therapeutics of the period. John Neill and Francis Gureny Smith's *A Hand-Book of Materia Medica and Therapeutics* is a good choice because it just happened to be published in the same year and city in which the American Pharmaceutical Association was established, namely, 1852 in Philadelphia.[4] Table II shows the classification scheme for remedies used by Neill and Smith, a classification that was not unlike that of many other books on materia medica of the period, such as George B. Wood's *A Treatise on Therapeutics and Pharmacology, or Materia Medica*.[5]

Space does not permit a discussion of this classification system in detail, nor is it necessary to do so to make my point about the differences in thinking about drug action between 1852 and 2002. Although of course we recognize some of the terms in this classification system, others are less familiar to us. More importantly, this is not the way that we would find drugs or-ganized and classified in a modern textbook of pharmacology. By and large, these terms describe broad physiological actions of the remedies, aimed at treating particular symptoms of disease. Cathartics purge and emetics vomit, while diaphoretics promote sweating and rubefacients inflame the skin. Terms such as "tonic" and "alterative" have broad and somewhat vague meanings.

Historian John Harley Warner has eloquently described the shift in therapeutics that occurred over the course of the nineteenth century, from what he calls "specificity" (or individualism) to "universalism."[6] Focusing on the United States, he shows that up to at least the 1860s, physicians viewed disease as essentially a systemic imbalance (much as their counterparts as far back as antiquity did). Although specific theories of pathology may have differed, Warner argues that they were all based on the general view that illness was usually due to either excessive excitement or enfeeblement of the body's systems. The body was viewed as an interconnected whole, and the role of the physician was to restore its natural balance. This was done primarily by stimulating or depressing the system as needed.

Treatment tended to be highly individualistic. The patient's health, or natural balance, was affected by such factors as climate, age, ethnicity, socioeconomic position, and habits. The idea of disease-specific remedies, which disregarded the idiosyncrasies of patient and place, was not generally accepted. Though physicians were increasingly recognizing the existence of specific diseases, they believed that various en-

TABLE II

Classification of Remedies (Neill and Smith, 1852)

General Remedies	Local Remedies	
Astringents	Emetics	Epispactics
Tonics	Cathartics	Rubefacients
Arterial Stimulants	Diuretics	Escharotics
Nervous Stimulants	Diaphoretics	Emollients
Cerebral Stimulants	Expectorants	Demulcents
Excito-Motor Stimulants	Emmenagogues	Diluents
Arterial Sedatives	Sialogogues	Antacids
Nervous Sedatives	Errhines	Anthelminitcs
Alteratives		

vironmental influences could change one disease into another and that a single disease could take on a variety of forms. They also believed that the physiological action of remedies could be modified by various influences. Warner notes that:

Two patients with the identical disease could require opposite treatments. This was precisely the point that Harvard professor John Ware made in admonishing his students to distinguish between 'a pathological and a therapeutic diagnosis.' The name that pathological diagnosis assigned to a disease was not a trustworthy guide in therapy, he urged, for 'cases of which the pathological character is precisely the same may require a treatment diametrically opposite.'[7]

Such views made it difficult to apply knowledge gained in one situation to another context. For example, Warner states, " . . . it was not at all clear that the findings of therapeutic research in urban hospitals were applicable to the vast majority of sick Americans."[8] The rapid growth of experimental medical science in the last decades of the nineteenth century, however, was to undermine the principle of specificity and usher in a more universalist approach to therapeutics.

Advances in chemistry and physiology, along with the emergence of such biomedical disciplines as pharmacology, bacteriology, and immunology, dramatically altered the understanding of disease and of the human body. Returning to Table II, we can see, for example, that there is no category for antimicrobial drugs in the classification scheme. This is not surprising, of course, given the fact that the germ theory of disease had not yet been established in 1852. A very few drugs that we now know to have antimicrobial action, most notably quinine, were in use at this time, but their therapeutic efficacy was empirically discovered and their mechanism of action was not understood. In the mid-nineteenth century, there was also no understanding of such vital components of the body as vitamins and hormones, although there was at least a vague recognition that certain factors in the diet could help prevent some diseases. The drugs that were available to the medical and pharmaceutical professions usually treated only the symptoms of disease rather than getting at the causes.

In an introductory lecture given to the medical class of 1856-1857 at Harvard University, Professor of Materia Medica Edward Clarke warned his students about the dangers of assuming that all they needed to cure disease was the right drug. He noted that one might get the impression from reading the treatises on materia medica of the day that one could find in these works all "the needful weapons with which to combat or manage disease." He went on to add:

It is true that experience and observation will soon disabuse you of your error. Before the first decade of your life as a practitioner has passed, perhaps before you have made a year's acquaintance with the sick room, you will have learned that though Senna will purge, and Ipecac vomit, and Calomel salivate, and Opium stupify, yet that neither Senna, Ipecac, Calomel or Opium will *cure* disease except in rare instances.[9]

Clarke, in fact, was pessimistic enough to express the view that not only did drugs not cure disease in most cases, but "judging from the discoveries of modern science, we have no reason to expect that they ever will."[10] Lest we be too harsh on Clarke for this judgement, let us remember that "modern science" had yet to substantially modify drug therapy in 1856, though it was on the eve of transforming medicine. What were the best medicines available to physicians in the mid-nineteenth century? Physician-historian Ronald Mann has summed up the most useful drugs of the mid-nineteenth century as follows:

The best of the first British Pharmacopoeia of 1864 must seem to be . . . digitalis, opium, atropine, a salt of morphine, quinine sulphate, ether, chloroform, ferrous sulphate, iodine, sodium bicarbonate, salt and a few other household remedies.[11]

Except for the then newly-discovered anesthetics ether and chloroform, most of these drugs had been used in Western medicine, at least in their crude natural form if not as pure chemical compounds, for centuries. For example, the use of opium to ease pain dates back to antiquity, and cinchona bark (the source of quinine) was introduced into European medicine to treat malaria and other intermittent fevers in the seventeenth century.

The second half of the nineteenth century, however, witnessed the beginnings of a biomedical revolution that was to eventually transform

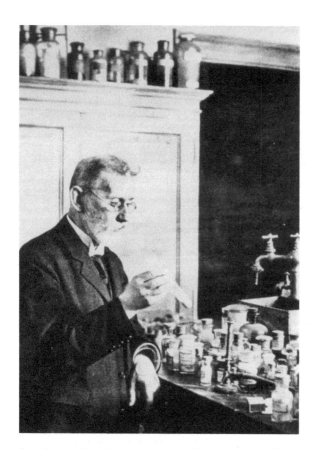

Paul Ehrlich, founder of modern chemotherapy, in his laboratory (courtesy of the National Library of Medicine).

drug therapy. Developments in the medical sciences led to the identification of specific causes for specific diseases and a better understanding of the action of drugs. So, for example, infectious diseases were shown to be caused by specific microorganisms. The cause of diphtheria is the same in everyone who contracts the disease, namely the diphtheria bacillus and the toxin it produces, and generally speaking the same remedy (in this case the diphtheria antitoxin that was developed in the 1890s) is used to treat the disease in each patient. Disease is not due to some general imbalance of the system, to be treated largely by stimulation or depression.

To the extent that space permits, let us briefly review some of these advances in medicine and the consequences for drug therapy. One

of the most important developments in this period was the demonstration that infectious diseases, which had long been the major medical causes of mortality, were caused by specific microorganisms. In the decades of the 1860s through the 1880s, Louis Pasteur in France and Robert Koch in Germany firmly established the germ theory of disease. A whole new science of microbiology grew up as a result of germ theory, and investigators began to isolate the pathogenic organisms that caused infectious diseases. For example, in 1882 Koch isolated the tubercle bacillus and demonstrated that it was the causal organism of tuberculosis.[12]

The science of immunology was another offshoot of the germ theory. Although smallpox inoculation had been practiced for centuries,

6

and Edward Jenner had introduced the safer technique of vaccination into medicine at the end of the eighteenth century, there was no understanding at the time of how immunization worked. Utilizing his knowledge of germ theory, Pasteur was able to develop vaccines against anthrax and rabies in the 1880s. Vaccines against other diseases followed in the ensuing decades. In the last decade of the nineteenth century, Emil von Behring and his colleagues in Germany used immunological principles to develop an antitoxin for the treatment of diphtheria, a major advance in drug therapy. The twentieth century witnessed the development of preventive vaccines against a host of illnesses, such as polio and measles, as well as the eradication of smallpox through a worldwide vaccination campaign.[13]

An understanding of the cause of infectious diseases also led to the development of chemotherapy in the early years of the twentieth century. German-Jewish physician Paul Ehrlich established the principles of the chemotherapy of infectious disease as he sought to discover compounds that would destroy pathogenic microorganisms in the human body without unduly harming the host cells. In 1910, he introduced Salvarsan, a specific chemical agent for the treatment of syphilis and the first synthetic chemical drug that proved efficacious against an infectious disease. Ehrlich was also instrumental, along with Englishman John Newport Langley, in developing the receptor theory of drug action at this time.[14]

The development of organic chemistry in the second half of the nineteenth century had already enabled biomedical researchers to unravel the chemical structure of some drugs, and there had even been some synthesis of new drugs, such as aspirin by the end of the century. Modern experimental pharmacology also was established as a discipline in the late nineteenth century, enabling researchers to better evaluate and understand the physiological action of

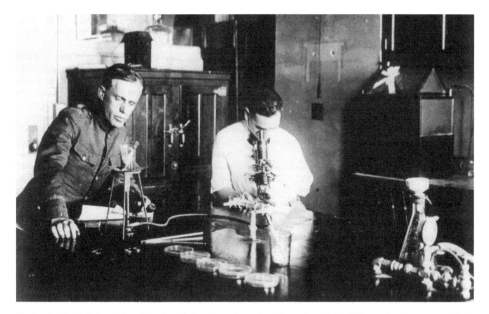

Beginning in the late nineteenth century, laboratory science transformed medicine. These scientists are at work in the Hygienic Laboratory, forerunner of the National Institutes of Health, in the early twentieth century (courtesy of the National Library of Medicine).

drugs. The symbiotic relationship between chemistry and pharmacology also promoted the beginnings of research on the relation between the chemical structure of a molecule and its pharmacological action. This kind of structure-activity thinking had played a crucial role in Ehrlich's work.[15]

In the early decades of the twentieth century, developments in physiology and biochemistry led scientific investigators to become more aware that disease could be caused not only by the presence of something in the body, namely germs, but also by the absence of some vital physiological constituent. Although there were earlier attempts to associate certain diseases with dietary deficiencies and earlier studies on glandular extracts, the concepts of hormones and vitamins did not clearly emerge until this time, when a number of such entities were isolated and used therapeutically. The first hormone to be isolated in a pure form was adrenaline (or epinephrine) in 1901, and the term "hormone" (from the Greek for "I excite") was introduced in 1905. One of the most dramatic examples of hormone therapy was insulin for the treatment of diabetes, introduced by Banting and Best and their colleagues at the University of Toronto in the early 1920s. The term "vitamin" (originally "vitamine") was coined in 1912, and researchers in the United States soon determined that one of these vitamins, what we now call vitamin A, was present in butterfat. Other vitamins were soon discovered and found their way into medical practice for the treatment of dietary deficiency diseases such as scurvy, rickets, and beriberi.[16]

After Ehrlich's success with Salvarsan, there followed a quarter of a century without much further progress in the discovery of drugs to treat infectious diseases. Then in 1935 there was a dramatic breakthrough when Gerhard Domagk in Germany announced that animal studies and clinical tests had demonstrated the curative action of Prontosil, an azo dye containing the sulfonamide group, against streptococcal infections. French scientists soon determined that Prontosil was broken down in the body, and that one of the products, sulfanilamide, was actually the active agent. This discovery paved the way for the synthesis of a whole series of compounds, the so-called "sulfa drugs," which proved efficacious against a variety of serious bacterial diseases.[17]

The sulfas were soon followed by the introduction of a yet more important class of "miracle drugs," the antibiotics. Following up on Alexander Fleming's 1929 paper reporting on the antibacterial effects of an extract from the *Penicillium* mold, Howard Florey, Ernst Chain and their co-workers at Oxford University isolated penicillin in relatively pure form in 1939. Animal tests and clinical trials demonstrated the remarkable efficacy of this drug in the treatment of infectious disease. The urgent need for penicillin for the war effort spurred the development of large-scale manufacturing procedures for the drug, with the United States leading the way. Even before the war had ended, another antibiotic, streptomycin, had been discovered in the laboratory of Selman Waksman at Rutgers University. Streptomycin was especially promising in the treatment of tuberculosis. In the late 1940s, a number of broad spectrum antibiotics were introduced, including chloramphenicol and the tetracyclines. The discovery of penicillin had ushered in the "era of antibiotics," the most useful drugs to date in the fight against infectious disease.[18]

The "era of antibiotics" was soon followed by the "era of psychopharmaceuticals." Although certain drugs, such as opium, had been used for centuries in the effort to treat mental illness, the first significant success in this area came with the introduction of chlorpromazine for the treatment of psychotic patients in 1952. Other psychoactive drugs that proved efficacious in the treatment of the mentally ill soon followed. Today we have a host of compounds, such as the selective serotonin uptake inhibitors, for the treatment of depression, anxiety, bipolar disorder, and other mental health problems.[19]

Heart disease, stroke, and cancer remain major killers in the United States, but there has been significant progress in the development of drug therapies against these diseases as we have increased our understanding of these illnesses. Taxol, for example, has proved efficacious in many cases in the treatment of breast and ovarian cancer. We have drugs available to help control the risk factors for heart disease and stroke, such as blood pressure and blood cholesterol level. Anticoagulants such as coumadin and diuretics such as Lasix are also valuable aids in dealing with cardiovascular illness.

In the limited space available, I have not been able to mention numerous other significant drugs introduced over the past 150 years. Whole categories of drug treatment have been omitted. For example, no mention has been made of the development of drugs that have proved useful in the treatment of asthma, Parkinson's disease, ulcers and other gastrointestinal problems, anemia, and a host of other medical conditions. Nor have I been able to do justice to the advances in our scientific understanding of the physiology and pathology of the human body and the mechanisms of drug action. I have also not discussed the changes that have taken place in our methods for evaluating drugs, especially the development of large-scale clinical trials to provide more reliable statistical evidence about the efficacy and toxicity of drugs. Finally, I have not touched upon some of the negative aspects of drug therapy, such as side effects and the development of drug resistance by microbes. The reader who wishes to learn more about these developments is invited to consult the references listed in the notes section of this paper.[20]

One other point that I would like to emphasize, however, is that while we have moved, in Warner's words, from specificity to universalism in terms of our theories of disease and drug action, we have become more specific with respect to our choice of medicinals to treat a given disease. That is, we do not rely as much on a polypharmaceutical "shotgun" approach, where a prescription might consist of many ingredients, as our predecessors did. Nor do we tend to use a particular remedy to treat a host of different diseases. We rely, as much as possible, on specific remedies for specific diseases, as I indicated above. By and large, these are single-entity remedies rather than combinations of ingredients, and they are generally chemically pure substances rather than plant or animal parts in their natural state. We have, for example, vitamins and hormones to treat specific deficiency diseases, antibiotics to attack specific microbes, and so on. This development has also occurred largely over the past 150 years.

Today we seem to be at the beginning of another new era in drug therapy, brought on by the rise of molecular biology as a result of the discovery of the helical nature of DNA and the breaking of the genetic code. Genetic engineering has allowed us to utilize microorganisms to manufacture drugs, for example, with the use of bacteria to produce human insulin. Our increased understanding of the human genome has opened the possibility of developing specific gene therapies to repair or compensate for genetic defects. Although we have not gone very far down this path yet, the potential for therapeutics is enormous. On the other hand, the ethical issues raised by genetic manipulation are a legitimate cause for concern, but that subject is beyond the scope of my paper.

These remarkable advances in drug therapy, coupled with the automation and large-scale manufacturing associated with industrialization, have had a profound impact on the role of the pharmacist. At the time that the APhA was founded in 1852, most prescriptions still involved more than one ingredient and required some compounding. Over time, the compounding function of the pharmacist has been eroded until it has virtually disappeared. Yet the introduction of all of these new and effective drugs has led to a dramatic increase in the number of prescriptions dispensed, fueling a continuing demand for pharmacists. The scientific complexities associated with modern drug therapy have forced the pharmacist to become more of an expert on the pharmacological action of drugs and the factors that affect such action. The pharmacist's responsibility no longer stops at the point where the patient takes the drug into his or her body. The pharmacy school curriculum of today contains substantial coursework in pharmacology and therapeutics, as well as clinical clerkship experiences. In many ways, the profession is still adjusting to these developments.

A recent publication of the American Chemical Society, entitled *The Pharmaceutical Century: Ten Decades of Drug Discovery*, makes the point that "the preponderance of drug development has taken place since 1900," for since that year "hundreds of drugs ranging from sulfanilamides to AZT have been developed, and many more are in the pipeline." Looking ahead, the publication states: "It appears that

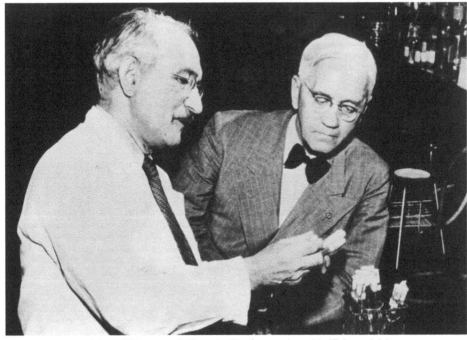

Antibiotic pioneers Selman Waksman and Alexander Fleming are pictured in Waksman's laboratory, in the 1940s.

the future will allow us to rationally attack the medical ills of the world."[21] In a resounding note of optimism, the editors predict:

"But at the rate that our knowledge is compounding, we shall soon know how to stop cancer from spreading, how to start the body's production of insulin, how to stop osteoporosis and grow new bone material, and possibly, how to regenerate the spinal cord."[22]

Given the dramatic developments that we have seen in the field of therapeutics since the APhA was founded in 1852, I hesitate to challenge these bold predictions. We have come a long way in the past 150 years with respect to drug therapy, and yet we still have a long way to go. While I do not want to rain on the parade, I think a note of caution, derived from history, is in order here. Towards the end of the nineteenth century, medical researchers buoyed by recent advances in understanding the relationship between the chemical structure of

drugs and their pharmacological activity got carried away in their enthusiasm for the near-term therapeutic potential of these developments. In lectures delivered in 1877, for example, British physician and pharmacologist Thomas Lauder Brunton expressed his belief that the time might not be far off when scientists would be able to synthesize substances that would act on the body in any given way, thus placing therapeutics on a completely rational basis.[23] In 1889, he reemphasized his hopes for therapeutics when he stated:

"The prospects of therapeutics appears to me very bright . . . .I think it is highly probable that before long we shall have a series of drugs which will stimulate the biliary secretion of the liver or modify its glycogenic function, arranged in order of comparative strength . . . .We may also look for a series of remedies which will modify the circulation by dilating the blood vessels not only temporarily but more or less permanently . . . .We may also, I think, fairly expect to obtain a series of remedies having an action upon the heart and vessels."[24]

In spite of the impressive advances made in drug therapy over the past century or so, we have not yet achieved the lofty goals envisioned by Brunton and some of his contemporaries. We still cannot predict the pharmacological action of any compound with certainty by merely inspecting its structural formula, nor can we yet design drugs at will for specific diseases. As Richard Klausner, former Director of the National Cancer Institute, reminded us in the celebratory publication about the "pharmaceutical century" mentioned above, predicting the future is still a risky business. In his words, with which I will close this paper:

"It's always amazing how, for some things, we dramatically underestimate how far they are in the future, and for other things, we dramatically overestimate them. We're not that bad at predicting things that might be part of the future, but we're really bad at predicting the timing and kinetics and path to them."[25]

Notes and References

1. O. W. Holmes, *Currents and Countercurrents in Medical Science, with Other Addresses and Essays* (Boston: Ticknor and Fields, 1861), p. 39.
2. Charles E. Rosenberg, "The Therapeutic Revolution: Medicine, Meaning, and Social Change in Nineteenth-Century America," in Morris J. Vogel and Charles E. Rosenberg, eds., *The Therapeutic Revolution: Essays in the Social History of Medicine* (Philadelphia: University of Pennsylvania Press, 1979), pp. 3-25 (quotation on p. 3).
3. The list of the top ten prescribed drugs is taken from the following two websites: www.rxlist.com (source: Scott-Levin, Newton, PA) and www.drugsandmeds.com (no source given).
4. John Neill and Francis Gurney Smith, a *Hand-Book of Materia Medica and Therapeutics* (Philadelphia: Blanchard and Lea, 1852).
5. George B. Wood, *A Treatise on Therapeutics and Pharmacology or Materia Medica*, second edition (Philadelphia: J. B. Lippincott, 1860).
6. John Harley Warner, "From Specificity to Universalism: Transformation in the Nineteenth-Century United States," in Yosio Kawakita, Shizu Sakai, and Yasuo Otsuka, eds., *History of Therapeutics: Proceedings of the 10ᵗʰ International Symposium on the History of Medicine—East and West* (Tokyo: Ishiyaku EuroAmerica, 1990), pp. 193-223. See also his *The Therapeutic Perspective: Medical Practice, Knowledge, and Identity in America, 1820-1885* (Cambridge, MA: Harvard University Press, 1986).
7. Warner, "From Specificity" (n. 6), p. 198.
8. *Ibid.*
9. Edward H. Clarke, *The Relation of Drugs to Treatment: An Introductory Lecture Before the Medical Class of Harvard University* (Boston: David Clapp, 1856), pp. 5-6.
10. *Ibid.*, p. 24.
11. Ronald D. Mann, *Modern Drug Use: An Inquiry on Historical Principles* (Lancaster, UK: MTP Press, 1984), p. 485.
12. On Pasteur, see Gerald Geison, *The Private Science of Louis Pasteur* (Princeton, NJ: Princeton University Press, 1995). On Koch, see Thomas D. Brock, *Robert Koch: A life in Medicine and Bacteriology* (Madison, WI: Science Tech Publishers, 1988).
13. On the history of immunology and immunization, see Arthur M. Silverstein, *A History of Immunology* (San Diego: Academic Press, 1989) and H. J. Parish, *A History of Immunization* (Edinburgh: E. & S. Livingstone, 1965).
14. On Ehrlich's chemotherapy and the receptor theory, see John Parascandola, "The Theoretical Basis of Paul Ehrlich's Chemotherapy," *J. Hist. Med.* 36 (1981): 19-43 and John Parascandola and Ronald Jasensky, "Origins of the Receptor Theory of Drug Action," *Bull. Hist. Med.* 48 (1974): 199-220.
15. See John Parascandola, "Structure-Activity Relationships: The Early Mirage," *Pharmacy in History* 13 (1971): 3-10 and John Parascandola, "The Controversy over Structure-Activity Relationships in the Early Twentieth Century," *ibid.* 16 (1974): 54-63.
16. See, e.g., Michael Bliss, *The Discovery of Insulin* (Chicago: University of Chicago Press, 1982) and Kenneth J. Carpenter, *The History of Scurvy and Vitamin C* (Cambridge: Cambridge University Press, 1986).
17. See John E. Lesch, "Chemistry and Biomedicine in an Industrial Setting: The Invention of the Sulfa Drugs," in Seymour H. Mauskopf, ed., *Chemical Sciences in the Modern World* (Philadelphia: University of Pennsylvania Press, 1993), pp. 158-215 and Marcel H. Bickel, "The Development of Sulfonamides (1932-1938) as a Focal Point in the History of Chemotherapy," *Gesnerus* 45 (1988): 67-86.
18. John Parascandola, "The Introduction of Antibiotics into Therapeutics," in Yosio Kawakita, Shizu Sakai, and Yasuo Otsuka, eds., *History of Therapy: Proceedings of the 10ᵗʰ International Symposium on the Comparative History of Medicine—East and West* (Tokyo: Ishiyaku EuroAmerica, 1990).
19. On the beginnings of psychopharmacology, see Judith P. Swazey, *Chlorpromazine in Psychiatry: A Study of Therapeutic Innovation* (Cambridge, MA: MIT Press, 1974) and Anne E. Caldwell, *Origins of Psychopharmacology from CPZ to LSD* (Springfield, IL: Charles C. Thomas, 1970).
20. Two books that give a good overview of the development of modern drug therapy are M. Weatherall, *In Search of a Cure: A History of Pharmaceutical Discovery* (Oxford: Oxford University Press, 1990) and Walter Sneader, *Drug Discovery: The Evolution of Modern Medicines* (Chichester, UK: John Wiley and Sons, 1985).
21. *The Pharmaceutical Century: Ten Decades of Drug Discovery* (Washington, D.C.: American Chemical Society, 2000), p. 7.
22. *Ibid.*, p. 11.
23. T. Lauder Brunton, *Pharmacology and Therapeutics: Gulstonian Lectures for 1877* (London: Macmillan, 1980), pp. 191-196.
24. T. Lauder Brunton, *An Introduction to Modern Therapeutics: Croonian Lectures for 1889* (London: Macmillan, 1892), p. 4.
25. Quoted by Celia M. Henry, "The Next Pharmaceutical Century," in *Pharmaceutical Century* (n. 21), pp. 239-240.

Chaulmoogra Oil and the Treatment of Leprosy

LEPROSY is perhaps the most feared, and the most misunderstood, disease in history. Although we have drugs today to control the disease, and we now know that it is one of the least contagious of the infectious diseases, the stigma attached to leprosy has still not been completely erased from the public mind. The connotations associated with the word leprosy have even led to an effort to rename the condition Hansen's disease, after the man who discovered the bacterial cause of the disease in the nineteenth century. Not surprisingly, many different substances were tried in an effort to treat this disease over the centuries, almost all of them worthless before the introduction of the sulfones in the 1940s. A 1964 monograph on the disease summarized past treatment efforts as follows:

A search of the literature during the past one hundred years or more reveals that almost every type of drug has been used in the attempt to bring about a cure of this disease. Very few remedies advocated during the past thirty or forty years are really new remedies. They have been tried by some workers at one time or another. These remedies include potassium iodide, arsenic, antimony, copper, sera, vaccines, and aniline dyes.[1]

An abridged version of this paper was presented at the annual meeting of the American Institute of the History of Pharmacy in New Orleans, LA, on 30 March 2003.

A quick perusal of the section on treatment in a 1925 book on the disease allows one to add another batch of failed remedies to the above list, including thymol, strychnine, baths of various kinds, X-rays, radium, and electrical currents.[2] The two distinguished authors of this volume then go on to discuss in some detail what they call the "one remedy which has been very generally recognized for many years as of value in leprosy, namely, Chaulmoogra oil."[3]

Chaulmoogra Oil Enters Western Medicine

Chaulmoogra oil entered Western medicine only in the nineteenth century, but it had been used in the East against leprosy and various skin conditions for many hundreds of years. One traditional story concerning the discovery of the use of the oil against leprosy is believed to be based on Burmese folklore. According to this tale, a Burmese prince contracted leprosy and was advised by the gods to withdraw from the world and to go into the forest to meditate. In the woods he was directed by the gods to a tree with a large fruit with many seeds. He was told to eat the seeds, which he did, and was thereupon cured of leprosy.[4] Another version of the origins of the oil attributes the discovery to Rama, who was once king of the Indian city of Benares (now Varanasi) but abdicated his

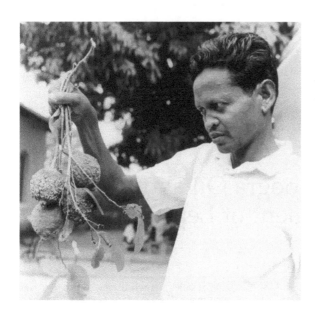

A man holds the fruit of the Chaulmoogra tree. (Photograph courtesy of The Leprosy Mission International.)

throne in favor of his son because he had contracted leprosy. Rama went into isolation in the jungle, where he lived off herbs and roots. He especially ate the fruit and leaves of the *Kalaw* tree, which cured him of leprosy. Next he met a young woman named Piya, who was living in a cave in the jungle. Piya, an Indian princess, had also been banished to the jungle because she had leprosy. Rama cured her of the disease with the *Kalaw*, and took her for his wife. The miraculous *Kalaw* tree, according to the legend, belonged to the genus *Hydnocarpus*, several species of which are the source of chaulmoogra oil.[5]

Whatever we think of this mythical explanation of the origin of the drug, it appears clear that chaulmoogra oil has a long history in Asia. The oil was long used in traditional Ayurvedic medicine in India for the treatment of leprosy and various skin conditions. It seems to also have been used for the treatment of leprosy in other Asian countries such as China and Burma.[6]

The oil was introduced into Western medicine by British physician Frederic John Mouat in 1854. Mouat, who came from a family of army surgeons, took his medical degree at

Edinburgh in 1839. The following year he entered the Indian Medical Service, where he served for 30 years. From 1841 to 1853, Mouat was professor at the Bengal Medical College, and it was during this period that he first became acquainted with chaulmoogra oil. He had an opportunity to try the remedy himself when he became first Physician to the Medical College Hospital in Calcutta in 1853.[7] In an 1854 paper in the *Indian Annals of Medical Science*, he wrote:

It is with considerable reluctance that I venture to submit for consideration of the profession in India, a few remarks upon the Chaulmoogra, as the opportunities which I have hitherto had of employing it are too few and restricted to enable me to recommend it with the confidence that I could wish. Its success was, however, so remarkable and indisputable in one well-marked case of the worst form of leprosy, that I venture to hope an external application of it to that most loathsome and intractable of diseases, may prove so successful, as to secure the general introduction of the remedy.[8]

Mouat notes that the oil comes from the seeds of the fruit of the tree known by the natives as chaulmoogra. The seeds are beat up with a clarified butter into a soft mass which is used in the treatment of cutaneous diseases. The seeds also yield by expression an oil with a peculiar and slightly unpleasant smell and taste. He goes on to say:

It appears to have been long known to, and prized by the Natives in the treatment of leprosy, and few of the faquirs traveling about the country are unacquainted with its properties. I was first informed of its properties by Mr. Jones, the Headmaster of the Hindoo College, a gentleman of eminent acquirements, who brought it to the notice of other practitioners in this city, and at whose recommendation it was tried at the Leper Asylum, with a favorable result.[9]

Mouat decided to try the oil on two cases of leprosy in his ward. He dressed the external ulcers of the patients with the oil, and also gave it to them internally in the form of a pill, made by beating the seeds into a pulp. He reported that the ulcers healed and the patients improved. He believed that the results were sufficiently encouraging to justify further trials.[10] He admitted that the remedy required "much more extended employment before any sound judgement can be framed of its *modus operandi*, and probable value." He added that his main objective in publishing these "crude notes" was to call the remedy to the attention of the profession. The oil was cheap and readily procurable, and might turn out to be efficient in the treatment of a large "and not unimportant class of cases met with in all Indian hospitals." In this connection, he mentioned that he had sent a quantity of the oil to a hospital in China and to a hospital in Mauritius to be tried against leprosy.[11]

Mouat indicates that the remedy and its use in cutaneous diseases was apparently first described by William Roxburgh under the name of *Chaulmoogra odorata*. In 1815, Roxburgh, a surgeon and naturalist, published a catalog of the plants in the East India Company's botanical garden in Calcutta. In this work, he mistakenly identified the seeds of the *Kalaw* tree, which according to the legend discussed above was a cure for leprosy, as those of the tree *Chaulmoogra odorata* under a different name.[12] The tree, indigenous to East India, was also known under the name of *Gynocardia odorata*. Throughout the nineteenth century, *Gynocardia* was believed to be the source of the seeds used to produce chaulmoogra oil. Then in 1901, Sir David Prain identified the true chaulmoogra

seeds of the Calcutta bazaar and of the Paris and London drugs sellers as coming from the tree *Taraktogenos kurzii*, which grows in Burma and Northeast India.[13] It appears that the chaulmoogra oil mentioned in early Ayurvedic texts, and available in South India, was from yet another tree. This tree, known as *Tuvakara* in Sanskrit, is *Hydnocarpus wightiana*, and is called "chaulmugra" in Hindu and Persian. It is a close relative of the *Taraktogenos* tree.[14]

Chaulmoogra oil was reintroduced as a treatment for leprosy in the Madras Leper Hospital in India in 1874. It had apparently been used there in the first half of the nineteenth century, but then abandoned for some reason. Although the oil continued to find some use, especially in India, it was not until the turn of the twentieth century that the remedy began to receive more attention from the medical profession in Europe and the United States.[15]

F. B. Power and the Chemistry of Chaulmoogra

Although there had been some work in the nineteenth century on the chemical constituents of chaulmoogra, the first comprehensive chemical analysis of the remedy was carried out by Frederick B. Power and his colleagues at the Wellcome Chemical Research Laboratories in London in the first decade of the twentieth century. Power had begun his career as a pharmacist, obtaining his pharmacy degree from the Philadelphia College of Pharmacy in 1874. After working for two years in the Philadelphia pharmacy of Edward Parrish, he went to Germany to undertake graduate studies. In 1880, he received his Ph.D. from the University of Strassburg for a thesis in plant chemistry under the direction of the eminent pharmacognosist Friedrich Flückiger. Upon returning to the United States he served for a year as professor of analytical chemistry at the Philadelphia College of Pharmacy before being called to the University of Wisconsin in 1883 to establish a school of pharmacy there.

Power served for ten years as head of the pharmacy program at Wisconsin, placing the new school on a sound scientific footing and establishing a tradition of research. He left Madison in 1892 to become scientific director of the newly-established laboratories of Fritzsche

Brothers of New Jersey, a firm devoted to the production of essential oils and fine organic chemicals. Over the next few years he published a series of important chemical studies on essential oils such as those of peppermint, cloves, bay, and wintergreen. Tragedy struck in late 1894 when Power's wife died after the birth of their third child, a son who himself lived for only a few days.[16]

Soon thereafter, Power's old friend and pharmacy school classmate, Henry Wellcome, contacted Power and offered him a job. Wellcome had left the United States in 1880 to partner with fellow American Silas Burroughs in founding the pharmaceutical firm Burroughs Wellcome and Company in London. After the death of Burroughs in 1895, Wellcome became the sole proprietor of the firm. Wellcome had always been more interested in scientific and medical research then his partner, and already in 1894 he had established the Wellcome Physiological Laboratories. Anxious to expand into chemical studies, Wellcome convinced Power to join the firm in 1896 to direct the newly-established Wellcome Chemical Research Laboratories.[17]

In London, Power continued his researches in plant chemistry. In 1904, Power obtained a large quantity of fresh chaulmoogra seeds from a London market and decided to make a complete investigation of the seeds. He identified the seeds as coming from the *Taraktogenos kurzii*. The shells were separated from the seeds, and the kernels were then subjected to hydraulic pressure yielding an oil. A residual "press-cake" was left behind. Each of the three components into which the seeds had been separated, the shells, the oil, and the "press-cake" made up about a third of the overall weight of the seeds.

Power and his colleagues subjected the oil and the press-cake to further chemical procedures, and isolated a number of compounds from these products. One of these was a new unsaturated fatty acid, isolated from the oil, which they named chaulmoogric acid. The acid was shown to have the formula $C_{18}H_{32}O_2$.[18]

The Wellcome investigators next turned their attention to two species of the *Hydnocarpus* tree which belonged to the same natural order as *Taraktogenos*, and which had also been long used in Western India and China for the same purposes for which chaulmoogra oil was employed. These species were *Hydnocarpus Wightiana*, mentioned above, and *Hydnocarpus anthelmintica*.

From the seeds of these trees, Power and his colleagues isolated fatty oils that were very similar in physical characteristics and chemical composition to chaulmoogra oil. When they subjected the oils from these two trees to further chemical analysis, they obtained chaulmoogric acid and a lower homologue of the same series. The new acid had the formula $C_{16}H_{28}O_2$ and was named hydnocarpus acid.[19] Power's laboratory also went on to investigate the seeds of *Gynocardia odorata*, which (as mentioned above) had long been erroneously believed to be the source of the chaulmoogra oil of commerce. The Wellcome group was able to clearly demonstrate that the oil from this tree was not chaulmoogric oil and contained neither chaulmoogric nor hydnocarpus acids.[20]

Power's group had thus established that two species of *Hydnocarpus* are sources of chaulmoogra oil, in addition to the *Taraktogenos* (later called *Hydnocarpus kurzii*) tree. They found that the oil from all three of these species yields two significant acids, which they named chaulmoogric acid and hydnocarpus acid, and they determined the chemical composition of these acids. They also confirmed that *Gynocardia odorata* was not a source of the oil. The two fatty acids and their derivatives were to come to play a significant role in the treatment of leprosy over the next few decades, and so their isolation and the determination of their chemical formulae were important contributions.

The Administration of Chaulmoogra

The question of the best form in which to administer chaulmoogra oil and its derivatives was one that troubled physicians who treated leprosy for some time. Originally the oil was either applied topically to leprous areas on the body or taken internally. External application had only limited value in treating the disease. Although oral administration of the remedy was more effective, this procedure was complicated by the fact that effective does of the oil tended to have a very nauseating effect on the patient. The effectiveness of the drug was limited by the digestive tolerance of the patient.[21] As one U. S. Public Health Service doctor reported in his autobiography, many patients would tell him, "Doctor, I'd rather have leprosy than take another dose."[22]

At the Louisiana Leper Home in Carville, Louisiana, the use of orally-administered chaulmoogra oil, in the form of drops, was begun in 1901 by Isadore Dyer.[23] In 1916, the attending physician at the Home, Ralph Hopkins, reported on the results of 170 patients treated with chaulmoogra oil. He divided these patients into two categories, incipient cases and advanced cases. With the 82 incipient cases, Hopkins reported results as follows: 17% discharged cured; 4% lesions disappeared; 24%

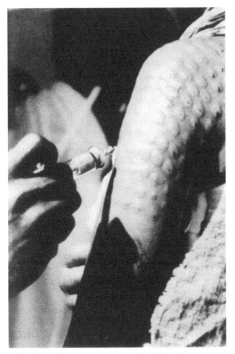

Administering chaulmoogra oil by injection. (Photograph courtesy of The Leprosy Mission International.)

improved and remaining at the Home; 24% absconded in improved condition; 8% worse; and 4% died. His results were less favorable with the advanced cases, where there were no cures and only about a quarter of the patients showed improvement or arrest.[24]

In the last decade of the nineteenth century, some clinicians began experimenting with the administration of the oil by intramuscular or subcutaneous injections. This method eliminated the nausea caused by oral administration of the drug, but could be very painful. The injections often produced severe local reactions and fever. In the early years of the twentieth century, a physician of the United States Public Health Service, Victor Heiser, found a way to diminish the pain and irritation caused by injection, as well as to secure greater absorption of the oil.[25]

Heiser was a career Public Health Service Officer who was serving as the Chief Quarantine Officer and Director of Health for the Philippine Island at the time of this work. Chaulmoogra oil had been used at the San Lazaro Hospital for lepers in Manila since the early years of the American occupation of the Philippines, but with limited success. In 1908, Heiser visited the Louisiana Leper Home and gained a favorable impression of the treatment of leprosy with chaulmoogra oil that was being carried out there. From Ralph Hopkins and Isador Dyer, Heiser learned better techniques for the oral administration of the oil. Upon his return to the Philippines, he arranged for the Louisiana method to be given a thorough trial at the San Lazaro Hospital in Manila under the immediate charge of the house physician, Elidoro Mercado.

The new method, which was initiated at San Lazaro in 1909, was much more successful than the former one, but still oral administration of the oil resulted in nausea and patient resistance to taking the drug. The physicians tried various methods to solve this problem, such as coating the chaulmoogra capsules with various substances and giving the oil by enema, but the results were unsuccessful. A review of the literature revealed that some physicians had tried hypodermic injection. So the hypodermic method was tried at San Lazaro, but it did not work well because the oil was not satisfactorily absorbed. Heiser then wrote to Merck and

Company in Germany to ask if they could suggest a substance that might increase the absorption of the oil when injected. The company replied that it had no definite knowledge on the subject, but that theoretically the addition of camphor or ether might have the desired result.[26]

Heiser and Mercado decided to add camphor to a prescription of chaulmoogra and resorcin which was typically given orally. To their great joy they found that the camphor-resorcin solution of chaulmoogra was readily absorbed.[27] Heiser wrote in his autobiography years later about the excitement of the first case treated:

Few can imagine with what a thrill we watched the first case to which chaulmoogra was administered in hypodermic form, how we watched for the first faint suspicion of eyebrows beginning to grow in again and sensation returning to paralyzed areas. We took photographs at frequent and regular intervals to compare progress and to check on our observations, fearing our imagination might be playing tricks upon us.[28]

Heiser published an account of the first two cases in *Public Health Reports* in 1913. These two patients had apparently been cured of the disease, i.e., leprosy bacilli were no longer found on clinical and microscopical examination, and were both released on probation. Because these patients were treated with a vaccine as well as the chaulmoogra oil, the results were compromised.[29] The following year, Heiser published an account of two more cases who had been successfully treated with chaulmoogra oil by hypodermic injection and released, and this time there was no other treatment given so that the results were clear.[30] In a supplement to the 1914 volume of *Public Health Reports*, Heiser reported on twelve more cases. The results were encouraging, but not definitive. Three of the patients stopped the treatment before any improvement could be seen. Of the remaining nine patients, one was considered microscopically negative and cured, four had progressed to the point where clinical evidence of the disease had practically disappeared, three showed marked improvement, and one showed only slight evidence of improvement.[31] Heiser concluded:

The present stage of development of the treatment herein described does not warrant a claim that anything like a specific for leprosy has been found, but experience does show that it gives more consistently favorable results than any other that has come to our attention, and it holds out the hope that further improvement may be brought about. It produces apparent cures in some cases, causes great improvement in many others, and arrests the progress of the disease in almost every instance.[32]

However, Heiser later stated that he was not completely satisfied with the continuing results. He thought that the treatment was too slow, and he admitted that "after the first flush of excitement, the interest of doctors, nurses, and patients all began to wane." The Public Health Service doctor recognized the need for a more effective cure.[33]

In 1915 Heiser visited Calcutta, India and met Sir Leonard Rogers of the Indian Medical Service. Heiser told Rogers about his results with chaulmoogra oil, and learned that one of Rogers' patients had nearly recovered from leprosy when treated with large does of gynocardic acid (a mixture of fatty acids from chaulmoogra oil). The acid seemed to be better tolerated by patients and more efficient than the oil itself. Rogers was apparently contemplating retiring and returning to England, but Heiser convinced him to remain in India and continue his work with chaulmoogra.[34] Rogers later recalled the next steps:

With the help of the Medical College Professor of Chemistry, Dr. Chuni Lal Bose, the soluble sodium salt or soap of gynocardic acid was made, which was easily soluble in water. From July 31, 1915 onwards, it was injected subcutaneously in a 3 per cent solution in leprosy patients with only slight local induration and pain. . . . By the end of the year I had satisfied myself that a definite advance had been made.

Progress was still slow and rather painful, so I next ascertained by means of a few painless animal experiments that sodium gynocardate could safely be injected intravenously (1916). It soon became apparent that by this route the drug was also more effective, so that a further advance had been made.[35]

Heiser claimed that on a visit to Hawaii, he alerted the authorities at the leper colony on Molakai to the work done in India, and suggested that they follow up on this research in the laboratory.[36] Whether or not it was actually Heiser who stimulated the effort, research on the treatment of leprosy with chaulmoogra derivatives was undertaken in Hawaii at about this time.

The sequence of events leading to the next development in the chaulmoogra story, namely the introduction of ethyl esters derived from the oil, is not entirely clear. It appears, however, that the work was begun by a young African-American woman named Alice Ball at the suggestion of Dr. Harry Hollmann, who was an Acting Assistant Surgeon at the Leprosy Investigation Station of the U. S. Public Health Service in Hawaii. It is possible that Hollmann learned of the work done in India through his Public Health Service colleague Victor Heiser, whether on his visit to Hawaii (the date of which is not known) or via some other contact.

Alice Ball was the first woman to earn a masters degree in science from the College of Hawaii in 1915, for a thesis dealing with the chemical constituents of *Piper methysticum*. She was then appointed to teach chemistry at the College of Hawaii. Either during her graduate work or shortly thereafter, she took up Hollmann's suggestion to experiment with the chemistry of chaulmoogra oil. Ball unfortunately became ill and died at the young age of 24 on December 31, 1916. Her work on chaulmoogra was then taken up by her supervisor, Arthur Dean, head of the College of Hawaii's chemistry department (and later the College's President).[37]

Since Ball did not have an opportunity to publish any of her research, it is not certain exactly how far she got on the problem. Dean and his coauthors do not credit Ball for any of the work that they reported in a series of publications on chaulmoogra between 1920 and 1922, but in an article in a medical journal in 1922, Hollmann clearly gives her credit for the discovery.

About the time that Rogers and Ghosh were starting their investigations in India, in Hawaii I interested Miss Alice Ball, M.S., an instructress in chemistry at the College of Hawaii in the chemical problem of obtaining for me the active agents in the oil of chaulmoogra.

After a great amount of experimental work, Miss Ball solved the problem for me by making the ethyl esters of the fatty acids found in chaulmoogra oil, employing the technic herewith described.[38]

Hollmann then goes on to describe the preparation of the esters by "Ball's Method." Stan Ali has led an effort in Hawaii to gain recognition for Ball for this work, and a plaque in her honor was placed on the campus of the University of Hawaii-Manoa in 2000 commemorating her work on chaulmoogra.[39] Nevertheless it was Dean and his co-workers who published on the subject and received credit for the work. They reported that they had investigated the fatty acids of chaulmoogra oil with the intent of trying to find a suitable form of the material for injection which would allow rapid absorption into the circulation. They stated that they found that the ethyl esters of the acids were thin fluid oils that lent themselves readily to intramuscular injections and were readily absorbed. They also described their methods for preparing the esters.[40] The ethyl esters came to be referred to as Dean's derivatives.[41]

Clinical trials were then carried out by Dean with the collaboration of J. T. McDonald, Director of the Public Health Service Leprosy Investigation Station and Superintending Physician to Kalihi Hospital in Honolulu. The esters were given in conjunction with other means of treatment, such as iodine, but eventually were given by themselves.[42] The results were encouraging, with 94 patients being "paroled" from the hospital in fiscal year 1921, although it was recognized that follow-up of these patients would be necessary to insure that the improvement was permanent rather than temporary. In the 1921 annual report of the Public Health Service, the report on the leprosy work in Hawaii stated that:

A few paroled patients going to their homes and describing the therapeutic and administrative methods of the station, has had a greater effect in inducing sufferers from leprosy to seek treatment than all the legal requirements or scientific discussions that can be invoked.

The morale of the patients in the hospital is excellent and in striking contrast to that of former days, when a leprous person was doomed to a long term of isolation, in most cases to be terminated only by death. All patients are zealously cooperating with the authorities of the hospital, intent upon becoming free of their afflictions and returning to their homes as useful members of society.[43]

The report went on to indicate that chaulmoogra oil derivatives (presumably the esters of the fatty acids) were being furnished by the Public Health Service to medical authorities in

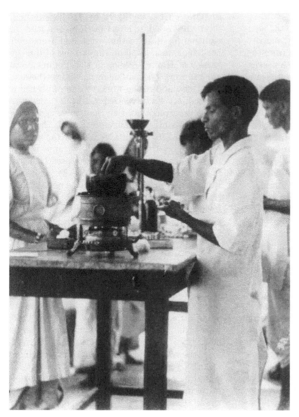

Preparing chaulmoogra oil, 1928 (courtesy of The Leprosy Mission International).

a variety of counties, from Bombay to China to Ecuador.

Hunting the Chaulmoogra Tree

As the use of chaulmoogra oil and its derivatives became more widespread, the demand for the oil increased. Concern about having an adequate supply of the oil led David Fairchild, head of the Division of Foreign Seed and Plant Introduction, Bureau of Plant Industry, U. S. Department of Agriculture to take action to prevent a shortage. For assistance, Fairchild turned to Joseph Rock, Professor of Systematic Botany at the College of Hawaii. Rock described his mission and the reasons for it as follows:

Owing to the high price of the oil on the United States and the probable scarcity of it in the near future, due to is successful application in the treatment of leprosy in Hawaii, I was authorized by the U. S. Department of Agriculture to obtain seeds of this species, to be introduced into Hawaii and our tropical possessions, with a view to establishing Chaulmoogra plantations.[44]

Rock was born in Vienna, Austria, in 1884. From early on he showed an interest in foreign lands and languages, and learned Arabic and Chinese while still a boy. After he graduated from the University of Vienna, he wandered around Europe for a time. In 1905, he traveled to the United States, settling briefly in New York. His health then forced him to seek a warmer and drier climate, so he soon moved to Texas, where he undertook further university studies to improve his English. In 1913, he became an American citizen.

Meanwhile, Rock had moved to Hawaii in 1907, where he taught school for a time. The following year he joined the Division of Forestry of the Board of Commissioners of Agriculture and Forestry for the Territory of Hawaii. Rock joined the faculty of the College of Hawaii and was placed in charge of its herbarium in 1911. Over the next few years he traveled to various parts of the world, collecting seeds and plants.[45]

Rock had always had a desire to travel in the Orient, and he got his opportunity when the Department of Agriculture asked him to go to Indo-China, Siam, Burma, and India to find seeds of the chaulmoogra tree. He first came across a genuine chaulmoogra tree in Burma, but it was not in fruit, so he could not collect any seeds. With the help of local villagers, he was finally led to a nearby forest with many chaulmoogra trees bearing fruit, and he was able to collect a large number of seeds. The seeds were then shipped to the United States, and eventually used to establish a plantation of 2,980 trees on the island of Oahu, Hawaii, in 1921-1922.[46]

The Fall Of Chaulmoogra

Chaulmoogra oil probably reached its height of popularity as a treatment of leprosy in the 1920s and 1930s. The oil, or perhaps more commonly the esters of its acids, had become the treatment of choice at facilities such as the Public Health Service leprosy hospital at Carville, LA, which had taken over the Louisiana Leper Home in 1921. Stanley Stein, who had entered the Carville hospital as a patient in 1931, recalled taking the oil for years without being cured of the disease, although he believed that it had once cleared up a cluster of nodules on his temple. He wrote of his experiences with the drug at Carville at follows:

Whether I was to take the oil externally, internally, or—as someone once said—eternally, was up to me. The oral doses were nauseously given out in the cafeteria at mealtime. The injections were administered in what to me was a distressingly public manner . . . the after effects were sometimes frightful—painful suppurating abscesses which would generate in the patient's backside. . . . I was hospitalized several times with chaulmoogra-induced, rear end ulceration.[47]

Even given the advances that had been

made with chaulmoogra, it was obviously not an ideal treatment for leprosy. Side effects still created problems, treatment was extended, and there was disagreement about how effective it really was. Although there were numerous reports in the literature about the drug's efficacy and many physicians swore by it, others were

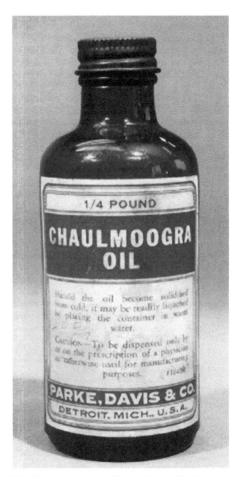

A bottle of chaulmoogra oil manufactured by Parke, Davis (from the G. W. Aimar Collection of the National Museum of American History, Smithsonian Institution).

skeptical about the therapeutic claims made for the drug. Then Director of the National Institute (later Institutes) of Health George McCoy, who had once headed the Leprosy Investigation Station in Hawaii and supported the use of chaulmoogra, had by 1942 come to doubt its therapeutic value. He published an attack on the drug in that year, noting that many experienced students of the disease expressed serious doubts about the value of the oil in treating leprosy, especially when discussing the subject in private. He quoted (anonymously) the views of four experts in leprosy whom he had consulted, all of them critical about the effectiveness of the drug.[48]

The downfall of chaulmoogra came about through the introduction of the sulfones to treat leprosy in the 1940s. Public Health Service Officer Guy Faget, Medical Director of the Carville hospital, was able to demonstrate through clinical trials the effectiveness of sulfone drugs against the disease. In 1947, chaulmoogra oil therapy was officially abandoned at Carville, and the sulfones became the treatment of choice. The sulfones also eventually led to a change of policy from one of isolation of leprosy victims to one of outpatient treatment with drugs. As early as 1948, the Carville hospital began to allow, under certain conditions, the medical discharge of patients who were still in the so-called "communicable state" (i.e., who were not bacteriologically negative).[49] As for chaulmoogra oil, by the 1950s it had essentially become just a colorful relic of pharmacy's past.

Notes and References

1. R. G. Cochrane and T. Frank Davey, *Leprosy in Theory and Practice*, second edition (Bristol: John Wiley & Sons, 1964), p. 374.
2. Leonard Rogers and Ernest Muir, *Leprosy* (Bristol: John Wright & Sons, 1925), pp. 245-254.
3. *Ibid.*, p. 254.
4. Cochrane and Davey, *Leprosy* (n. 1), p. 374.
5. O. K. Skinsnes, "Origin of Chaulmoogra Oil—Another Version," *Int. J. Leprosy* 40 (1972): 172-173.
6. Jane Buckingham, *Leprosy in Colonial South India: Medicine and Confinement* (Houndmills, UK: Palgrave, 2002), pp. 91-92; J. C. Ghosh, *A Monograph on Chaulmoogra Oil and Its Use in the Treatment of Leprosy as Explained in Ayurveda* (Madras, 1917), reprinted in J. C. Ghosh, *New Industries, With Numerous Suggestions Intended for Educationists and Capitalists Throughout India* (Calcutta: Butterworth, 1919);

Norman Taylor, *Plant Drugs That Changed the World* (New York: Dodd, Mead: 1965), pp. 219-227; Scott A. Norton, "Useful Plants of Dermatology. I. *Hydnocarpus* and Chaulmoogra," *J. A. Acad. Dermatol.* 31 (1994): 683-686.
7. On Mouat, see Donald McDonald, *Surgeons Two and a Barber: Being Some Account of the Life and Work of the Indian Medical Service (1600-1947)* (London: William Heinemann, 1950), p. 145; biographical sketch of Frederic John Mouat in Appendix A of "Lonely Islands: The Andamanese," an online documentation by George Weber (URL = andaman.org/book/app-a/a-mouat.htm).
8. F. J. Mouat, "Notes on Native Remedies. No. 1. The Chaulmoogra," *Indian Ann. Med. Sci.* 1 (1854): 646-652, p. 646.
9. Mouat, "Notes on Native Remedies" (n. 8), p. 648.
10. Mouat, "Notes on Native Remedies" (n. 8), pp. 648-651.
11. Mouat, "Notes on Native Remedies" (n. 8), pp. 651-652.
12. Mouat, "Notes on Native Remedies" (n. 8), p. 647; Buckingham, *Leprosy* (n. 6), pp. 91-92.
13. Rogers and Muir, *Leprosy* (n. 2), p. 254.; Buckingham, *Leprosy* (n. 6), p. 92.
14. Buckingham, *Leprosy* (n. 6), p. 92.
15. Buckingham, *Leprosy* (n. 6), pp. 93-94.
16. For biographical information on Power, see John Parascandola, "Frederick Belding Power," *Dict. Sci. Biog.* XI (1975): 120-121; Max Phillips, "Frederick Belding Power, Most Distinguished American Phytochemist," *J. Chem. Ed.* 31(1954): 258-261.
17. On Wellcome and his company, see Robert Rhodes James, *Henry Wellcome* (London: Hodder and Stoughton, 1994).
18. Frederick Belding Power and Frank Howorth Gornall, "The Constituents of Chaulmoogra Seeds," *J. Chem. Soc.* 85 (1904): 838-851.
19. Frederick Belding Power and Marmaduke Barrowcliff, "The Constituents of the Seeds of Hydnocarpus Wightiana and of Hydnocarpus Anthelmintica. Isolation of a Homologue of Chaulmoogric Acid," *J. Chem. Soc.* 87 (1905): 884-896.
20. Frederick Belding Power and Marmaduke Barrowcliff, "The Constituents of the Seeds of Gynocardia Odorata," *J. Chem. Soc.* 87 (1905): 897-900.
21. Rogers and Muir, *Leprosy* (n. 2), p. 254; Ernest Muir, *Handbook on Leprosy: Its Diagnosis, Treatment and Prevention* (Cuttack: R. J. Grundy, 1921), p. 41.
22. Victor Heiser, *An American Doctor's Odyssey: Adventures in Forty-five Countries* (New York: W. W. Norton, 1936), p. 250.
23. Isadore Dyer, "The Cure of Leprosy," *Medical News* 87 (1905): 199-206. See also Rogers and Muir, *Leprosy*, p. 254.
24. Ralph Hopkins, "Observations on the Treatment of Leprosy with Special Reference to Chaulmoogra Oil," *New Orleans Med. Surg. J.* 69 (1916-1917): 223-232.
25. Rogers and Muir, *Leprosy* (n. 2), p. 255.
26. Heiser, *American*, pp. 250-251; Victor Heiser, "Leprosy. Its Treatment in the Philippine Islands By the Hypodermic Use of a Chaulmoogra Oil Mixture," Supplement No. 20 to *Pub. Health Rep.*, volume 29, 1914, p. 23. Excerpt of this supplement were also published in *Pub. Health Rep.* 29 (1914): 2763-2767 because of the "general interest" of the conclusions.
27. Heiser, *American* (n. 22), p. 250.
28. Heiser, *American* (n. 22), p. 251.
29. Victor Heiser, "Leprosy. A Note Regarding the Apparent Cure of Two Lepers in Manila," *Pub. Health Rep.* 28 (1913): 1855-1856.
30. Victor Heiser, "Leprosy. Treatment of Two Cases with Apparent Cure," *Pub. Health Rep.* 29 (1914): 21-22.

31. Heiser, "Leprosy. Its Treatment in the Philippines" (n. 30). There appears to be an error in the statistical summary on p. 22, but the net results shown in percentage terms and a review of the 12 individual cases confirms the figures I have given.

32. Heiser, "Leprosy. Its Treatment in the Philippines" (n. 30), p. 25.

33. Heiser, *American*, p. 251.

34. *Ibid.*, p. 251; Leonard Rogers, *Happy Toil: Fifty-Five Years of Tropical Medicine* (London: Frederick Muller, 1950), pp. 189-193; lecture by Leonard Rogers as quoted in Frank Oldrieve, *India's Lepers: How to Rid India of Leprosy* (London: Marshall Brothers, 1924), pp. 77-78.

35. Rogers, *Happy Toil*, pp. 190-191.

36. Heiser, *American* (n. 22), pp. 251-252.

37. Charles J. Dutton, *The Samaritans of Molokai: The Lives of Father Damien and Brother Dutton Among the Lepers* (New York: Dodd, Mead, 1932), p. 231; Susan Kreifels, "Alice Ball Made a Stunning Find in Her Early 20s," *Honolulu Star-Bulletin*, February 18, 2000; Susan Kreifels, "Ground Breaking African-American UH Chemist Finally Recognized," *Honolulu Star-Bulletin*, March 1, 2000. The *Star-Bulletin* is online at starbulletin.com. See also n. 36.

38. Harry T. Hollmann, "The Fatty Acids of Chaulmoogra Oil in the Treatment of Leprosy and Other Diseases," *Arch. Dermatol. Syph.* 5 (1922): 94-101, p. 95. I am grateful to Margaret Brynes and Karen Sinkule of the National Library of Medicine for assistance in locating the journal volume and obtaining a copy of this article for me when the volume had been removed from the shelves for microfilming.

39. Kreifels, "Ground Breaking" (n. 37).

40. See, for example, Arthur L Dean and Richard Wrenshall, "Fractionation of Chaulmoogra Oil," *J. Amer. Chem. Soc.* 42 (1920): 2626-2645; Arthur L. Dean and Richard Wrenshall, "Fractionation of Chaulmoogra Oil," *Pub. Health Rep.* 36 (1921): 641-660; Arthur L. Dean and Richard Wrenshall, "Preparation of Chaulmoogra Oil Derivatives for the Treatment of Leprosy," *Pub. Health Rep.* 37 (1922): 1395-1399.

41. See, for example, G. L. Hagman, "On the Treatment of Leprosy with Dean's Derivatives of Chaulmoogra Oil," *China Med. J.* 37 (1923): 568-571; J. T. McDonald, "Treatment of Leprosy with the Dean Derivatives of Chaulmoogra Oil," *J. Amer. Med. Assoc.* 75 (1920): 1483-1487.

42. J. T. McDonald and A. L. Dean, "The Treatment of Leprosy. With Especial Reference to Some New Chaulmoogra Oil Derivatives," *Pub. Health Rep.* 35 (1920): 1959-1974; J. T. McDonald and A. L. Dean, "The Constituents of Chaulmoogra Oil Effective in Leprosy," *J. Amer. Med. Assoc.* 76 (1921): 1470-1474.

43. *Annual Report of the Surgeon General of the Public Health Service of the United States*, 1921, p. 79. For further information on the Public Health Service leprosy investigations in Hawaii, see O. A. Bushnell, "The United States Leprosy Investigation Station as Kalawao," *Hawaiian J. Hist.* 2 (1968): 76-94; Jerrold M. Michael, "The Public Health Service Leprosy Investigation Station on Molokai, Hawaii, 1909-13 - An Opportunity Lost," *Pub. Health Rep.* 95 (1980): 203-209.

44. J. F. Rock, "Hunting the Chaulmoogra Tree," *Nat. Geog.* 41 (1922): 242-276, p. 242.

45. For biographical information on Rock, see Alvin K. Chock, "Joseph F. Rock, 1884-1962," *Amer. Horticul. Mag.* 42 (1963): 158-167; Mike Edwards, "Our Man in China: Joseph Rock," *Nat. Geog.* 191 (1997): 65-81.

46. Rock, "Hunting" (n. 44); Chock, "Rock" (n. 45), p. 162. See also Norman Taylor, *Plant Drugs that Changed the World* (Dodd, Mead: 1965), pp. 219-227.

47. Stanley Stein (with Lawrence G. Blochman), *Alone No Longer: The Story of a Man who Refused to Be One of the Living Dead* (New York: Funk and Wagnalls, 1963), pp. 38-39.

48. G. W. McCoy, "Chaulmoogra Oil in the Treatment of Leprosy," *Pub. Health Rep.* 57 (1942): 1727-1733.

49. For the story of the discovery of the sulfones, see John Parascandola, "Miracle at Carville: The Introduction of the Sulfones for the Treatment of Leprosy," *Pharm. Hist.* 40 (1998): 59-66.

From Mercury to Miracle Drugs: Syphilis Therapy over the Centuries

SHORTLY after Columbus had arrived in the New World, as the fifteenth century drew to a close, a terrible new disease which we now call syphilis appeared in Europe. A controversy developed over whether or not the disease had been imported to Europe from the Americas, beginning with Columbus and his crew, or had existed in Europe earlier, perhaps in a different form. The question of the origin of syphilis is still not firmly resolved today, as there is evidence both for and against the American origin theory. The venereal nature of syphilis was recognized relatively early.

Once the venereal nature of syphilis was understood, people could be (and were) warned against having intimate relations with individuals who were infected, assuming they could identify the infected. But once one had contracted the disease, what remedies were available to alleviate, if not cure, the malady? Some of those who believed that the pox was the just rewards of immoral behavior questioned whether or not those afflicted with the disease even deserved to be treated.[1]

An earlier version of this paper was delivered as a plenary lecture at the 38th International Congress for the History of Pharmacy, Seville, Spain, September 19–22, 2007.

Not surprisingly, when this terrible new disease first appeared, all sorts of remedies were recommended for dealing with it. For example, Torella advised such strange treatments as applying a cock or pigeon flayed alive, or a live frog cut in two, to an infected penis.[2] A major aim of most treatment was to remove the morbid matter causing the disease from the patient. This could be done in various ways, for example, by blood-letting or the use of laxatives. An alternative method involved having the patient bathe in a mixture of wine and herbs, or in olive oil. Syphilitics could also be placed in an enclosed heated space, causing them to sweat, another mechanism for eliminating corrupt matter from the body.[3]

The two remedies that eventually came to be by far the most popular, however, were mercury and guaiacum. Mercury had long been used, especially by the Arabs, in the treatment of skin diseases and even leprosy. Therefore it seemed reasonable to try it against syphilis, which generally involved skin lesions and was thought to resemble leprosy. Numerous physicians in the early sixteenth century advocated the use of mercury in the forms of ointments or rubs. Even anti-venereal underpants, coated on the inside with a mercurial ointment, were available in Italy. It was recognized, however, that excess mercury could be harmful. Overdosing with mercury could lead to such toxic side effects as shaking, paralysis, and the loosening and loss of teeth. Sometimes the mercury was applied to the body and the patient was then placed in a heated area for long periods of time. This introduced the possibility of mercury vapors entering the respiratory tract, which could be very dangerous.[4]

At first mercury was only given externally, for example, in the form of an ointment. The internal administration of mercury seemed to be too dangerous. At the end of the eighteenth century, however, the internal administration of mercury began to overtake the external methods. The mercury could be administered in the form of enemas, or taken orally in a gum form or as calomel (the salt mercurous chloride). Van Swieten's liquor, consisting of grains of corrosive sublimate (mercuric chloride) dissolved in a solution of water and alcohol, became popular in the late eighteenth century. Mercury poisoning was probably not uncommon, but side effects that were probably due to the treatment were often attributed to the disease itself. Mercury remained the preferred treatment for syphilis up into the twentieth century.[5]

The principal challenger to mercury in the early history of syphilis was guaiacum (or guaiac) wood. The guaiacum tree was native to the Indies, and the Spanish and the Portuguese began using the wood to treat syphilis by the early fifteenth century. At the time, it was widely believed that God often placed remedies for a disease in the areas where that disease flourished. Since many Europeans began to ascribe the origins of syphilis to the Americas, it did not seem unreasonable that a cure for the disease might exist in that part of the world.[6]

The wood was administered by grinding it into a powder and then boiling it in water. The resulting decoction (the liquid remaining when the wood is removed) was then ingested by the patient. But typically treatment with guaiacum involved much more than simply drinking a decoction made from the wood. The patient was generally placed in a warm room and put on a strict diet with limited food intake. He or she was also given mild laxatives. The patient then drank a large dose of the decoction daily, after which he or she was wrapped in blankets to induce sweating. This regimen was carried out for thirty days, and was undoubtedly quite debilitat-

ing to the patient. A 1519 book by the German humanist and religious reformer Ulrich von Hutten on guaiacum, which was translated into several languages, helped to popularize the drug. Hutten himself suffered from syphilis and was convinced that he had been cured by guaiacum (although he appears to have eventually died of syphilis). As someone who was opposed to the medical establishment, he was delighted to recommend an empirical remedy that came from a "barbarian" land with no doctors.[7]

Historian Sheldon Watts has suggested that the Spaniard Oviedo, who was the first to ascribe the origins of syphilis to the New World in his 1526 book about the Indies, helped to popularize guaiacum for financial reasons. While in the Indies, Oviedo learned that the wood was a reputed cure for syphilis. According to Watts, Oviedo knew that the public accepted the doctrine that for every disease or poison God had placed a cure nearby, and so he claimed that

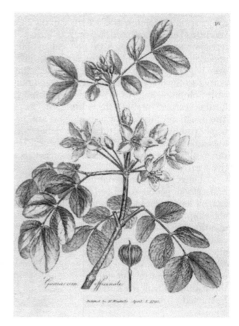

Guaiacum. From William Woodville, Medical Botany, *volume 1 (London, 1790). Courtesy of the National Library of Medicine.*

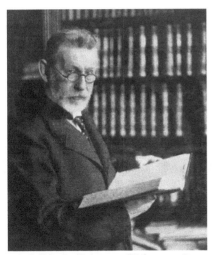

Paul Ehrlich, the discoverer of Salvarsan. Courtesy of the National Library of Medicine.

the people of the Indies had long suffered from syphilis but were able to cure the disease with guaiacum. He arranged for his partners, the Fugger family of bankers, to obtain monopoly rights from the King of Spain to import and market the wood throughout the Spanish Empire. This arrangement resulted in handsome profits for Oviedo and the Fuggers.[8]

Mercury and guaiacum were also not infrequently used together in the treatment of syphilitics by doctors anxious to cover all bases. In the sixteenth century, the efficacy of guaiacum was challenged by Paracelsus, and its use began to progressively decline. Sometimes it was replaced by other woods and roots, included sarsaparilla, another American import. Mercury temporarily lost some of its credibility around the beginning of the nineteenth century, but made a comeback by the 1860s. Although there were certain new treatments that were employed in the nineteenth century, such as potassium iodide and certain preparations of arsenic, Quétel has concluded that other forms of treatment had a hard time competing with mercury. Mercury remained king in the treatment of syphilis until the twentieth century, although it left much to be desired as a remedy.[9]

While Mercury continued to dominate the

treatment of syphilis, in desperation many physicians tried a host of other methods as well. The chancres or ulcers of syphilis victims were sometimes cauterized (burned with a heated instrument or caustic substance). Steam baths were combined with mercury vapor. One doctor even tried using smallpox vaccination as a treatment for syphilis. Thomas Lowry wrote about the case of one poor soldier in the Union Army during the American Civil War in the 1860s as follows:

Surgeon E. A. Tomkins of Fort Yamhill, Oregon, described an unfortunate soldier with syphilis who, over a period of about four month, was treated with potassium iodide in sarsaparilla, corrosive sublimate, lunar caustic, calomel, black draught, emetics, blistering, iron, quinine, and external chloroform. At the end of the treatment, he was in severe pain, with one leg badly swollen and cold, barely able to walk.[10]

In the early years of the twentieth century the cause of syphilis was uncovered and a diagnostic test for its detection became available. Soon another major advance occurred that was to transform the treatment of the disease. Paul Ehrlich, who had been devoting much of his research in the 1890s to immunology, returned in the first decade of the twentieth century to a subject that had interested him earlier, the development of chemical agents to treat infectious disease. Ehrlich and his coworkers in Frankfurt began a search for chemical substances that would attack disease-causing microorganisms within the body. The hope was to find chemical drugs that acted like "magic bullets" that would specifically destroy the microorganisms without injury to human cells. His work initially focused on a group of microorganism called trypanosomes, which caused such diseases as sleeping sickness.

Ehrlich learned in 1905 that two British researchers had found that the arsenic-containing organic compound atoxyl could eliminate trypanosomes from the blood of infected animals. Unfortunately, it was soon found that relapses commonly occurred and that the large therapeutic doses required could damage the optic nerve and produce blindness. Ehrlich reasoned, however, that he might be able to modify the structure of atoxyl in a way that reduced or eliminated its effect on the optic nerve while still retaining its toxicity towards trypanosomes. Over the next few years, hundreds of arsenic compounds were synthesized and tested in his laboratory.

After the discovery of the spirochete that caused syphilis in 1905, Ehrlich began trying arsenical drugs against syphilis as well because there appeared to be a similarity between trypanosomes and spirochetes. In 1909, the Japanese scientist Sahachiro Hata, working in Ehrlich's laboratory, discovered that compound number 606 was effective in treating syphilis infections in rabbits. After extensive animal tests, Ehrlich arranged for the drug to be distributed to selected medical specialists for human clinical trials. The results were promising, and in 1910 Ehrlich announced the new drug to the world. Demand for 606 soon outgrew the ability of Ehrlich's laboratory to produce it, and he arranged with a German chemical company to produce the drug under the trade name Salvarsan.[11]

Salvarsan represented the first effective treatment for syphilis, and hence was hailed as a major medical breakthrough. Although the drug was indeed a major advance in the treatment of the disease, it was by no means an ideal therapeutic agent. Salvarsan, as an arsenical compound, had serious side effects. It also had to be administered by injection, and treatment was prolonged, sometimes involving an injection a week for a year or more. Ehrlich did introduce a somewhat improved form of the drug, Neosalvarsan, within a few years, and other arsenicals were introduced later. In spite of the problems with arsenical therapy, it remained the primary form of treatment of syphilis from its introduction until the discovery of the effectiveness of penicillin against the disease in the 1940s.

Initially the length of treatment with arsenical drugs generally extended from several weeks to perhaps two months. Treatment regimens varied, however, and the high cost of the drug meant that there was a tendency to stop its use once the Wasserman test, measuring the presence in the blood of the spirochete that caused syphilis, was negative. As a result of experience during the First World War and immediately thereafter, however, it became clear that it was necessary to continue treatment for a significantly longer period of time in order to avoid relapse.

In 1921, the use of bismuth to enhance the efficacy of the arsenicals was introduced. Like arsenic and mercury, however, bismuth had certain toxic side effects. During the 1920s, the standard therapy for syphilis involved weekly injections of arsenic preparations, frequently rotated with mercury and bismuth compounds, for a period of one to two years. In the United States, the most widely accepted schedule was that developed by the Cooperative Clinical Group, organized in 1928 by five large American syphilis clinics. Their protocol for acute syphilis involved weekly injections of Neosalvarsan and bismuth, on an alternating schedule, for a period of 68 weeks. This regimen was complicated to administer, expensive, prolonged, and potentially dangerous, and patients did not always complete the full course of therapy.[12]

Although this therapy was reasonably effective in the treatment of primary and secondary syphilis, side effects ranged from relatively minor ones, such as nausea and headache, to serious problems such as necrosis (death of skin cells) at the site of injection, kidney failure, and acute hepatitis, occasionally resulting in death. In addition, arsenical therapy had little or no effect in cases of advanced neurosyphilis, a late stage of the disease affecting the nervous system. This was especially true in patients who had developed general paresis, involving brain damage and characterized by dementia and paralysis.[13]

In 1917, however, an Austrian physician began experimenting with a form of therapy for paresis that became widespread in the 1920s and after. A medical graduate of the University of Vienna, Julius Wagner-Jauregg accepted an appointment in a psychiatric clinic. Although he had no formal training in psychiatry, which was still in its infancy as a discipline, he became professor of psychiatry at the University of Graz in 1893. He also continued clinical research in mental health in his hospital practice. Early in his career, he developed an interest in investigating the effects of inducing fevers in patients with psychoses, based on empirical observations from early times that patients with mental illness sometimes seemed to improve when attacked by a fever.

In 1917, Wagner-Jauregg decided to try using malaria as a form of fever therapy in patients with paresis. He injected nine patients suffering from this condition with tertian malaria, a form of the disease which was relatively innocuous and could generally be cured by drug therapy with quinine. He found that six of the cases showed significant remission, and in three of these cases the remission proved to be enduring. In 1919, he began this experimental treatment on a large scale. Others also began to carry out clinical trials with malaria therapy, which proved to be far more successful than any previous treatment for paresis. In 1922, the treatment was used on the first American patient at St. Elizabeths Hospital in Washington, DC. The method was soon widely accepted and Warner-Jauregg received the Nobel Prize in Physiology or Medicine in 1927 for his discovery of the therapeutic value of malaria inoculation in the treatment of paresis.[14]

Joel Braslow has argued that we cannot answer the question of whether malaria fever therapy actually worked with any degree of certainty. No randomized clinical trails of the sort that would be accepted as evidence today were ever performed on the method. With the discovery of the effectiveness of penicillin against syphilis in 1943, malaria therapy was eventually phased out, although it remained the treatment of choice until the late 1940s and early 1950s, and continued to find some use even after that time. In its heyday, it was certainly widely believed to be effective. In addition, Braslow has pointed out that it resulted in a decided improvement in the relationship between physicians and paresis patients. Whereas previously, both the patients and their doctors had viewed the condition of the patients as hopeless, there was now some cause for optimism. Braslow wrote:

The advent of malaria therapy restructured patients' and physicians' perceptions of themselves and each other. Irrespective of whether the treatment worked, not only did these physicians believe that they could act decisively against the syphilitic spirochete, but their belief in its efficacy allowed them to write more sympathetically about their patients and, perhaps, to care for them in a less objectified and more humane way. Furthermore, this new technology not only allowed patients to seek hospitalization voluntarily but permitted even those who were there against their will to become active participants in their treatment.[15]

Developments in the 1930s resulted in some modifications in the treatment of syphilis in its earlier stages. As Kampmeier has pointed out, the stumbling block to adequate treatment with arsenicals continued to be the issue of compliance on the part of the patients. A course of weekly injections for over a year was too much of a burden for many patients, and so often the full treatment was not carried out. Experiments reported by Harold Hyman at Mount Sinai Hos-

pital in New York in 1933 demonstrated that active medications could be delivered relatively safely by means of slow intravenous drip. This work led Hyman's colleague Louis Chargin to speculate that the intravenous drip procedure might be applied to arsenic therapy, with the possible result of curing syphilis in a matter of days or weeks, instead of a year or more. However, the procedure required hospitalization of the patients.

Chargin, Hyman and their coworkers began clinical testing of the intravenous drip method of Neoarsphenamine therapy for syphilis at Mount Sinai Hospital in 1933. Although the results were promising, the death of a patient led the team to look for a drug that might be less toxic and more stable. At about this time, other investigators had shown that Mapharsen (arsenoxide) was much less toxic than Neoarsphenamine but equally as effective. The Mount Sinai group switched to Mapharsen and continued their studies with good results and a substantial decrease in toxic effects in a five-day treatment regimen. Large-scale clinical trials at a number of institutions confirmed these early results, demonstrating that at the most effective dose intravenous Mapharsen therapy yielded satisfactory results in 85 to 90 percent of cases of primary syphilis and 70 percent of cases of secondary syphilis.[16]

Of course, there was also no shortage of quack doctors and patent medicines supposedly able to cure syphilis, as had been the case for centuries. In nineteenth century America such nostrums as Swaim's Panacea and Helmbold's Extract of Buchu had been advertised as cures for syphilis.[17] So-called medical or anatomy museums, generally aimed at men, also were often fronts for quacks who claimed to treat venereal disease and sexual dysfunctions. Brooks McNamara described a typical American museum of this type as follows:

Once inside the main room, the assault on the patron's nerves began in earnest. Everywhere about him were glass cases filled with hideously diseased organs modeled in death-like wax or luridly painted papier-mâché. The lights were low, the atmosphere hushed and funereal. Case after case displayed gaping sores and hideous deformities attributed to syphilis, gonorrhea, or that nameless terror of the nineteenth century, the "secret vice," masturbation. . . . At this point a solicitous "floor man" would appear from nowhere and begin to talk to the frightened patient. If it appeared that the customer was in need of medical aid–or could be convinced that he was–he

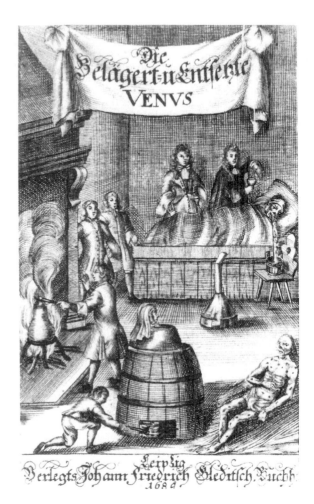

Various methods of treating syphilis, including fumigation. From Steven Blankaart, Die belägert- und entsetzte Venus *(Augsburg, 1710). Courtesy of the National Library of Medicine.*

was steered upstairs to the "medical institute" run by an "eminent specialist" in the various secret diseases.[18]

In the twentieth century, as regulation of the advertising and labeling of medicines increased in the United States and other countries, the marketers of syphilis remedies turned to using euphemisms for the disease in an attempt to disguise their claims. Everyone knew, for example, that "blood poisoning" in an advertisement meant syphilis. Products sold as "blood purifiers" had been used by some people as rem-

edies for syphilis in the nineteenth century. Sarsaparilla tonics, such as Ayers and Hoods, were popular in this regard, as this plant (as we have seen) was originally thought to be a remedy for syphilis. Such products continued to be used in the 1920s and beyond. For example, Compound Syrup of Sarsaparilla and Burdock with Iodide of Potassium was being sold as a treatment for "blood poisoning resulting from syphilis" in the 1930s.[19]

By the late nineteenth century, however, sarsaparilla had largely fallen into disuse for this purpose in orthodox medicine, although syrup of sarsaparilla was still being used as a vehicle for delivering drugs such as mercury and iodine (which were used to treat syphilis). Textbooks of pharmacology of the early twentieth century generally dismiss the value of sarsaparilla as a remedy for syphilis. Arthur Cushny's popular textbook of pharmacology, for example, stated that the drug "has some reputation in the treatment of syphilis, but there is no reason to believe that it is of any service here."[20]

Patent medicine quacks were not hesitant to don the mantle of science to sell their wares. Not long after Ehrlich discovered Salvarsan, for example, a New York charlatan marketed a cure for "blood poison" (syphilis) in which he used both Ehrlich's name and the number 606 (a term by which Salvarsan was also known). In the 1930s, a practitioner opened the "606 Medical Laboratory" in Chicago for the treatment of "men's disease" – a euphemism for syphilis and gonorrhea. The advertisement for this establishment could easily have given one the impression that Dr. Ehrlich himself was in charge. Another twentieth century "cure" for syphilis was named Ricord's Specific, drawing on the name of a famous nineteenth-century syphilologist.[21]

Dr. Sayman's Wonder Herbs was another patent medicine of the twentieth century that supposedly cured syphilitic "taints." The remedy consisted of a mixture of various plant products, such as ginger, rhubarb, licorice and senna, along with sodium bicarbonate or sodium carbonate. The Chief of Drug Control of the United States Food and Drug Administration noted in 1933 that while the medicine might be of some value in relieving gas in the stomach and bowel, it was worthless in the treatment of syphilis. Furthermore, he added:

Yet this concoction was recommended for syphilitic 'taints,' as if you could have just a little bit of this dread disease! But when you have syphilis you have it. It is as impossible to have a mere taint of it as it would be to fire off a cannon a little bit at a time."

Quack devices were also used for the supposed diagnosis and cure of syphilis. Albert Abrams, "the dean of twentieth century charlatans" in the United States, built a series of machines which he claimed could diagnose the disease of a patient from a sample of dried blood, even if the patient were miles away. In

time, Abrams stated that the patient's autograph would work just as well, which enabled him to diagnose syphilis in famous persons of the past such as Henry Wordsworth Longfellow and Edgar Allan Poe. A New York "clinic" used an electrical device to treat young men who had been led to believe that they might be infected with syphilis. The patient sat naked on a kind of toilet throne with his back against a metal plate and his scrotum suspended in a whirling pool of liquid. Both the liquid and the metal plate were hooked to a battery, and the patient received a shock, presumably convincing him that the treatment was working.[23]

The introduction of penicillin as a therapeutic agent in the 1940s revolutionized the treatment of syphilis. Alexander Fleming had accidentally discovered the anti-bacterial properties of the *Penicillium* mold in 1928, and realized that a substance produced by the mold (which he called penicillin) might have therapeutic value as a topical agent against disease-causing bacteria. It was not until the early 1940s, however, that researchers at Oxford University in England isolated a relatively pure form of Fleming's penicillin and were able to demonstrate its therapeutic efficacy in animals and then in human clinical trials. The United States government gave high priority to the development of penicillin on a large-scale for use in the war effort, as the drug was proving to be the most potent anti-bacterial substance known to date. At first supplies were limited and mostly reserved for military use, but by 1944 innovations introduced in American government, university and industry laboratories had greatly increased the yield and available supply of penicillin. In April 1945, all restrictions on its distribution in the United States were removed.[24]

In 1943, investigators at the Mayo Clinic showed that penicillin was effective against gonorrhea bacilli that were resistant to the sulfa drugs, thus giving physicians another weapon against this venereal disease. PHS physician John Mahoney and his colleagues at the Venereal Disease Research Laboratory in the PHS hospital at Staten Island, New York, soon confirmed these results. But Mahoney also decided to divert a small amount of his limited supply of the drug from the gonorrhea research to test it against syphilis. According to a coworker of Mahoney, the drug was first tried against the spirochetes that cause syphilis *in vitro* (i.e., outside of the body in a test tube or other apparatus) and failed to show any activity. Fortunately, the Staten Island investigators proceeded to the next step in trying penicillin *in vivo* (i.e., in the living body) in syphilitic rabbits.[25]

The results of limited animal tests were so encouraging that Mahoney decided to move ahead to clinical experiments. He justified this early move to testing on humans because penicillin appeared to be generally non-toxic and no harm would be done if the drug did not work and he had to return to arsenic therapy. In 1943, it has not yet been recognized that penicillin could produce serious allergic side effects in some patients.[26]

In June 1943, Mahoney and his colleagues began their clinical study with four patients. The results were promising, and the Staten Island group gave a preliminary report of the work at a national meeting. Although they were cautious in their report of the results, especially since the study had involved only four patients, their paper created great excitement. Microbiologist Gladys Hobby, who heard the presentation of the paper, later recalled:

I have a mental image of the room where I first heard Mahoney and his associates describe their results on the use of penicillin in the treatment of syphilis. The room was crowded. Loudspeakers and projection equipment were not as sophisticated then as now. Everyone strained to hear what was said, and the impact was electrifying. By then much had been written on penicillin, but no one had expected that an antibacterial agent would be active against spirochetes as well. Hearing John Mahoney describe the effect of penicillin on the course of syphilitic lesions was overwhelming.[27]

The story was picked up by the popular press as well. In an article headed "New Magic Bullet," *Time* discussed how Mahoney, in a "jam-packed session" of the meeting, announced that "penicillin had apparently cured four cases of early penicillin." Dr. Mahoney, according to the story, was "stunned" by the results. The magazine also reported Mahoney's cautious statement that penicillin would have to be tested in a large number of cases over a long period of time before it could be considered a cure for syphilis, but even given the limitations of the study, the results generated high hopes for this new drug against an old disease. One doctor who took to the floor to comment on the paper at the meet-ing was carried away by his enthusiasm to exult: "This is probably the most significant paper ever presented in the medical field."[28] At another conference a month later, a PHS physician referred to the work of Mahoney and his colleagues as "overshadowing anything that has happened in syphilis control since the days of Ehrlich."[29]

The results of the limited study at Staten Island were promising enough to lead to the organization of a large-scale, national clinical trial of penicillin in the treatment of syphilis. Initially, eight civilian venereal disease clinics, along with one each from the Army, Navy and Public Health Service, participated in the study, but additional facilities were later included. Not surprisingly, the Staten Island PHS hospital, where Mahoney and his colleagues were located, was one of the original sites for the study. In September 1944, Mahoney and other participants in the study published papers describing their results with over 1400 cases. They were able to demonstrate that penicillin treatment led to the disappearance of the spirochete from open lesions, the healing of those lesions, and a reversal of the blood serologic response from positive to negative (presumably due to the elimination of spirochetes from the blood). Further clinical trials confirmed the place of penicillin as the treatment of choice for syphilis.[30]

On 26 June 1944, the U. S. Army adopted penicillin as the routine treatment for syphilis. Penicillin allowed military physicians to get men suffering from venereal disease back to being available for combat quickly. The infected men remained ambulatory and began to convalesce almost immediately after treatment was begun, so they could be kept close to the front lines and returned to combat as soon as the therapy was completed. At first, however, there was not enough penicillin available to treat all cases that might potentially benefit from it. Penicillin of course had therapeutic value of the treatment of war wounds and various infections diseases other than syphilis and gonorrhea.[31] Physician-ethicist Henry Beecher called attention in a 1969 paper to the problem that military surgeons faced in this situation:

Allocation of penicillin within the Military was not without its troubles: When the first sizable shipment arrived at the North African Theatre of Operations, U.S.A., in 1943, a decision had to be made between using it for 'sulfa-fast' [sulfa-resistant] gonorrhea or for infected war wounds [its effectiveness against syphilis had not been fully established at the time]. Colonel Edward D. Churchill, Chief Surgical Consultant for that Theatre, made the decision to use the available penicillin for those "wounded" in brothels. Before indignation takes over, one must recall the military manpower shortage of those days. In a week or less, those overcrowding the military hospitals with venereal disease could be restored to health and returned to the battle line.[32]

A moral issue of a different sort was raised by those concerned about the impact of penicillin on sexual mores. As it became more and more obvious that syphilis and gonorrhea could be cured relatively quickly and painlessly with penicillin, some feared that this situation would encourage sexual promiscuity and immorality. One historian had cited a theologian of the period who worried that venereal disease would come to be regarded as strictly a medical problem, with its sociological and moral implications ignored. A graduate student in social work, who completed a research project at a rapid treatment center in 1947, admitted in her dissertation that she could not answer the question of "whether penicillin will be a help or a hindrance to the control of venereal disease; whether by making the treatment so short and effective patients will lose the fear of contracting the disease and will show more laxness in their sexual behavior." A number of public health officials suggested that the quicker and less arduous penicillin treatment could actually lead to an increase in venereal disease. Johns Hopkins bacteriologist Thomas B. Turner, for example, gave a talk at the 1948 ASHA meeting entitled "Penicillin: Help or Hindrance?" in which he discussed the successes of the drug against venereal disease, but also cited the loss of fear as a deterrent to exposure. Similar concerns about the undermining of standards of morality had been voiced when Ehrlich's Salvarsan had been introduced to treat syphilis in the early twentieth century.[33]

Concerns about the impact that penicillin might have on sexual behavior did not materially slow the adoption of the drug for the treatment of syphilis and gonorrhea. Nor, however, did the advent of this more effective drug therapy eliminate these diseases or the social and moral issues surrounding them.

Notes and References

1. Kevin Siena, "The Clean and the Foul: Paupers and the Pox in London Hospitals, c. 1550 - c. 1700," in Kevin Siena, ed., *Sins of the Flesh: Responding to Sexual Disease in Early Modern Europe* (Toronto: Centre for Reformation and Renaissance Studies, 2005), pp. 261-84.
2. Claude Quétel, *History of Syphilis*, translated into English by Judith Braddock and Brian Pike (Baltimore: Johns Hopkins University Press, 1990), p. 23.
3. Jon Arrizabalaga, John Henderson, and Roger French, *The Great Pox: The French Disease in Renaissance Europe* (New Haven, CT: Yale University Press, 1997), pp. 29-30.
4. Quétel, *History of Syphilis* (n. 2), pp. 30-32, 84; Owsei Temkin, "Therapeutic Trends and the Treatment of Syphilis before 1900," *Bulletin of the History of Medicine* 29 (1955): 309-16.
5. Quétel, *History of Syphilis* (n. 2), pp. 85-86.
6. Deborah Hayden, *Pox: Genius, Madness, and the Mysteries of Syphilis* (New York: Basic Books, 2003), pp. 48-49.
7. Quétel, *History of Syphilis* (n. 2), pp. 27-30; Arrizabalaga, et. al., Great Pox, pp. 99-103.
8. Sheldon Watts, *Epidemics in History: Disease, Power and Imperialism* (New Haven, CT: Yale University Press, 1997), p. 130.
9. Quétel, *History of Syphilis* (n. 2), pp. 63, 83-86, 116-17.
10. Thomas P. Lowry, *The Story the Soldiers Wouldn't Tell: Sex in the Civil War* (Mechanicsburg, PA: Stackpole Books, 1994), pp. 105-06.
11. John Parascandola, "The Theoretical Basis of Paul Ehrlich's Chemotherapy," *Journal of the History of Medicine* 36 (1981): 19-43.
12. Janice Dickin McGinnis, "From Salvarsan to Penicillin: Medical Science and VD Control in Canada," in *Essays in the History of Canadian Medicine*, ed. Wendy Mitchinson and Janice Dicken McGinnis (Toronto: McClelland and Stewart, 1988), pp. 126-47; R. H. Kampmeier, "Syphilis Therapy: An Historical Perspective," *Journal of the American Venereal Disease Association* 3 (1976): 99-108; *Milestones in Venereal Disease Control: Highlights of a Half-Century* (Washington, DC: U. S. Department of Health, Education, and Welfare, 1957); Jay Casell, *The Secret Plague: Venereal Disease in Canada 1838-1939* (Toronto: University of Toronto Press, 1987), p. 56.
13. Jeffrey S. Sartin and Harold O. Perry, "From Mercury to Malaria to Penicillin: The History of the Treatment of Syphilis at the Mayo Clinic—1916-1955," *Journal of the American Academy of Dermatology* 32 (1995): 255-61.
14. *Nobel Lectures, Physiology or Medicine 1922-1941* (Amsterdam: Elsevier, 1965; Paul Weindling, "Julius Wagner-Jauregg," in *Nobel Laureates in Medicine or Physiology: A Biographical Dictionary*, ed. Daniel M. Fox, Marcia Meldrum, and Ira Rezak (New York: Garland Publishing, 1990), pp. 545-48; Sartin and Perry, "From Mercury" (n. 13); Joel Braslow, "The Influence of a Biological Therapy on Physicians' Narratives and

Interrogations: The Case of General Paralysis of the Insane and Malaria Fever Therapy, 1910-1950," *Bulletin of the History of Medicine* 70 (1996): 577-608.

15. Braslow, "The Influence" (n. 14), pp. 606-07.

16. Kampmeier, "Syphilis Therapy" (n. 12), p. 105; Louis Chargin and William Leifer, "Massive Dose Arsenotherapy of Early Syphilis by Intravenous 'Drip Method'," *A. M. A. Archives of Dermatology* 73 (1956): 482-84; Harold Thomas Hyman, "Massive Arsenotherapy in Early Therapy by the Continuous Intravenous Drip Method," *Archives of Dermatology and Syphilology* 42 (1940): 253-61; "Massive Arsenotherapy for Syphilis," *Journal of the American Medical Association* 126 (1944): 554-57.

17. James Harvey Young, *The Toadstool Millionaires: A Social History of Patent Medicines in America before Federal Regulation* (Princeton, NJ: Princeton University Press, 1961), pp. 58-66, 114-17.

18. Brooks McNamara, *Step Right Up: An Illustrated History of the American Medical Show* (Garden City, NY: Doubleday, 1976), p. 42.

19. James Harvey Young, *The Medical Messiahs: A Social History of Health Quackery in Twentieth-Century America* (Princeton, NJ: Princeton University Press, 1967), p. 84; Ruth deforest Lamb, *American Chamber of Horrors: The Truth about Food and Drugs* (New York: Farrar and Rinehart, 1936), p. 71; F. J. Cullan, "Federal Control of Venereal Disease Nostrums Through Proposed Legislation," *Journal of Social Hygiene* 19 (1933): 513-522.

20. Arthur Oslo, George E. Farrar, Jr., and Robertson Pratt, *Dispensary of the United States of America 1960 Edition* (Philadelphia: J. B. Lippincott, 1960), p. 1215; David M. R. Culbreth, *A Manual of Materia Medica and Pharmacology*, sixth edition (Philadelphia: Lea and Febiger, 1917), p. 121; Arthur R. Cushny, *A Textbook of Pharmacology and Therapeutics*, third edition (Philadelphia: Lea Brothers, 1903), p. 355.

21. Young, *Toadstool Millionaires* (n. 17), p. 168; Casell, *Secret Plague* (n. 12), p. 63; Suzanne Poirier, *Chicago's War on Syphilis, 1937-1940: The Times, the Trib, and the Clap Doctor* (Urbana, IL: University of Illinois Press, 1995), pp. 61-63.

22. Cullan, "Federal Control" (n. 19), p. 519.

23. James Harvey Young, "Device Quackery in America," *Bulletin of the History of Medicine* 39 (1965): 154-162.

24. The literature on the history of penicillin is extensive. See, e.g., Robert Bud, *Penicillin: Triumph and Tragedy* (Oxford: Oxford University Press, 2007); Gladys Hobby, *Penicillin: Meeting the Challenge* (New Haven, CT: Yale University Press, 1985); Kevin Brown, *Penicillin Man: Alexander Fleming and the Antibiotic Revolution* (Stroud, UK: Sutton, 2004).

25. John Parascandola, "John Mahoney and the Introduction of Penicillin to Treat Syphilis," *Pharmacy in History* 43 (2001): 3-13; Hobby, *Penicillin* (n. 24), p. 152.

26. J. F. Mahoney, R. C. Arnold, and Ad Harris, "Penicillin Treatment of Early Syphilis: A Preliminary Report," *American Journal of Public Health* 33 (1943): 1387-91.

27. Mahoney and Harris, "Penicillin Treatment" (n. 26);

Hobby, *Penicillin* (n. 24), pp. 155-56.

28. "New Magic Bullet," *Time Magazine* 42 (25 October 1943): 38, 40.

29. J. R. Heller, Jr., "Syphilis Control in Wartime," *Southern Medical Journal* 37 (1944): 219-223 (quotation on p. 222).

30. A. N. Richards, "Production of Penicillin in the United States (1941-1946)," *Nature* 201 (1964): 441-45; J. E. Moore, "Preliminary Statement," in National Research Council—U. S. Public Health Service, *Meeting of Penicillin Investigators*, February 7 and 8 1946, p. 1 (copy at National Library of Medicine); J. F. Mahoney, R. C. Arnold, Burton L. Sterner, Ad Harris, and M. R. Zwally, "Penicillin Treatment of Early Syphilis: II," *Journal of the American Medical Association* 126 (1944): 63-67; Joseph Earle Moore, J. F. Mahoney, Walter Schwartz, Thomas Sternberg, and W. Barry Wood, "The Treatment of Early Syphilis with Penicillin: A Preliminary Report of 1,418 Cases," *Journal of the American Medical Association* 126 (1944): 67-72.

31. Richards, "Production of Penicillin," p. 444; Odin W. Anderson, *Syphilis and Society—Problems of Control in the United States, 1912-1964* (Chicago: Center for Health Administration Studies, Health Information Foundation, 1965), pp. 20-21; R. A. Vonderlehr and J. R. Heller, Jr., *The Control of Venereal Disease* (New York: Reynal and Hitchcock, 1946), p. 3.

32. Henry K. Beecher, "Scarce Resources and Medical Advancement," *Daedalus* 98 (1969): 275-313 (quotation on pp. 280-81).

33. McGinnis, "From Salvarsan to Penicillin" (n. 12), pp. 145-46; Judith Torregrosa, "A Study of Forty-Four Syphilitic Patients Under Treatment at the Louisville Rapid Treatment Center from March 1, 1947 to April 15, 1947," M.S. in Social Work dissertation, University of Louisville, 1947 (quotation on p. v); Richard A. Koch and Ray Lyman Wilbur, "Promiscuity as a Factor in the Spread of Venereal Disease," *Journal of Social Hygiene* 30 (1944): 517-29; Vonderlehr and Heller, *Control of Venereal Disease* (n. 31), p. 65; Elizabeth Fee, "Sin vs. Science: Venereal Disease in Baltimore in the Twentieth Century," *Bulletin of the History of Medicine* 43 (1988): 141-64; Allan M. Brandt, *No Magic Bullet: A Social History of Venereal Disease in the United States Since 1880*, expanded edition (Oxford: Oxford University Press, 1987), p. 46.

The research for this paper was part of a larger project on the history of syphilis that resulted in the publication of Dr. Parascandola's book on *Sex, Sin, and Science: A History of Syphilis in America* (Westport, CT: Praeger, 2008).

INDEX OF PROPER NAMES OF PERSONS AND INSTITUTIONS

Note: Names that are mentioned only once in passing have been excluded from the index.